Dermatology: A Case Study Approach

Dermatology: A Case Study Approach

Editor: Malia West

AMERICAN
MEDICAL PUBLISHERS
www.americanmedicalpublishers.com

AMERICAN
MEDICAL PUBLISHERS
www.americanmedicalpublishers.com

Cataloging-in-Publication Data

Dermatology: a case study approach / edited by Malia West.
p. cm.
Includes bibliographical references and index.
ISBN 979-8-88740-634-3
1. Dermatology. 2. Skin--Diseases. I. West, Malia.
RL72 .C55 2023
616.5--dc23

American Medical Publishers,
41 Flatbush Avenue,
1st Floor, New York,
NY 11217, USA

ISBN 979-8-88740-634-3 (Hardback)

Contents

Preface

This book was inspired by the evolution of our times; to answer the curiosity of inquisitive minds. Many developments have occurred across the globe in the recent past which has transformed the progress in the field.

The area of medicine that focuses on the diagnosis, treatment, and management of diseases and conditions affecting the skin, hair, nails, and mucous membranes is known as dermatology. A few of the common skin diseases which are treated within this field are eczema, psoriasis and dermatitis. Eczema refers to a chronic inflammatory condition that leads to itchy, red, and dry skin. Psoriasis is an autoimmune skin condition characterized by red, scaly patches on the skin. Dermatitis is an inflammation of the skin caused by contact with irritants or allergens. Treatments for these conditions may use topical medications, moisturizers or systemic medications, depending on the disease and its severity. This book contains some path-breaking studies in the field of dermatology. The various advancements in this field are glanced at and their applications as well as ramifications are looked at in detail. For all those who are interested in dermatology, this book can prove to be an essential guide.

This book was developed from a mere concept to drafts to chapters and finally compiled together as a complete text to benefit the readers across all nations. To ensure the quality of the content we instilled two significant steps in our procedure. The first was to appoint an editorial team that would verify the data and statistics provided in the book and also select the most appropriate and valuable contributions from the plentiful contributions we received from authors worldwide. The next step was to appoint an expert of the topic as the Editor-in-Chief, who would head the project and finally make the necessary amendments and modifications to make the text reader-friendly. I was then commissioned to examine all the material to present the topics in the most comprehensible and productive format.

I would like to take this opportunity to thank all the contributing authors who were supportive enough to contribute their time and knowledge to this project. I also wish to convey my regards to my family who have been extremely supportive during the entire project.

Editor

1

Coexistence of Pemphigus Vulgaris and Lichen Planus following COVID-19 Vaccination

Zeinab Aryanian,[1,2] Kamran Balighi,[1,3] Arghavan Azizpour,[1,3] Kambiz Kamyab Hesari,[1,4] and Parvaneh Hatami[1]

[1]Autoimmune Bullous Diseases Research Center, Tehran University of Medical Sciences, Tehran, Iran
[2]Department of Dermatology, Babol University of Medical Sciences, Babol, Iran
[3]Department of Dermatology, Razi Hospital, Tehran University of Medical Sciences, Tehran, Iran
[4]Department of Dermatopathology, Razi Hospital, Tehran University of Medical Sciences, Tehran, Iran

Correspondence should be addressed to Parvaneh Hatami; p_hatami2001@yahoo.com

Academic Editor: Henry Wong

SARS-CoV-2 vaccines were approved without long-term monitoring due to emergent situation and might have several side effects. Herein, we describe the first case with development of both LP and PV following COVID-19 vaccination. Immunological alteration due to COVID-19 vaccination and its potential role in triggering autoimmune disorders were also dealt with.

1. Introduction

Coronavirus disease 2019 or COVID-19 caused by SARS-CoV-2 was first reported in December 2019 and soon became a pandemic in March 2020 [1]. Since serious health issues were raised regarding COVID-19 outbreak, SARS-CoV-2 vaccines were approved without long-term monitoring and it turned out that they can cause several adverse effects including mucocutaneous manifestations [2–5].

tLichen planus (LP) is a chronic inflammatory dermatosis, involving skin, appendages, and mucous membranes [6, 7].

Pemphigus vulgaris (PV) is a rare blistering disorder with mucocutaneous involvement characterized by the production of autoantibodies against desmogleins (Dsg), which play an important role in the maintenance of cell-to-cell adhesion [8].

There are some reports of development of lichen planus-like lesions in pemphigus patients [9–11].

Although the presence of LP or PV following COVID-19 or its vaccines has been rarely reported, their coexistence following COVID-19 vaccination has not been reported yet.

Here, we present the first case of coexistence of LP and PV following COVID-19 vaccination.

2. Case Presentation

A 43-year-old man was referred to our clinic for evaluation of mouth sores and dark spots on the face from three months ago. He was otherwise healthy and had no notable drug history. His initial symptom was dysphonia which developed quite abruptly within 48 hours of receiving the second dose of the Oxford-AstraZeneca COVID-19 vaccine, though he did not report any adverse effect following receiving the first dose of the same vaccine. He had progressed to develop sore throat and erosive buccal lesions. Curiously, he also noted increasing dark spots on his face at this time which were not proceeded by blisters or ulcers. Histopathologic sampling and direct immune fluorescence evaluation of a dorsal tongue ulcer by an outside dermatologist confirmed the diagnosis of pemphigus vulgaris (PV). Treatment had been initiated with 80 mg/day prednisolone and 150 mg/day azathioprine with partial control of the disease. The patient was subsequently referred to our clinic for further management.

Upon examination, residual PV erosions were found on oral palatal mucosa and scalp (Figures 1(a) and 1(b)). We

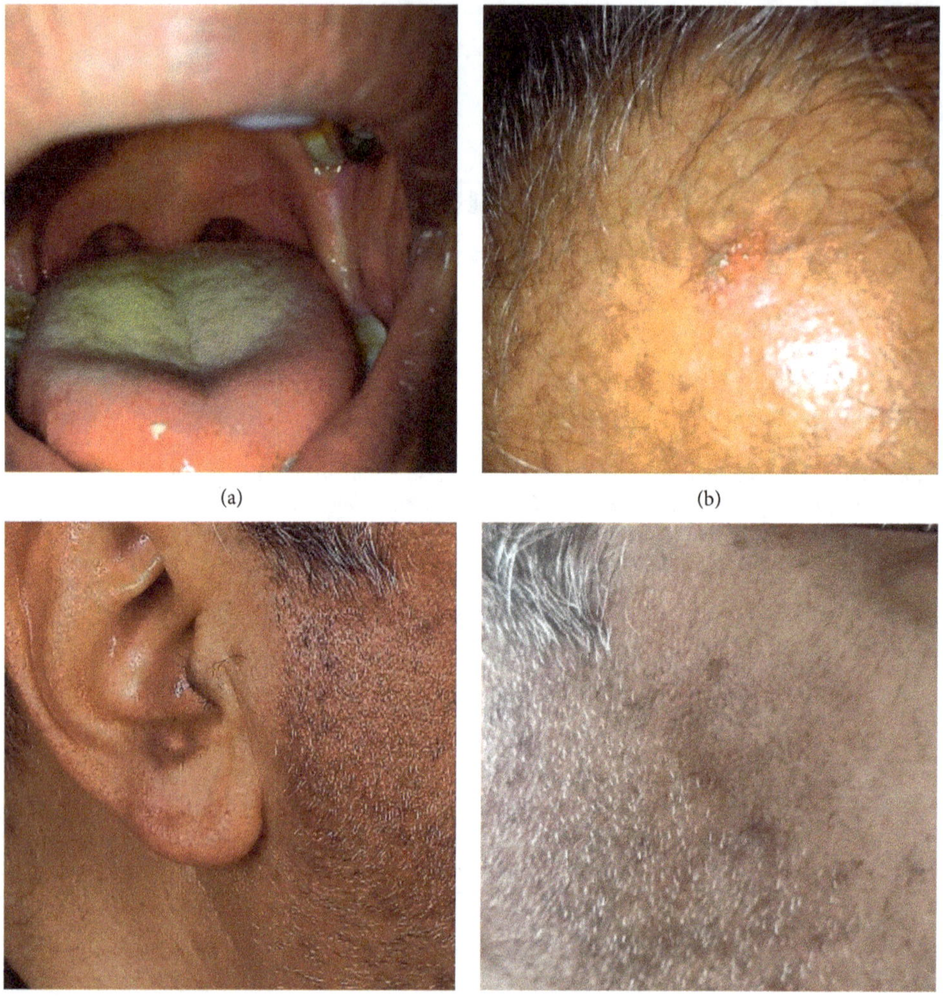

(a) (b) (c) (d)

Figure 1: Oral mucosal lesions (a) and scalp erosion (b) due to pemphigus and hyperpigmented macules on ear (c) and cheek (d) due to lichen planus pigmentosus following COVID-19 vaccination.

also noticed multiple well-defined grey-brown hyperpigmented macules on the ears, cheeks, and chin (Figures 1(c) and 1(d)). He denied exposure to any topical medications or potential for personal care product/occupational contact dermatitis. Since the nature of this pigmentation was unclear, we performed a punch biopsy of a representative chin lesion which showed typical findings of lichen planus (LP) pigmentosus (Figure 2).

We started a topical corticosteroid (mometasone cream qhs) for the LP lesions with recommendation for diligent sun protection. Considering the incomplete response of PV to azathioprine, rituximab was initiated (500 mg every week for 4 sessions) which resulted in considerable clinical response and tapering the prednisolone. At present, his old PV lesions have been healed without developing any new lesion on 5 mg/day prednisolone and his LP lesions, although partially, have been improved.

Figure 3 shows the exact time points regarding the history of the patient. It is worthy to note that patient did not have any positive personal or family history regarding other immunological disorders such as rheumatoid arthritis, type 1 diabetes, autoimmune thyroid disease, irritable bowel disease, and systemic lupus erythematosus. Moreover, no one in his family showed any immunologic reaction following COVID-19 vaccination.

3. Discussion

Coexistence of LP and PV has rarely been reported. Most previously reported cases had the oral forms of both diseases [9–11]. PV and LP share some immune pathogenic features including aberrant immune responses. LPP is mainly derived by cell-mediated immunity while the major mechanism of developing PV is auto antibody formation against desmoglein (Dsg) 1, 3 [12, 13]. T cells, however, are implicated in the pathogenesis of PV. Furthermore, circulating anti-Dsg 1, 3 in some patients with oral LP has been reported, suggesting possible shared immunogenic pathways [13].

Whenever a mixed picture of PV is concurrent with LP-like features, one should consider the critical paraneoplastic pemphigus [14]. However, our patient did not have severe refractory stomatitis which is the clinical hallmark of

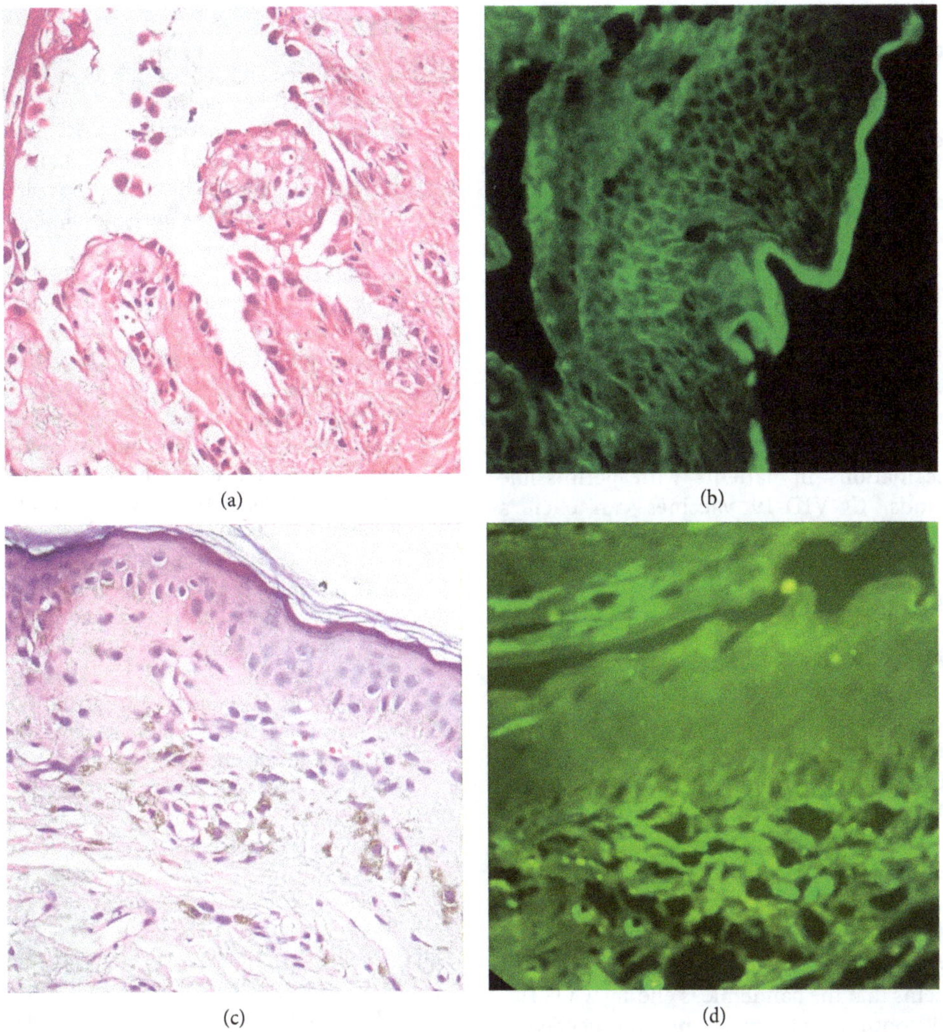

FIGURE 2: Suprabasal epidermal acantholysis and cleft containing inflammatory cells and rounded acantholytic cells with intensely eosinophilic cytoplasm and a perinuclear halo. DIF shows intercellular deposition throughout the epidermis compatible with diagnosis of PV (a, b). Hyperkeratosis, atrophic epidermis with vacuolar alteration of the basal cell layer, and pigmentary incontinence and negative. DIF, compatible with diagnosis of LP pigmentosus (c, d)

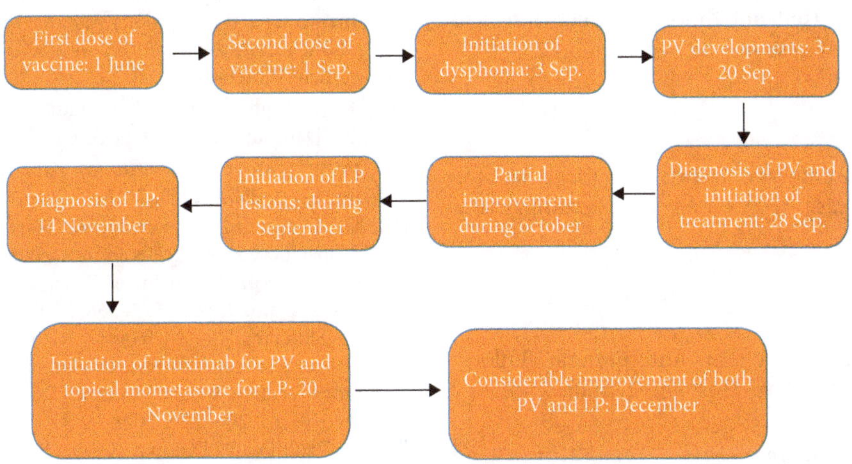

FIGURE 3: The exact time points of events.

paraneoplastic pemphigus. The histopathology and DIF pattern were also not suggestive of paraneoplastic pemphigus.

The new-onset occurrence of LP or PV, individually, has been reported following COVID-19 infection or various COVID-19 vaccine platforms including AstraZeneca or Pfizer, which was presented both after first or second dose of vaccine [15–17]. This might reflect that the dose of vaccine is not of a great importance in triggering autoimmune condition.

The simultaneous occurrence of cutaneous LP pigmentosus and PV triggered by COVID-19 vaccination in our case, to the best of our knowledge, has not been previously reported in the literature.

It has been long known that autoimmune disorders can be triggered by various environmental factors such as viral infections or vaccinations in patients with permissible genetic backgrounds. COVID-19 vaccines can elicit a T-helper type 1(Th1) response, increasing pro-apoptotic mediators such as interferon gamma (IFN γ), thereby explaining occurrence of LP following vaccination [18]. Though PV is supposed to be a Th2-dominant disease, some studies suggested a possible role of CD8+ T cells via Fas/Fas ligand pathway in the pathogenesis of PV [19]. On the other hand, COVID-19 vaccines have been shown to have a high capability to elicit critical immune regulators like cytotoxic CD8+ T cells and memory cells [20] which might explain the occurrence of PV in this setting. Moreover, COVID-19 vaccines, especially adenovirus-containing ones, might render an environmental trigger for induction of autoimmune disorders such as PV in genetically susceptible patients possibly through epitope spreading or bystander activation phenomenon [21].

Although it seems that the pandemic is ending, COVID-19 vaccination will continue in future. Hence, it is needed to know more about COVID-19 vaccine-associated dermatologic reactions. Logically among them, we may encounter some rare but important and even life-threatening reactions that should be better studied and managed. We recommend a strict workup and report of development of new autoimmune disorders and unusual dermatologic conditions to better understand immune system work frame and early treatment of disorders (but not too early which interfere with immunologic body response to vaccination).

Consent

Written informed consent was obtained from the patient for publication of this case report and any accompanying images.

Disclosure

This study was performed at the Autoimmune Bullous Diseases Research Center, Razi Hospital, Tehran, Iran.

Authors' Contributions

All the authors have equally participated in preparing the manuscript.

References

[1] A. P. Munro and S. N. Faust, "COVID-19 in children: current evidence and key questions," *Current Opinion in Infectious Diseases*, vol. 33, no. 6, pp. 540–547, 2020.

[2] G. Bogdanov, I. Bogdanov, J. Kazandjieva, and N. Tsankov, "Cutaneous adverse effects of the available COVID-19 vaccines," *Clinics in Dermatology*, vol. 39, no. 3, pp. 523–531, 2021.

[3] M. Burlando, A. Herzum, C. Micalizzi, E. Cozzani, and A. Parodi, "Cutaneous reactions to COVID-19 vaccine at the dermatology primary care," *Immunity, Inflammation and Disease*, vol. 10, no. 2, pp. 265–271, 2021.

[4] Y. Kalantari, A. Sadeghzadeh-Bazargan, Z. Aryanian, P. Hatami, and A. Goodarzi, "First reported case of delayed-type hypersensitivity reaction to non-hyaluronic acid Polycaprolactone dermal filler following COVID-19 vaccination: a case report and a review of the literature," *Clinical Case Reports*, vol. 10, no. 2, Article ID e05343, 2022.

[5] P. Hatami, Z. Aryanian, H. Nicknam Asl, and A. Goodarzi, "Mucocutaneous adverse effects following COVID-19 vaccination: a comprehensive review of the literature with a presentation of some cases from Iran," *Iranian Journal of Dermatology*, vol. 24, no. 4, pp. 331–338, 2021.

[6] Z. M. Wang, J. Zhang, F. Wang, and G. Zhou, "The tipped balance of ILC1/ILC2 in peripheral blood of oral lichen planus is related to inflammatory cytokines," *Frontiers in Cell and Developmental Biology*, vol. 9, Article ID 725169, 2021.

[7] Z. Aryanian, A. Shirzadian, P. Hatami, and H. Dadras, "High incidence of metabolic syndrome components in lichen planus patients: a prospective cross-sectional study," *International Journal of Clinical Practice*, vol. 2022, Article ID 7184678, 6 pages, 2022.

[8] K. Balighi, P. Hatami, M. J. Sheikh Aboli et al., "Multiple cycles of rituximab therapy for pemphigus: a group of patients with difficult- to-treat disease or a consequence of late rituximab initiation?" *Dermatologic Therapy*, vol. 35, no. 2, Article ID e15249, 2022.

[9] N. Kianfar, S. Dasdar, H. Mahmoudi, S. Tavakolpour, K. Balighi, and M. Daneshpazhooh, "Lichen planus-like lesions in 36 patients with pemphigus: a cross-sectional study," *Oral Diseases*, vol. 27, no. 4, pp. 947–951, 2021.

[10] F. Mohaghegh, Z. Talebzadeh, M. Bahraminejad, and M. Rezaei, "Coexistence of periorbital lichen planus pigmentosus and pemphigus vulgaris: report of an unusual case and a rare association," *Clinical Case Reports*, vol. 9, no. 7, Article ID e04480, 2021.

[11] K. Balighi, H. Mahmoudi, S. Tavakolpour, and M. Daneshpazhooh, "Coexistence of oral lichen planus and pemphigus vulgaris," *Clinical Oral Investigations*, vol. 22, no. 8, pp. 2953–2955, 2018.

[12] H. Takahashi, M. Kouno, K. Nagao et al., "Desmoglein 3–specific CD4+ T cells induce pemphigus vulgaris and interface dermatitis in mice," *Journal of Clinical Investigation*, vol. 121, no. 9, pp. 3677–3688, 2011.

[13] T. Shiohara, Y. Mizukawa, R. Takahashi, and Y. Kano, "Pathomechanisms of lichen planus autoimmunity elicited by cross-reactive T cells," *Current Directions in Autoimmunity*, vol. 10, pp. 206–226, 2008.

[14] G. Paolino, D. Didona, G. Magliulo et al., "Paraneoplastic pemphigus: insight into the autoimmune pathogenesis, clinical features and therapy," *International Journal of Molecular Sciences*, vol. 18, no. 12, p. 2532, 2017.

[15] I. Hiltun, J. Sarriugarte, I. Martinez-de- Espronceda et al., "Lichen planus arising after COVID-19 vaccination," *Journal of the European Academy of Dermatology and Venereology: JEADV*, vol. 35, no. 7, pp. e414–e415, 2021 Jul.

[16] K. Thongprasom, N. Pengpis, E. Phattarataratip, and L. Samaranayake, "Oral pemphigus after COVID-19 vaccination," *Oral Diseases*, 2021.

[17] V. L. S. De Medeiros, A. U. Monteiro-Neto, D. D. T. Franca, R. Castelo Branco, E. O. de Miranda Coelho, and D. M. Takano, "Pemphigus vulgaris after COVID-19: a case of induced autoimmunity," *SN Comprehensive Clinical Medicine*, vol. 3, no. 8, p. 1768, 2021.

[18] J. E. Lemieux, A. Li, M. Gentili et al., "Vaccine serologic responses among transplant patients associate with COVID-19 infection and T peripheral helper cells," *medRxive*, vol. 2021.07.11, Article ID 21260338, 2021.

[19] F. Giurdanella, L. Fania, M. Gnarra et al., "A possible role for CD8+ T lymphocytes in the cell-mediated pathogenesis of pemphigus vulgaris," *Mediators of Inflammation*, vol. 2013, Article ID 764290, 5 pages, 2013.

[20] N. Kumar, N. Admane, A. Kumari et al., "Cytotoxic T-lymphocyte elicited vaccine against SARS-CoV-2 employing immunoinformatics framework," *Scientific Reports*, vol. 11, no. 1, p. 7653, 2021.

[21] C. Galván Casas, A. Català, G. Carretero Hernández et al., "Classification of the cutaneous manifestations of COVID-19: a rapid prospective nationwide consensus study in Spain with 375 cases," *British Journal of Dermatology*, vol. 183, no. 1, pp. 71–77, 2020.

2

A Case of Secondary Syphilis with the Extragenital Chancre on the Nipple

Xiao Yan Wang, Juliandri, Zi Jing Liu, Jia Wen Zhang, Yun Yi Liu, Da-Guang Wang and Yang Xu

Department of Dermatology, The First Affiliated Hospital of Nanjing Medical University, Nanjing 210029, China

Correspondence should be addressed to Yang Xu; cardioos@163.com

Academic Editor: Ravi Krishnan

Syphilis is a sexually transmitted disease caused by *Treponema pallidum*. The signs and symptoms of syphilis vary depending on which of the four stages it presents. The primary stage of syphilis classically presents with a painless ulcer (chancre). We report a case of the extragenital chancre on the nipple which is examined from skin biopsy and immunohistochemistry. This case showed that it is important to identify the special site's pruritus erythema by pathology and serological examination.

1. Introduction

Syphilis is a common sexually transmitted or blood contracted, congenital transmission disease. It can be divided into primary syphilis, secondary syphilis, tertiary syphilis, and neurosyphilis. The diagnosis is based on the clinical manifestations and serological methods. In this article, we report a case of secondary syphilis with extragenital chancre on the nipple.

2. Case Presentation

A 56-year-old male was presented to our dermatology department on June 12, 2018, with complaints of the right nipple erosion and discomfort for a week. Diagnosis of "eczema" was made and the patient was treated with topical zinc oxide oil and traditional Chinese herbal cream. Physical examination showed local erythematous erosion with a few exudations on the right nipple (Figure 1) and a skin biopsy was performed. The histopathological results showed epidermal hyperplasia, cutaneous protrusion, migration of small amount of inflammatory cells, infiltration of large number of cells around the blood vessels of the dermis, and some of the nucleus were large, with scattered cells such as the lymphocytes and plasma cells (Figure 2). Immunohistochemistry was recommended to confirm the diagnosis. The results revealed the (the right papillary skin) proliferation of lymphocytes: CD20(+), CD3(+), CD5(+), Pax-5(+), CD38(+), Bcl-2(+), CD10(−), Bcl-6(−), MUM1(−), Cyclin D1(−), CD163(+), Igκ(+), and Igλ(+), combined with hematoxylin-eosin (H-E) staining, showed numerous lymphoplasmacytes infiltration in the cutaneous dermal layer (Figure 3). On the follow-up, the patient complained of painless itchy erythema on bilateral soles. Physical examination showed that bilateral palms and soles had multiple copper-red macula and papules, some of which were desquamated on the surface (Figure 4). The syphilis serology examination showed that TPPA was positive, RPR was positive, and the titer was >1 : 32, so the diagnosis was confirmed for syphilis. Then the patient was treated with IM injection of 2.4 million units of benzathine penicillin. Following a week later for follow up, the papillary erosion scab desquamation and the erythema subsided, the bilateral palms and the soles of dark erythema also subsided. And the 2.4 million units of benzathine penicillin were administered intramuscularly once a week for three weeks totally. The patient is still in further follow-up.

3. Discussion

Syphilis is a sexually transmitted disease caused by *Treponema pallidum* [1]. The primary-stage of syphilis is mainly characterized by painless ulcers (chancre), which occur mostly in the genitals, anus, oral cavity [2], lips, pharyngeal, and nipple-areola [3]. There have been several reports of primary syphilis

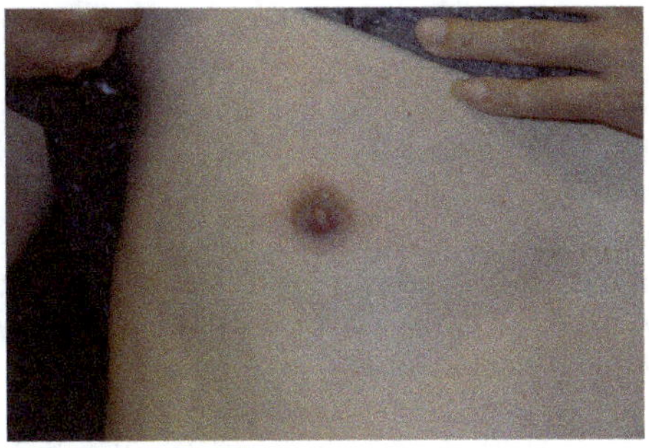

Figure 1: An erythematous erosion with a few exudation on the right nipple before treatment.

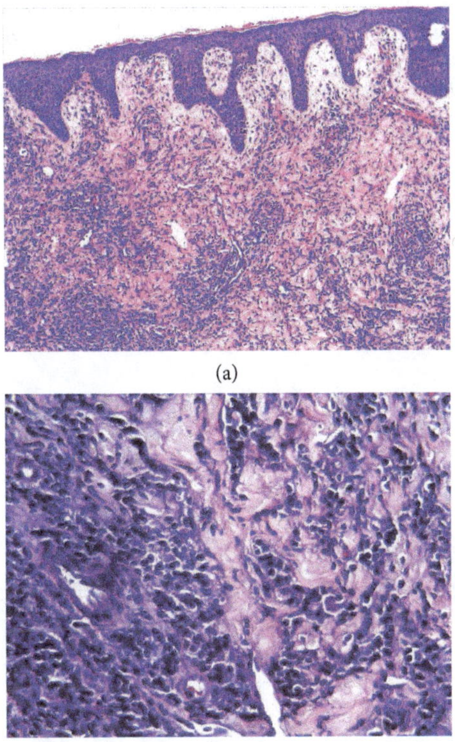

(a)

(b)

Figure 2: Biopsy of the nipple showed that epidermal hyperplasia, cutaneous protrusion, a migration of small amount of inflammatory cells, an infiltration of large number of cells around the blood vessels of the dermis (a). The inflammatory cells in the dermis were majorly lymphocytes and plasma cells (b). (H-E staining, original magnification: (a) ×100; (b) ×400)

occurring on the nipple and, its clinical manifestations vary [4–7], such as erythema nodules on the nipple, swelling, erosion, indolent ulcers, asymptomatic scaly erythematous or crusted plaque, etc. This case is a unilateral nipple erythematous exudation change, which can be easily misdiagnosed as eczema, Paget's breast disease and so on. Histopathological and immunohistochemical results suggested that lymphocytes and plasma cells infiltrate the dermis, and the diseases of intradermal plasma cell infiltration are common in plasmacytosis, plasmacytoma, syphilis, and fungal infections. The dermis may have plasma cells, neutrophils, and lymphocytes infiltrated in primary syphilis. In immunohistochemistry Pax5, CD20 are

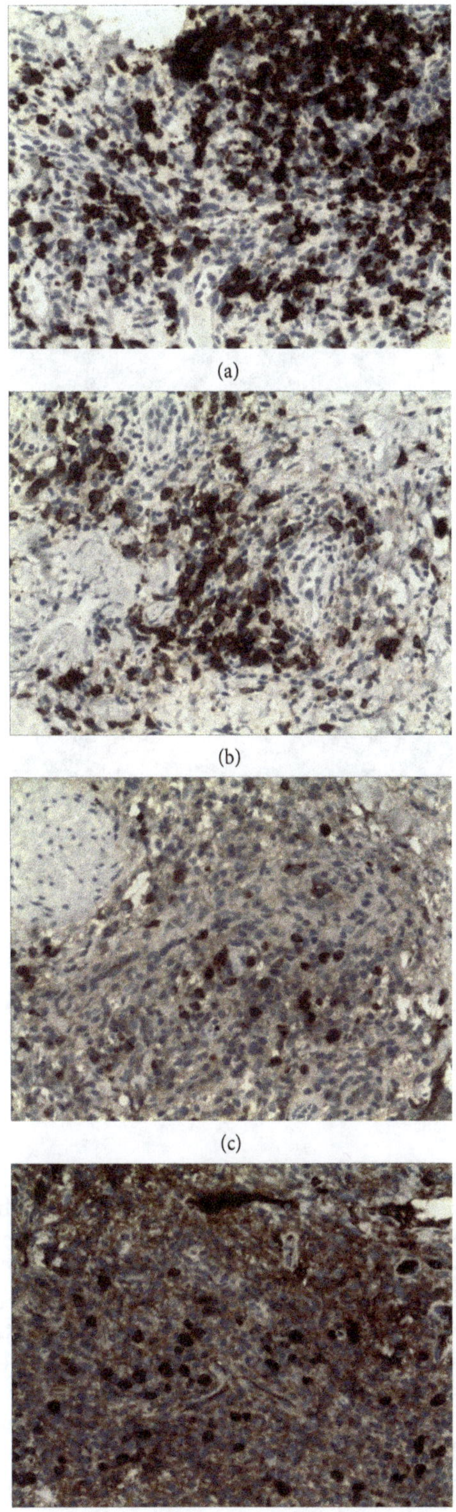

(a)

(b)

(c)

(d)

Figure 3: Immunohistochemical staining showed that lymphocplasmocytes infiltration in the cutaneous dermal layer. (a: CD20(+), b: CD38(+), c: lgκ(+), d: Igλ(+), original magnification: ×400)

expressed on the surface of B cells, CD3, are CD5 are the T cells markers. CD163 is expressed by the macrophages, CD38 is most strongly expressed in plasmocytes; however, Bcl-2(+), CD109(−), Bcl-6(−), MUM1(−), Cyclin D1(−), Alk(−), Igκ(+),

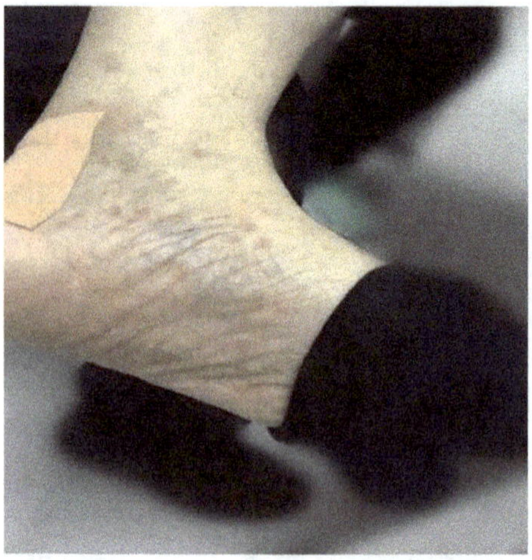

(a)

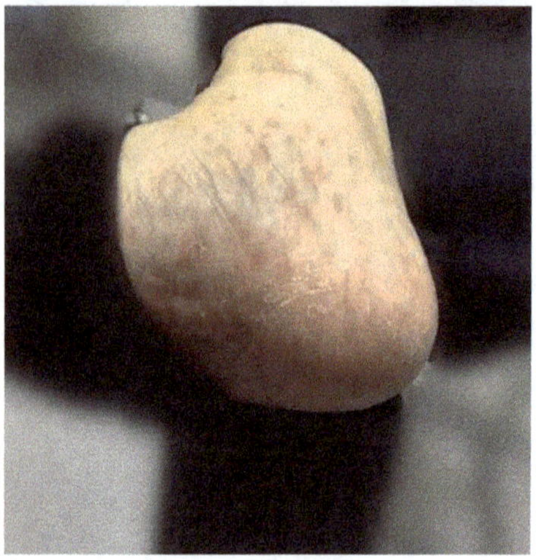

(b)

FIGURE 4: Bilateral palms and soles had multiple copper-red macula and papules some of which were desquamated on the surface. ((a): left sole, (b): right sole)

and Igλ(+) could exclude the neoplastic lesion. The pathological results are consistent with clinical manifestations, highly indicating the diagnosis of syphilis. During the visit, the patient developed a typical second-stage syphilis change on the palm toe, which was characterized by a palm-toe rose rash. Further serological tests confirmed the final diagnosis. This patient was more unusual that there was an atypical syphilis and a typical second-stage syphilis during the visit. Due to no itchy erythema on skin or mucosa without related allergic history, it is necessary to consider the possibility of noncommon infection or tumor, thus pathological and serological examination are required.

References

[1] R. W. Peeling, D. Mabey, M. L. Kamb, X. S. Chen, J. D. Radolf, and A. S. Benzaken, "Syphilis," *Nature Reviews Disease Primers*, vol. 3, no. 1, pp. 17–73, 2017.

[2] P. J. Read and B. Donovan, "Clinical aspects of adult syphilis," *Internal Medicine Journal*, vol. 42, no. 6, pp. 614–620, 2012.

[3] H. Fukuda, M. Takahashi, K. Kato, T. Oharaseki, and H. Mukai, "Multiple primary syphilis on the lip, nipple-areola and penis: an immunohistochemical examination of *Treponema pallidum* localization using an anti-*T. pallidum* antibody," *The Journal of Dermatology*, vol. 42, no. 5, pp. 515–517, 2015.

[4] S. Podlipnik, P. Giavedoni, M. Alsina, A. Garcia-Herrera, J. Ferrando, and J. J. Mascaro, "An erythematous nodule on the nipple: an unusual presentation of primary syphilis," *Journal of Cutaneous Pathology*, vol. 42, no. 4, pp. 239–243, 2015.

[5] J. Y. Lee, M. H. Lin, and Y. C. Jung, "Extragenital syphilitic chancre manifesting as a solitary nodule of the nipple," *Journal of the European Academy of Dermatology and Venereology*, vol. 20, no. 7, pp. 886–887, 2006.

[6] H. Y. Chiu and T. F. Tsai, "A crusted plaque on the right nipple," *JAMA*, vol. 308, no. 4, pp. 403–404, 2012.

[7] S. Zheng, J. Liu, X. Xu, X. Gao, and H. Chen, "Primary syphilis presenting as bilateral nipple-areola eczematoid lesions," *Acta Dermato Venereologica*, vol. 94, no. 5, pp. 617–618, 2014.

3

New-Onset Lichen Planus Induced by the Pfizer COVID-19 Vaccine

Fadi A. Alghamdi,[1] Shahad T. Khayyat,[2] Mohammed M. Alshareef,[3] and Wala'a Felemban[4]

[1]*Department of Dermatology, King Fahad Armed Forces Hospital, Jeddah, Saudi Arabia*
[2]*College of Medicine and Surgery, King Abdulaziz University, Jeddah, Saudi Arabia*
[3]*Department of Dermatology, King Abdulaziz Hospital, Makkah, Saudi Arabia*
[4]*Department of Pathology, King Fahad Armed Forces Hospital, Jeddah, Saudi Arabia*

Correspondence should be addressed to Shahad T. Khayyat; shahadt2010@gmail.com

Academic Editor: Hristo Dobrev

Objective. Coronavirus disease 2019 (COVID-19) vaccine distribution continues to expand; however, increased cutaneous reactions have been reported. Several recent studies suggest a link between COVID-19 vaccination and the development of various cutaneous complications. Lichen planus is a chronic, immune-mediated, inflammatory dermatological illness with an unclear etiology. In this case report, we assessed the relationship between COVID-19 vaccination (Pfizer) and lichen planus diagnosis and evaluated the link between additional doses of the vaccine and disease progression. *Methods.* Complete clinical, laboratory, and histopathological assessment of a patient was performed with ethical and privacy considerations. Written informed consent for all clinical data, images, and publication was obtained from the patient. *Results.* New-onset lichen planus appeared 48 hours after the first dose of the Pfizer vaccine. The symptoms worsened following the second dose. The patient responded gradually to topical corticosteroids, and lichen planus was controlled within 21 days. *Conclusion.* Our case significantly contributes to the literature by highlighting that additional doses of the Pfizer vaccine can contribute to disease progression. Therefore, reporting the patient's condition associated with COVID-19 vaccination should be considered. Future studies should be performed to investigate the combined onset of lichen planus and multisystem COVID-19 vaccine-related complications.

1. Introduction

The coronavirus disease 2019 (COVID-19) pandemic was announced in March 2020 by the World Health Organization. Healthcare, social, and economic disturbances became widespread in most countries [1], encouraging further investigation and development of vaccines against severe acute respiratory syndrome coronavirus 2, as to date, no effective management existed [1]. As the COVID-19 vaccines became widely distributed, cutaneous reactions were increasingly observed. Previously, 414 registry individuals with dermatologic responses after receiving mRNA COVID-19 vaccines from Moderna (83%) and Pfizer (17%) were evaluated, of which systemic manifestations—including fatigue, headache, fever, and muscle and joint pain—were reported [2]. A wide range of documented skin conditions was identified following COVID-19 immunization, including local responses at the injection site, urticaria, and morbilliform eruptions with unexpected adverse events (including pityriasis-rosea-like rashes) [2]. Moreover, a case of lichen planus (LP) caused by COVID-19 vaccination was reported [2]. The prevalence of LP, a mucocutaneous, inflammatory dermatosis [3] is approximately 1% in the United States. It mainly affects individuals aged 40–60 years; however, LP has also been identified in younger individuals, and males and females are equally affected [3]. Polygonal, flat-topped, violaceous papules and plaques are typical characteristics of LP. Physical assessment of oral or cutaneous LP may reveal "Wickham's striae," superimposed, reticulated white scales [3]. The clinical findings based on lesion morphology include hypertrophic, bullous, actinic, and erosive types of LP. Hypertrophic LP, defined as scaly, hyperkeratotic, pruritic flat-topped plaques, are frequently found on the anterior distal lower limbs. Bullous LP appears as vesicles or bullae inside LP lesions. Actinic LP is characterized as atrophic, hyperpigmented lesions with a rolling edge that occur in sun-exposed areas and are suspected to be caused by ultraviolet radiation. Erosive LP refers to painful, eroded, or ulcerated lesions that usually include mucosal tissues and can cause scarring. The appearance of violaceous plaques with central clearing and atrophy is the characteristic of annular atrophic LP, an uncommon variant of LP. LP pigmentosus is described as hyperpigmented, lichenoid plaques distributed in sun-exposed or flexural regions [3].

Topical corticosteroids of medium to high potency are used as a first-line treatment for cutaneous LP. Based on the severity of the condition and the physician's expertise, other methods, such as intralesional injection, may be applied [3]. As a second-line therapy, systemic corticosteroids (oral or intramuscular injection) are commonly administered. Oral retinoid and phototherapy are other treatment options. Additional medications are being evaluated to treat this illness, including griseofulvin, oral metronidazole, efalizumab, thalidomide, sulfasalazine, mycophenolate mofetil, ciclosporin, and azathioprine [3].

While the correlation between LP and COVID-19 vaccinations should be determined, no studies investigating this relationship exist, making case reports a valuable source of information on the influence of additional vaccine doses on disease progression.

Thus, this case is the first to report new-onset LP following Pfizer vaccine administration, demonstrating a positive correlation between subsequent doses of the Pfizer vaccine and the progression of LP.

2. Case Presentation

A 67-year-old woman with hypertension, diabetes mellitus, and hypercholesterolemia presented to our dermatology outpatient clinic with chief complaints of multiple, new-onset, red to purple, itchy skin lesions after receiving her first dose of the Pfizer COVID-19 vaccine 5 months before attending our clinic. Skin lesions initially appeared on her back 2 days after vaccination. She received the second Pfizer vaccine dose after 30 days and gradually developed a new and similar skin manifestations associated with pruritus over the bilateral shoulders and chest. There was no bloody or purulent discharge observed, and no similar previous episodes had occurred. The patient was a nonsmoker, and when queried about possible provoking factors, she confirmed that there was no evidence of infection or alteration in medication, no recent social or emotional imbalances, negative history of food or drug allergies, and no family history of similar complaints.

Physical examination showed multiple annular, hypertrophic, scaly, violaceous, and well-demarcated polygonal papules and plagues on her back (Figure 1), chest (Figure 2), and bilateral shoulders. No scalp, oral, genital, or nail involvement was noted. Hepatitis serology showed negative results. A papule biopsy on her back was performed, revealing a separated epidermis from the underlying dermis; hyperkeratosis, hypergranulosis, and superficial, dermal, band-like lymphocytic infiltrates were observed. Dysplasia and malignancy were not evident. Considering these factors and test results, we diagnosed the patient with LP.

The patient was followed up after 14 days (Figure 3), during which she gradually responded to topical corticosteroids without new active skin lesions developing, and the disease was controlled within 21 days.

Informed written consent for the publication of all patient photographs and medical information was provided to the authors at the time of article submission to the journal, with the understanding that this information may be publicly available. The study was approved by the responsible research and ethics committee at King Fahd Armed Forces Hospital (approval number: REC 489).

3. Discussion

COVID-19 immunizations and related adverse effects are new to the medical field; therefore, early detection and management of rare COVID-19 vaccination-related dermatological cases and consideration of the third vaccination dose are vital.

Our patient developed new-onset cutaneous LP 2 days after receiving the first Pfizer dose, and progression occurred following the second dose. Another case of cutaneous LP was reported within 2 days; however, symptoms appeared after the second Pfizer dose [4]. Conversely, another case of cutaneous LP related to the Pfizer vaccine occurred 2 weeks after the second dose [5]. Two other patients were previously observed. The first patient suffered a relapse of lichen planopilaris 14 days after the second AstraZeneca vaccine dose, and the second suffered an LP flare-up 3 days after the first Sinopharm vaccine dose [6]. All previously mentioned cases [4–6] included middle-aged women, similar to our case. However, these participants had a controlled LP that was provoked by the COVID-19 vaccine [4–6].

LP is an inflammatory disorder of the skin, hair, nails, and mucous membranes; while its pathogenesis is not fully understood, it represents a T-cell-mediated autoimmune disease [3]. In addition, this condition is associated with previous exposure to triggering agents, including viruses, vaccines, and drugs [3].

In July 2020, a patient tested positive for COVID-19 and was diagnosed with annular LP 5 days later [7]. The author of that study concluded that LP appeared to directly correlate with the positivity rate of hepatitis C in a given population, in addition to vaccines for hepatitis B, influenza, rabies, diphtheria, tetanus, pertussis, measles, mumps, and rubella [7]. Clinical experiments showed that these vaccines activate a Th1 response, increasing interleukin 2, tumor necrosis factor (TNF), and interferon (IFN) serum levels (cytokines that play a role in LP development) [8]. Although the pathogenesis remains unknown, upregulation of the Th1 response increases the levels of proapoptotic cytokines, such

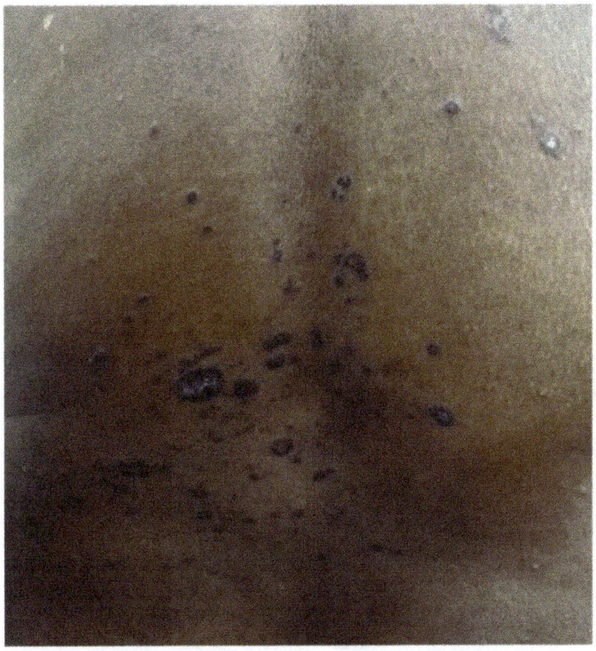

Figure 1: Multiple annular, hypertrophic, violaceous, well-demarcated papules and plaques over the back.

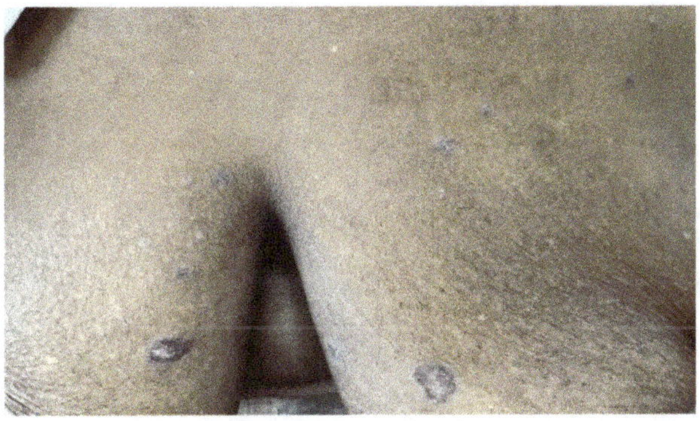

Figure 2: Multiple annular, hypertrophic, violaceous, well-demarcated papules and plaques on the chest.

as TNFα and IFNγ, which have been identified as critical factors for basal keratinocyte apoptosis in LP [3]. Furthermore, antimalarials, angiotensin-converting enzyme inhibitors, thiazide diuretics, nonsteroidal anti-inflammatory drugs, quinidine, beta-blockers, TNFα inhibitors, and gold are among the medications linked to LP [9, 10]. The LP onset in our patient might be attributable to the COVID-19 vaccine, as the first episode of cutaneous symptoms emerged after receiving the first Pfizer vaccine dose. Moreover, the patient confirmed that she had progressively developed multiple, new, similar pruritic skin lesions over the chest and bilateral arms 30 days after receiving the second vaccine dose, thus indicating a positive correlation between increased dosage and disease progression.

The limitation of our study was the time constraints that hindered detailed examination and analysis.

As COVID-19 immunizations and related side effects are new to the medical field, dermatologists play a crucial role in diagnosing COVID-19 vaccination-related cutaneous sequelae. Our case is relevant for further understanding this relationship, highlighting that additional doses of the Pfizer vaccine contribute to the LP disease progression. Therefore, this should be addressed by institutions administering COVID-19 vaccinations. We suggest further research investigating the concurrent LP onset and multisystem COVID-19 vaccine-related problems due to insufficient current literature, especially regarding COVID-19 vaccination complications on the cutaneous system and other involved systems.

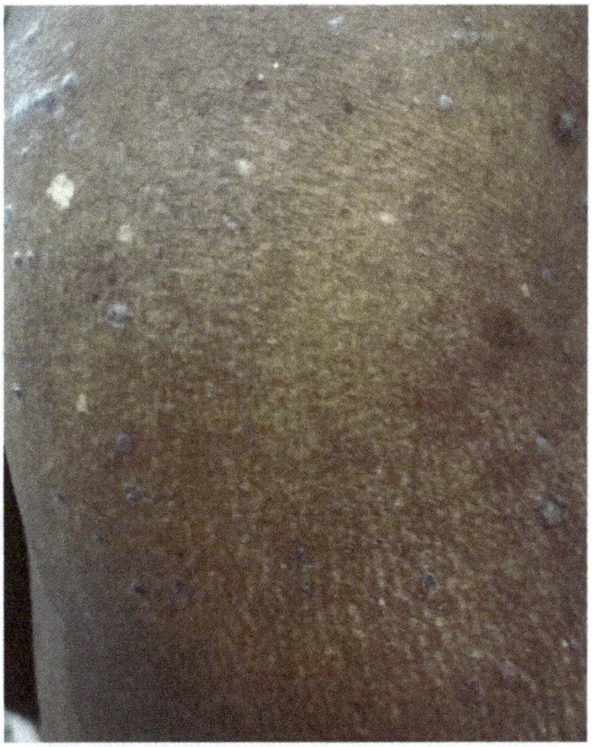

Figure 3: Improvement of the lichen planus lesions over the shoulders.

Disclosure

The funder was involved in writing, editing, and approval of the manuscript and in the decision to publish.

Acknowledgments

This work was supported by King Fahad Armed Forces Hospital, Jeddah, Saudi Arabia, and the funding was acquired by Dr. Fadi A. Alghamdi.

References

[1] A. K. Dutta, "Vaccine against Covid-19 disease-present status of development," *Indian Journal of Pediatrics*, vol. 87, no. 10, pp. 810–816, 2020.

[2] D. E. McMahon, E. Amerson, M. Rosenbach et al., “Cutaneous reactions reported after Moderna and Pfizer COVID-19 vaccination: a registry-based study of 414 cases,” *Journal of the American Academy of Dermatology*, vol. 85, no. 1, pp. 46–55, 2021.

[3] J. S. Lehman, M. M. Tollefson, and L. E. Gibson, “Lichen planus,” *International Journal of Dermatology*, vol. 48, no. 7, pp. 682–694, 2009.

[4] I. Hiltun, J. Sarriugarte, I. Martínez-de-Espronceda et al., “Lichen planus arising after COVID-19 vaccination,” *Journal of the European Academy of Dermatology and Venereology: JEADV*, vol. 35, no. 7, pp. e414–e415, 2021.

[5] A. Herzum, M. Burlando, M. F. Molle, C. Micalizzi, E. Cozzani, and A. Parodi, “Lichen planus flare following COVID-19 vaccination: a case report,” *Clinical Case Reports*, vol. 9, Article ID e05092, 12 pages, 2021.

[6] R. Diab, F. Araghi, M. Gheisari, Z. A. Kani, and H. Moravvej, “Lichen planus and lichen planopilaris flare after COVID-19 vaccination,” *Dermatologic Therapy*, vol. 35, no. 3, Article ID e15283, 2022.

[7] B. Diaz-Guimaraens, M. Dominguez-Santas, A. Suarez-Valle, D. Fernandez-Nieto, J. Jimenez-Cauhe, and A. Ballester, “Annular lichen planus associated with coronavirus SARS-CoV-2 disease (COVID-19),” *International Journal of Dermatology*, vol. 60, no. 2, pp. 246-247, 2021.

[8] U. Sahin, A. Muik, E. Derhovanessian et al., “COVID-19 vaccine BNT162b1 elicits human antibody and T_H1T cell responses,” *Nature*, vol. 586, pp. 594–599, 2020.

[9] A. Asarch, A. B. Gottlieb, J. Lee et al., “Lichen planus-like eruptions: an emerging side effect of tumor necrosis factor-α antagonists,” *Journal of the American Academy of Dermatology*, vol. 61, no. 1, pp. 104–111, 2009.

[10] S. Halevy and A. Shai, “Lichenoid drug eruptions,” *Journal of the American Academy of Dermatology*, vol. 29, no. 2, pp. 249–255, 1993.

4

Mycosis Fungoides: Analysis of Ophthalmologic Findings in a Series of Cases

Carina G. Colossi,[1] Juliano Mondadori,[2] Pedro K. M. Barreto,[2] Felipe M. Valença,[2] Rodrigo Duquia,[2] and Manuel A. P. Vilela[1,2]

[1] *Institute of Cardiology/University Cardiology Foundation and Post-Graduation Program, Ivo Corrêa-Meyer Institute of Ophthalmology, Porto Alegre-RS, Brazil*
[2] *Federal University of Health Sciences of Porto Alegre, Brazil*

Correspondence should be addressed to Manuel A. P. Vilela; mapvilela@gmail.com

Academic Editor: Alireza Firooz

Background. Ophthalmic findings in mycosis fungoides (MF) can be highly variable. It seems that the prevalence of ophthalmic findings could be much more common than previously assumed. *Objective.* To present case series examined in the last 12 months, together with a literature review. *Methods.* Symptomatic patients with biopsy-proven mycosis fungoides were examined ophthalmologically in a 12-month period. The medical records of affected patients were reviewed. *Results.* Eight patients were examined. Of these, 75% were male, all were Caucasian, and average age was 58.2 years. Blepharitis (50.0%), thickened eyelids (37.5%), and flaking (25.0%) were the most prevalent findings. *Conclusion.* Incidence of MF affecting the eyes and surrounding structures may be greater than estimated. Early case management offers means to reduce difficulties experienced with later diagnosis. Regular monitoring by an ophthalmologist is justified, including that of asymptomatic cases.

1. Introduction

Mycosis fungoides (MF) is a rare primary T-cell cutaneous lymphoma. Its annual estimated incidence is 6.4-9.6 cases per one million inhabitants in the USA [1–3]. Clinical diagnosis is usually difficult, especially at early stages. Diagnosis often requires multiple biopsies and is commonly performed quite late, given its similarities with other conditions and the scarcity of typical clinical or histopathologic signs [2–5]. Blotches or flaking erythematous plaques are usually the initial manifestation, making the condition similar to other skin disorders such as eczemas, atopic dermatitis, psoriasis, and pityriasis lichenoides. In the next stage infiltrative lesions appear as the disease progresses. Following this, tumorous lesions appear and lymph nodes and other organs are affected. It is a disease mostly affecting White adults. As a rule the disease is indolent and controllable. Available treatment is for the most part palliative, although it is free from risks and serious side effects and improves long-term control and survival [1–5]. Bone marrow transplant is the only treatment that cures the disease but is rarely adopted [6, 7].

MF involving the eyes and their surrounding structures is considered to be rare (2% of affected cases) and is probably underestimated owing to difficulties in diagnosing it in the early stages [1]. Only three sizeable series can be found in the accounts available in the literature. Among the 30 patients described by Stenson & Ramsay [8], 36.7% had ophthalmological changes and eyelid tumours were the most common finding (26.7%). Leib et al. [9] described 17 cases and eyelids were the most frequently affected region by blepharitis or ectropion. Cook et al. [10] assessed 210 cases, whereby the most prevalent condition was ectropion (40.4%).

Our aim is to present case series examined over the last 12 months, to review the literature, updating manifestation in the eyes and their surrounding structures, as well as possibilities for case management.

2. Case Report

In the period comprising October 2016 to October 2017, eight cases with clinical and histopathologic diagnosis of MF were referred by the Dermatology Service of a University in Southern Brazil. These were only visually symptomatic patients and did not account for all patients examined in that period (total number of cases with MF: 40). The ophthalmological examination consisted of corrected Snellen visual acuity, extrinsic motricity, pupil reflexes, applanation tonometry (Perkins), anterior and posterior biomicroscopy (Topcon SL 1E, Tokyo, Japan and 90-D Volk lens, USA), and indirect binocular ophthalmoscopy with mydriasis (Eyetec model ODS 6.0, São Paulo, Brazil). All eight cases were examined. Average age was 58.2 years (29–77), the majority (75.0%) were male and 100% were Caucasian. All patients examined signed a free and informed consent form and this study was approved by the institution's Research Ethics Committee. Burning eyes (50%), progressive impaired vision (37.5%), and redness (37.5%) were the most common symptoms, followed by itchy, watery, and crusts on eyelashes and eyebrows (25%). Average corrected visual acuity was 0.90 in both eyes. Findings directly linked to MF were blepharitis (50.0%), eyelid thickening (37.5%), flaking skin (25.0%), and filamentary keratitis (12.5%). Age-associated findings were cataract (37.5%), pingueculae (37.5%), and macular RPE changes (12.5%). 62.5% were undergoing phototherapy (PUVB) whilst the remainder were only receiving symptomatic maintenance therapy. Demographic characteristics and ophthalmic findings are shown in Table 1.

3. Discussion

MF can be the result of chronic antigenic stimulation, possibly owing to occupational or infectious factors or genetic mutations, triggering uncontrolled clonal growth and accumulation of T helper lymphocytes on the skin. It usually progresses slowly and 70% of cases are diagnosed at this stage, having erythematous plaques distributed in regions of the body usually protected from the sun (buttocks, breasts, and lower torso). In 30% of cases the disease is more aggressive and forms infiltrative or tumorous lesions and in some cases tends to develop with erythroderma [2–5, 11].

In terms of histopathology, MF consists of multiplication of $CD4^+$CD45RO T lymphocytes, with some cases of $CD8^+$ expression (20%). Neoplastic cells are commonly atypical small or intermediate lymphocytes with hyperchromatic nuclei and having a cerebrum-like aspect surrounded by clear cytoplasm (10%). Infiltrate occurs along the dermoepidermal junction, with lymphocytic epidermotropism present in 96% of cases in the form of clusters or isolated cellularity, with no spongiosis in 25% of cases (Pautrier's microabscess). Specific cytopathic modifications, keratinocyte apoptosis, Civatte bodies, and colloid bodies also often occur. Molecular markers generally do not show positive cellularity enabling disease definition, especially in its initial stages. Presence of the TOX gene in the cells may assist confirmation of diagnosis. These difficulties have led to the creation of a diagnostic algorithm that integrates clinical, histologic, immunophenotypic, and molecular criteria by the International Society for Cutaneous Lymphomas [3–5, 12].

Estimated MF prevalence in the eyes and surrounding structures is low (2%) and among those having visual symptoms it is 26.7%–40.4% [7–11, 13, 14]. Incidence is possibly underestimated given the difficulty in diagnosing it and late diagnosis, in addition to clinical variants. Primary eye conditions, prior to skin repercussions, are extremely rare. The eyelids and eye surface are usually the most affected areas, particularly in more advanced stages. Ectropion is the most common manifestation on the eyelids, caused by tumours or cutaneous infiltration. Case management is complicated regardless of the mechanism and may compromise eye surface integrity [7–11, 13, 14].

In our series flaking blepharitis was the most common finding, followed by eyelid thickening and eyelash and eyebrow flaking. The most prevalent complaints were burning, impaired vision, redness, itching, and crust on eyelashes and eyebrows. The signs and symptoms found by Leib et al. [9] in their series were similar. Other regions directly affected by the process are the conjunctiva, sclera (episcleral infiltrate), corneas (punctuate keratitis, stromal opacification, melts, and subepithelial infiltrates), retina, choroid and vitreous body (infiltrates, uveitis, and vascular occlusions), and the optic nerve (infiltration and neuropathy) [8, 14–22].

Nonspecific manifestations include dry eyes, cataracts, corneal ulcers, glaucoma, chorioretinal scars, peripheral nerve palsy, and campimetric defects, among others. In our series, cataracts, exuberant pingueculae, and pigment change in the macular region were detected and associated with age. The most prevalent dermatological complaints were pruritus, erythematous-scaling plaques or rash on nonexposed areas, and infiltrative plaques.

Systemic case management is palliative. Evidence collected through systematic review concluded that monotherapy and different combinations showed similar results [23]. PUVA, in isolation or combined with interferon-alpha or retinoids, has been found to be beneficial in many situations [24]. PUVA may be a confounder, but all cases reported here used towels and goggles to protect the eye region. Systemic methotrexate or methotrexate associated with interferon-alpha or bexarotene in more advanced stages has produced favourable evidence. At local level, care of chronic eyelid edge infections, corneal exposure, and surface lubrication tend to be the most adopted measures. Eyelid thickening can be alleviated by using PUVA, but severe ectropion and tumours require surgical repair. Infiltrative conjunctival envelopment can be managed with radiotherapy and topical corticosteroids [16]. Choroid, retina, vitreous or optic disc infiltrations are associated guarded prognoses and may be treated with intravitreal methotrexate or other systemic chemotherapy drugs (5-fluorouracil, leucovorin) and/or localized radiation [25].

Our study is cross-sectional, small, and not representative of all MF cases we cared for during the period. Its strength lies in the description of ocular manifestations in cases that have not yet developed into visceral disease. Functional morbidity of the eyes at this stage is relevant and as such paying careful attention to patient complaints and early case management can reduce the severity of eye impairment.

Table 1: MF case demographic, clinical, and examination characteristics.

Case	Age (years)	Sex	Clinical signs	Complaints	VA	Examination	General management
1	67	M	infiltrative plaques, scaly lesions	IMPAIRED VISION ITCHING, EYELASH CRUSTS, WATERY EYES	OD 0.7 OE 0.6	Eyelid thickening, blepharitis/conjunctivitis, eyelash and eyebrow flaking, filamentary keratitis, nuclear 2+ cataract	
2	77	M	erythema patches, pruritus	IMPAIRED VISION	OD 0.6 OE 0.6	Eyelid thickening, PSC cataract	
3	56	M	maculopapular rash and itchy lesions	BURNING	OD 1.0 OE 1.0	Exuberant pingueculae	PH
4	72	F	erythema patches, pruritus	BURNING IMPAIRED VISION	OD 0.6 OE 0.6	Exuberant pingueculae Mild axial cataract	PH
5	62	F	erythema patches, scale, pruritus	REDNESS; BURNING	OD 0.9 OE 0.9	Exuberant pingueculae, Macular RPE change	PH
6	29	M	Fine scale, itchy macules	REDNESS WATERY EYES	OD 1.0 OE 0.9	Blepharitis, eyelash flaking	
7	51	M	erythema patches, pruritus	ITCHING	OD 1.0 OE 1.0	Blepharitis	PH
8	52	M	maculo-papulomatous and itchy lesions	BURNING; CRUSTS, REDNESS	OD 1.0 OE 1.0	Blepharitis, eyelid thickening	PH
Average	58.2	M (75%)	Erythematous-scaling plaques or rash 87.5% Pruritus 62.5% Infiltrative plaques: 12%	BURNING 50% IMPAIRED VISION 37.5% REDNESS 37.5% ITCHING 25% CRUSTS 25% WATERY EYES 25%	OD 0.9 OD 0.9	Blepharitis 50% Cataract 37.5% Eyelid thickening 37.5% Pingueculae 37.5% Eyelash flaking 25.0% Filamentary keratitis 12.5% Macular RPE change 12.5%	PH 62.5%

M = male, F = female, VA = corrected visual acuity, PH = phototherapy, PSC = posterior subcapsular cataract, RPE = retinal pigment epithelium.

In conclusion, the incidence of MF affecting the eyes and their surrounding structures may be greater than estimated. Early case management offers means to reduce difficulties experienced with later diagnosis. Regular monitoring by an ophthalmologist is justified and may contribute to reducing sequelae, including regular monitoring of asymptomatic cases when the likelihood of conversion to eye symptoms over time is still unknown.

References

[1] V. D. Criscione and M. A. Weinstock, "Incidence of cutaneous T-cell lymphoma in the United States, 1973–2002," *JAMA Dermatology*, vol. 143, no. 7, pp. 854–859, 2007.

[2] C. S. Ahn, A. ALSayyah, and O. P. Sangüeza, "Mycosis fungoides: an updated review of clinicopathologic variants," *American Journal of Dermatopathology*, vol. 36, no. 12, pp. 933–951, 2014.

[3] S. I. Jawed, P. L. Myskowski, S. Horwitz, A. Moskowitz, and C. Querfeld, "Primary cutaneous T-cell lymphoma (mycosis fungoides and Sézary syndrome): part I. Diagnosis: clinical and histopathologic features and new molecular and biologic markers," *Journal of the American Academy of Dermatology*, vol. 70, no. 2, pp. 205.el–205.e16, 2014.

[4] K. Olek-Hrab and W. Silny, "Diagnostics in mycosis fungoides and Sezary syndrome," *Reports of Practical Oncology and Radiotherapy*, vol. 19, no. 2, pp. 72–76, 2014.

[5] N. Pimpinelli, E. A. Olsen, M. Santucci et al., "Defining early mycosis fungoides," *Journal of the American Academy of Dermatology*, vol. 53, no. 6, pp. 1053–1063, 2005.

[6] E. Atilla, P. A. Atilla, S. C. Bozdag et al., "Allogeneic hematopoietic stem cell transplantation for refractory mycosis fungoides (MF) and Sezary syndrome (SS)," *International Journal of Hematology*, vol. 106, no. 3, pp. 426–430, 2017.

[7] M. Criscuolo, L. Fianchi, P. Chiusolo, S. Giammarco, A. Bacigalupo, and L. Pagano, "Allogeneic Transplant for Mycosis Fungoides in Patient with Wiskott-Aldrich Syndrome," *Journal of Clinical Immunology*, vol. 38, no. 1, pp. 7–9, 2018.

[8] S. Stenson and D. L. Ramsay, "Ocular findings in mycosis fungoides," *JAMA Ophtalmology*, vol. 99, no. 2, pp. 272–277, 1981.

[9] M. L. Leib, H. Lester, R. E. Braunstein, and R. L. Edelson, "Ocular findings in cutaneous T-cell lymphoma," *Annals of Ophthalmology*, vol. 23, no. 5, pp. 182–186, 1991.

[10] B. E. Cook Jr., G. B. Bartley, and M. R. Pittelkow, "Ophthalmic abnormalities in patients with cutaneous T-cell lymphoma," *Ophthalmology*, vol. 106, no. 7, pp. 1339–1344, 1999.

[11] S. I. Jawed, P. L. Myskowski, S. Horwitz, A. Moskowitz, and C. Querfeld, "Primary cutaneous T-cell lymphoma (mycosis fungoides and Sézary syndrome): part II. Prognosis, management, and future directions," *Journal of the American Academy of Dermatology*, vol. 70, no. 2, pp. 223.el–223.e17, 2014.

[12] G. A. Levy-Clarke, D. Greenman, P. C. Sieving et al., "Ophthalmic Manifestations, Cytology, Immunohistochemistry, and Molecular Analysis of Intraocular Metastatic T-Cell Lymphoma: Report of a Case and Review of the Literature," *Survey of Ophthalmology*, vol. 53, no. 3, pp. 285–295, 2008.

[13] H. C. Foerster, "Mycosis fungoides with intraocular involvement," *Transactions of the American Academy of Ophthalmology and Otolaryngology*, vol. 64, pp. 308–313, 1960.

[14] R. J. Leitch, I. G. Rennie, and M. A. Parsons, "Ocular involvement in mycosis fungoides," *British Journal of Ophthalmology*, vol. 77, no. 2, pp. 126-127, 1993.

[15] D. Jusufbegovic and D. H. Char, "Clinical variability of ocular involvement in Mycosis fungoides," *JAMA Ophthalmology*, vol. 133, no. 3, pp. 341–343, 2015.

[16] S. S. Aldrees, P. Zoroquiain, S. A. Alghamdi, P. T. Logan, S. Callejo, and M. N. Burnier Jr., "Conjunctival Involvement of T-Cell Lymphoma in a Patient with Mycosis Fungoides," *Case Reports in Ophthalmological Medicine*, vol. 2016, Article ID 4786498, 5 pages, 2016.

[17] M. Ralli, J. W. Goldman, E. Lee, L. C. Pinter-Brown, B. J. Glasgow, and D. Sarraf, "Intraocular involvement of mycosis fungoides," *JAMA Ophtalmology*, vol. 127, no. 3, pp. 343–345, 2009.

[18] B. C. Erny, P. R. Egbert, I. M. Peat, K. Shorrock, and A. R. Rosenthal, "Intraocular involvement with subretinal pigment epithelium infiltrates by mycosis fungoides," *British Journal of Ophthalmology*, vol. 75, no. 11, pp. 698–701, 1991.

[19] G. C. Williams, E. Holz, A. G. Lee, and R. L. Font, "T-cell lymphoproliferative disorder of vitreous associated with mycosis fungoides," *JAMA Ophtalmology*, vol. 118, no. 2, pp. 278–280, 2000.

[20] M. J. Wan, T. G. Sheidow, G. W. Jones, and J. G. Heathcote, "Vitritis as the initial manifestation of recurrent mycosis fungoides," *Retinal Cases & Brief Reports*, vol. 3, no. 3, pp. 240–242, 2009.

[21] J. L. Keltner, E. Fritsch, R. C. Cykiert, and D. M. Albert, "Mycosis Fungoides: Intraocular and Central Nervous System Involvement," *JAMA Ophtalmology*, vol. 95, no. 4, pp. 645–650, 1977.

[22] D. M. Pariser, "Mycosis Fungoides Involving the Brain and Optic Nerves," *JAMA Dermatology*, vol. 114, no. 3, pp. 397–399, 1978.

[23] D. Humme, A. Nast, R. Erdmann, S. Vandersee, and M. Beyer, "Systematic review of combination therapies for mycosis fungoides," *Cancer Treatment Reviews*, vol. 40, no. 8, pp. 927–933, 2014.

[24] E. Hodak and L. Pavlovsky, "Phototherapy of Mycosis Fungoides," *Dermatologic Clinics*, vol. 33, no. 4, pp. 697–702, 2015.

[25] R. Reddy and S. J. Kim, "Intraocular T-cell lymphoma due to mycosis fungoides and response to intravitreal methotrexate," *Ocular Immunology and Inflammation*, vol. 19, no. 4, pp. 234–236, 2011.

5

Lymphomatoid Papulosis Type A: A Case Report of the "Wait-and-See Strategy" in a 27-Year-Old Male Patient with Extensive Disease

Eirini Kavvalou ,[1] Maria Stefanidou,[1] Sabine Elke Krueger-Krasagakis,[1] George Evangelou,[1] Dimitra Koumaki,[1] Leonidas Marinos,[2] Maria Tzardi,[3] and Konstantinos Krasagakis[1]

[1]*Department of Dermatology, University General Hospital of Heraklion, 71500 Heraklion, Greece*
[2]*Department of Haematopathology, Evaggelismos General Hospital of Athens, Ipsilantou 45-47, 10676, Athens, Greece*
[3]*Department of Pathology, University Hospital of Heraklion, 71500 Heraklion, Greece*

Correspondence should be addressed to Eirini Kavvalou; ekavvalou@hotmail.com

Academic Editor: Ravi Krishnan

This is the case of a 27-year-old male patient with a newly diagnosed extensive lymphomatoid papulosis type A involving cosmetically sensitive areas (e.g. face), who refused to be treated with a low dose of methotrexate, as recommended by the published literature. The natural course of the disease was proved to be strikingly satisfying though, with a complete regression of all skin lesions at the 4-week follow-up, including an ulcerated nodule 3 x 3 cm in dimension, which was expected to heal at least in months. We report this case to reconsider weighting the risks and the short-term benefits of methotrexate treatment, even in the case of an extensive disease.

1. Introduction

Lymphomatoid papulosis is a rare, recurrent, self-healing papulonodular skin eruption and part of the group of cutaneous $CD30^+$ lymphoproliferative disorders (LPDs). It is associated with a lifelong increased incidence of malignant lymphoma [1]. In case of an extended disease, treatment with methotrexate in a low dose is recommended in order to hasten the regression of the lesions [2]. In this case report a 27-year-old patient with extensive disease refused to take methotrexate because of its potential harmful side effects. The result in the 4-week follow-up was strikingly satisfying with the majority of papulonodular lesions having regressed, living hyperpigmented scarred lesions. Of interest has been the spontaneous regression of a nodular, ulcerated lesion with a diameter of 3 × 3 cm. Our case highlights the significance of weighting the potential harmful effects of methotrexate treatment against the possibility of a spontaneous regression even in terms of an extensive lymphomatoid papulosis.

2. Case Presentation

A 27-year-old male patient with a history of expanding skin lesions was referred to us for further management, after having received a 7-day per os antibiotic treatment with cefuroxime with no improvement. On physical examination there was a nodular, incipiently ulcerated, crumbly lesion 3 × 3 cm in dimension on the extensor surface of the left thigh, as well as crops of multiple elevated dome-shaped nodules and papules of reddish color and shiny, smooth surface on the trunk, the upper and lower extremities, the neck, periorbital and on the genitalia (Figures 1(a) and 1(b)). At some sites there was also a perilesional scaling. No pruritus was mentioned. The palms, the soles, and the mucous membranes were not involved. Moreover, a history of tiredness feeling in the previous months was mentioned. The history revealed though no consistent systemic B symptoms. The differential diagnosis included lymphomatoid papulosis, other cutaneous lymphomas, sarcoidosis, histiocytosis, and cutaneous

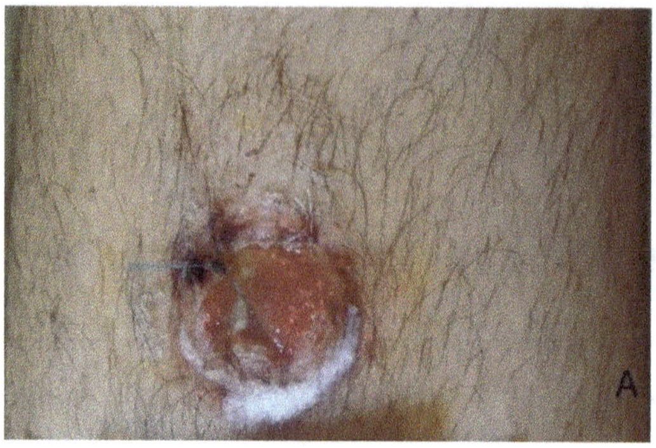

(a)

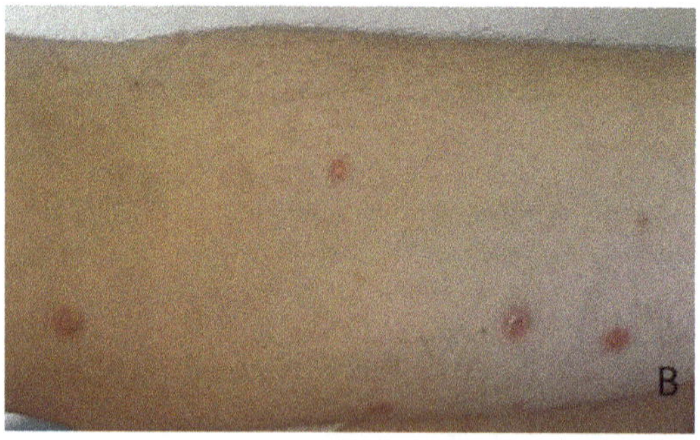

(b)

FIGURE 1: A large ulcerated 3×3 cm tumor on the extensor surface of the left thigh at presentation (a); a widespread erythematous papulonodular eruption involving the face, the trunk and the extremities with occasional scaling at the periphery of the lesions (b).

infections (cutaneous leishmaniasis, atypical mycobacterial infection, and bacillary angiomatosis). Laboratory examination revealed an increased serum title of Bartonella quintana (1/80) and the patient received doxycycline 100 mg 1×2 for 2 weeks, with no change in a 2-week control examination. No other abnormal laboratory results were found (serology for CMV, EBV, HIV, HBV, HCV, Toxoplasma, Treponema pallidum, Leishmania, Coxiella burnetii, Mycoplasma pneumonia, Chlamydia pneumonia, Quantiferon test, RF, IgA, IgG, IgM, C3, C4, ANA, and ENA Screen). In the context of a possible histiocytosis we ordered an ophthalmological and an ENT consultation, both of which revealed no pathological signs. We performed two biopsies, one from the ulcerated lesion on the left thigh and another one from a dome-shaped but not ulcerated lesion on the left back. Bacterial, fungal, and mycobacterial cultures from the specimens were negative. Histology revealed a diffuse lymphocytic infiltration in the reticular dermis by small, medium, and large sized lymphocytes, some of which with anaplastic nuclei, accompanied by a variable number of neutrophils and histiocytes (Figures 2(a)–2(c)). Immunophenotypically the lymphocytes were CD3+ (Figure 3(a)), CD30+ (>75%, Figures 3(b) and 3(c)), CD4+, MUM1+, CD8-, ALK-1-, CD15-, and TIA-1-/+ (20% positive). The cellular marker for proliferation, Ki-67, was estimated ~ 80%. The epidermis was spared and showed a psoriasiform hyperplasia. Peripheral blood smear as well as immunophenotypic analysis of peripheral blood and bone marrow was performed with normal findings. The bone marrow biopsy showed absence of neoplastic infiltration, with minor deviations of the hemopoietic series of no particular significance. CT-scan of neck-thorax-abdomen showed no lymphadenopathy. The proposed diagnosis, based upon the correlation of clinical, histological, and immunophenotypical (expression of CD30) findings, was primary cutaneous CD30+ lymphoproliferative disorder with multifocal signs classified as lymphomatoid papulosis type A. According to the NCCN v2.2019 guidelines for primary cutaneous CD30+ T-cell lymphoproliferative disorders for adult patients with extensive disease, observation is preferred for asymptomatic patients [3]. Methotrexate (10 to 35 mg per week by oral or subcutaneous administration) is opted among other treatments in symptomatic patients and has been proposed to our patient due to the large ulcerative lesion on the left thigh and the extensive multifocal disease involving cosmetically important body areas. However, the patient refused to take any medication because of the potential adverse reactions of the therapy. At 4-week follow-up a striking improvement was observed, with the total of the lesions having regressed. Of notice was the regression of the ulcerated nodular lesion on the left thigh (Figures 4(a) and 4(b)). No new lesions were found. A complete response was observed at the follow-up visits, which remained in the last 6 month follow-up.

3. Discussion

Lymphomatoid papulosis is a rare, chronic, recurrent, self-healing disease with excellent prognosis in the majority of cases [4]. The list with the available treatment

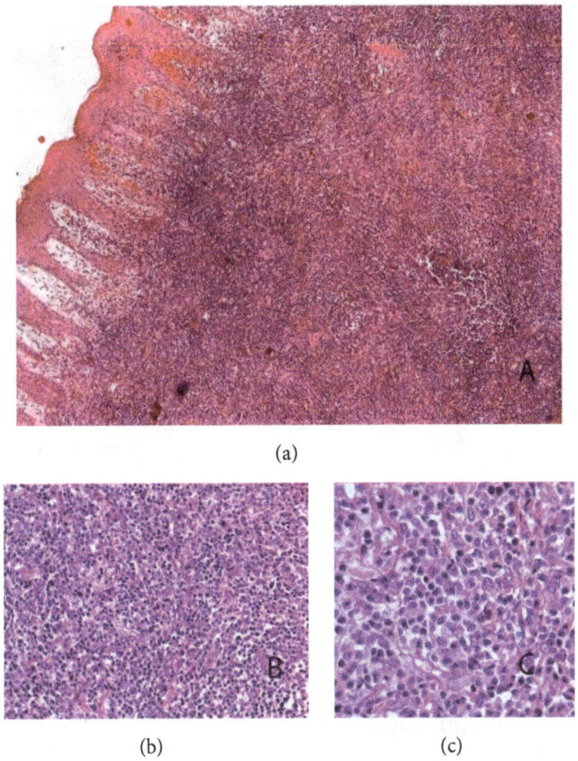

FIGURE 2: Histology revealed a diffuse lymphocytic infiltration in the reticular dermis by small, medium, and large sized lymphocytes, some of which with anaplastic nuclei, accompanied by a variable number of neutrophils and histiocytes (hematoxylin-eosin stain x 20 (a), x 40 (b), x 60 (c)).

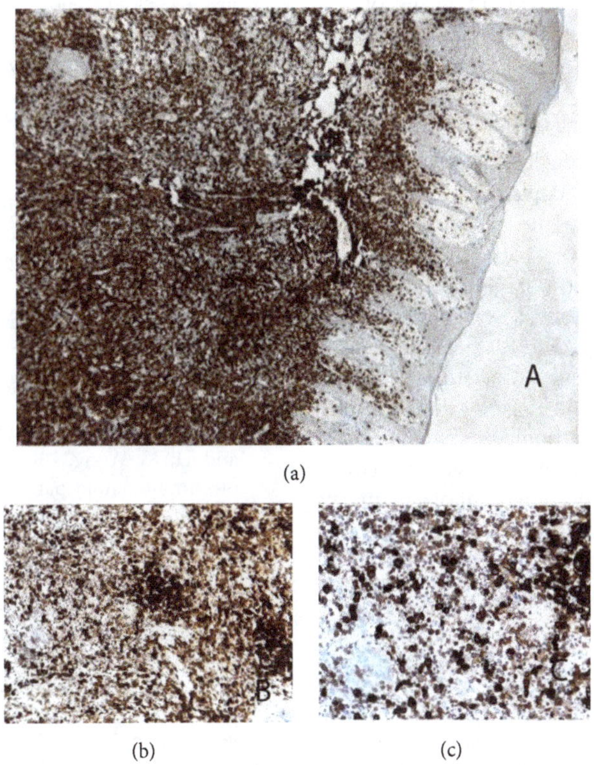

FIGURE 3: Immunophenotypically the lymphocytes were CD3+ (x20) (a) and >75% CD30+ (x40) (b) and (x60) (c) (Immunohistochemistry with Envision Detection System Peroxidase/DAB, Rabbit/Mouse).

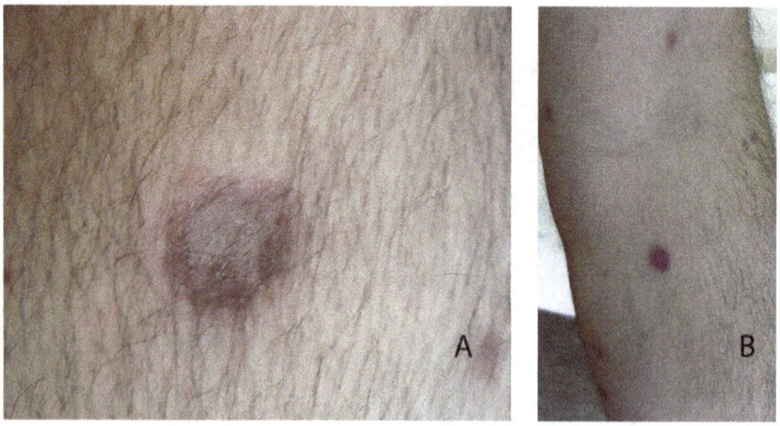

(a) (b)

Figure 4: Complete remission of the eruption leaving depressed scars, including the previous tumor on the left thigh (a) and the papulonodular eruption at other body sites (b).

modalities includes apart from topical steroids [3], topical mechlorethamine [3], methotrexate [2, 5–7], targeted phototherapy [8], photodynamic therapy[9], oral or topical retinoids [10], and anti-CD30 monoclonal antibody-drug-conjugate (brentuximab vedotin) [11]. None of them changes actually the natural history of the disease or reduces the risk of developing an associated lymphoma [2]. However, they may hasten the healing of the lesions and prevent the eruption of new lesions [2]. In case of a limited or asymptomatic disease, a wait-and-see strategy is recommended. In terms of an extensive disease or a disease involving cosmetically sensitive areas (e.g. face)—as in our case—a low-dose methotrexate treatment is initiated, followed by a maintenance treatment [2]. Regarding our case of a 27-year-old male patient with extensive disease, involving cosmetically sensitive areas, a low-dose-methotrexate treatment was planned, in order to hasten the healing and preventing the eruption of new lesions, but was not accepted by the patient. The course of the untreated lesions, including the large ulcerated one, which usually may take months to heal, was impressively satisfying at the 4-week follow-up. The case should make us consider weighting the risks and the short-term benefits of methotrexate treatment, even in the case of an extensive disease. However, a situation like this should be systematically followed by the possibility of a relapse, the risk for second hematological neoplasia, and even development of a primary cutaneous anaplastic large cell lymphoma.

References

[1] J. H. Kunishige, H. McDonald, G. Alvarez, M. Johnson, V. Prieto, and M. Duvic, "Lymphomatoid papulosis and associated lymphomas: a retrospective case series of 84 patients," *Clinical and Experimental Dermatology*, vol. 34, no. 5, pp. 576–581, 2009.

[2] W. Kempf, K. Pfaltz, M. H. Vermeer et al., "EORTC, ISCL, and USCLC consensus recommendations for the treatment of primary cutaneous CD30-positive lymphoproliferative disorders: lymphomatoid papulosis and primary cutaneous anaplastic large-cell lymphoma," *Blood*, vol. 118, no. 15, pp. 4024–4035, 2011.

[3] National Comprehensive Cancer Network, "Primary cutaneous CD30+ lymphoproliferative disorders," https://www.nccn.org/professionals/physician_gls/pdf/primary_cutaneous.pdf, 2019.

[4] M. W. Bekkenk, F. A. M. J. Geelen, P. C. van Voorst Vader et al., "Primary and secondary cutaneous CD30+ lymphoproliferative disorders: a report from the Dutch Cutaneous Lymphoma Group on the long-term follow-up data of 219 patients and guidelines for diagnosis and treatment," *Blood*, vol. 95, no. 12, pp. 3653–3661, 2000.

[5] E. C. Vonderheid, A. Sajjadian, and M. E. Kadin, "Methotrexate is effective therapy for lymphomatoid papulosis and other primary cutaneous CD30-positive lymphoproliferative disorders," *Journal of the American Academy of Dermatology*, vol. 34, no. 3, pp. 470–481, 1996.

[6] M. Bruijn, B. Horváth, P. van Voorst Vader, R. Willemze, and M. Vermeer, "Recommendations for treatment of lymphomatoid papulosis with methotrexate: a report from the Dutch Cutaneous Lymphoma Group," *British Journal of Dermatology*, vol. 173, no. 5, pp. 1319–1322, 2015.

[7] K. M. Newland, C. J. McCormack, R. Twigger et al., "The efficacy of methotrexate for lymphomatoid papulosis," *Journal of the American Academy of Dermatology*, vol. 72, no. 6, pp. 1088–1090, 2015.

[8] A. P. Kontos, H. A. Kerr, F. Malick, D. P. Fivenson, H. W. Lim, and H. K. Wong, "308-nm Excimer laser for the treatment of lymphomatoid papulosis and stage IA mycosis fungoides," *Photodermatology, Photoimmunology & Photomedicine*, vol. 22, no. 3, pp. 168–171, 2006.

[9] M. Rodrigues, C. McCormack, L. Yap et al., "Successful treatment of lymphomatoid papulosis with photodynamic therapy," *Australasian Journal of Dermatology*, vol. 50, no. 2, pp. 129–132, 2009.

[10] R. A. Krathen, S. Ward, and M. Duvic, "Bexarotene is a new treatment option for lymphomatoid papulosis," *Dermatology*, vol. 206, no. 2, pp. 142–147, 2003.

[11] M. Duvic, M. T. Tetzlaff, P. Gangar, A. L. Clos, D. Sui, and R. Talpur, "Results of a phase II trial of brentuximab vedotin for cd30+ cutaneous t-cell lymphoma and lymphomatoid papulosis," *Journal of Clinical Oncology*, vol. 33, no. 32, pp. 3759–3765, 2015.

6

A Rare Case of Checkerboard-Like Becker Nevi with a Unique Distribution of Abnormalities

Chanidapa Wongtada,[1] Pravit Asawanonda,[2] and Marisa Pongprutthipan[2]

[1]*M.D., Graduated from Chulalongkorn University, Bangkok, Thailand*
[2]*Division of Dermatology, Department of Medicine, King Chulalongkorn Memorial Hospital, Bangkok, Thailand*

Correspondence should be addressed to Chanidapa Wongtada; parwongtada21@gmail.com

Academic Editor: Alireza Firooz

Becker nevus syndrome refers to a rare disorder comprising the typical pigmented lesion and its associated developmental abnormalities. Becker nevus itself is typically localized on the upper trunk, scapular or upper arm unilaterally; however, it can occasionally occur as multiple or bilateral lesions on any parts of the body. In this report, a rare case of multiple Becker nevi arranged in a unique checkerboard-like pattern is presented. More uniquely, the associated abnormalities found in this patient, breast hypoplasia and leg lipodystrophy, seem to be regionally correlated with the nevi. In closing, we would like to raise an easy-to-remember 6B's mnemonic, which stands for Becker, Breast, Bone, Bowen's disease, Basal cell carcinoma, and Beta-actin, for the cases of Becker nevus syndrome.

1. Introduction

Becker nevus is a well-defined, irregular border, tan to dark brown hyperpigmented cutaneous hamartoma, which is commonly associated with hypertrichosis and presented in unilateral localized fashion on upper trunk. Less common sites are extremities, face/neck, abdomen, and lower back, respectively [1]. There are various malformations that are in association with Becker nevi, contributing to Becker nevus syndrome. The common associated malformations include breast hypoplasia, musculoskeletal malformation, and scoliosis [1]. Interestingly, according to a systematic literature review by Schneider et al., Becker nevi and the malformations seem to have a regional correspondence [1]. In this case report, we present an uncommon case of Becker nevus syndrome with a unique checkerboard mosaic pattern and regional corresponding breast hypoplasia and leg lipodystrophy.

2. Case Report

A 20-year-old woman presented with multiple hyperpigmented patches involving the entire right hemibody and left upper back since birth. The patches were asymptomatic and became darker during puberty. There was no family history of similar disorders. On skin examination, multiple well-defined, irregular-border hyperpigmented patches were observed on the entire right side of the body with alternate areas of pigmentary change and sharp demarcation at anterior midline, resembling a checkerboard mosaic pattern. Moreover, there were dark brown patches on left upper back extending towards left shoulder and left chest. Further examination showed left breast hypoplasia and a slight smaller circumference of right leg comparing to the left (Figure 1). Ultrasonography of breasts confirmed relatively small size of left breast with normal appearance of fibroglandular tissue. Plain-film X-rays of both legs found no bony abnormalities with an equal leg length and similar shadow of muscle masses. Considering this evidence, the smaller right leg most likely results from subcutaneous fat hypoplasia.

On histopathology of the skin biopsy from left upper back and right abdomen, both sites exhibited acanthosis, slightly increased number of melanocytes along the basal layer of epidermis, mild elongation, and bridging of hyperpigmented rete ridges, compatible with Becker nevus.

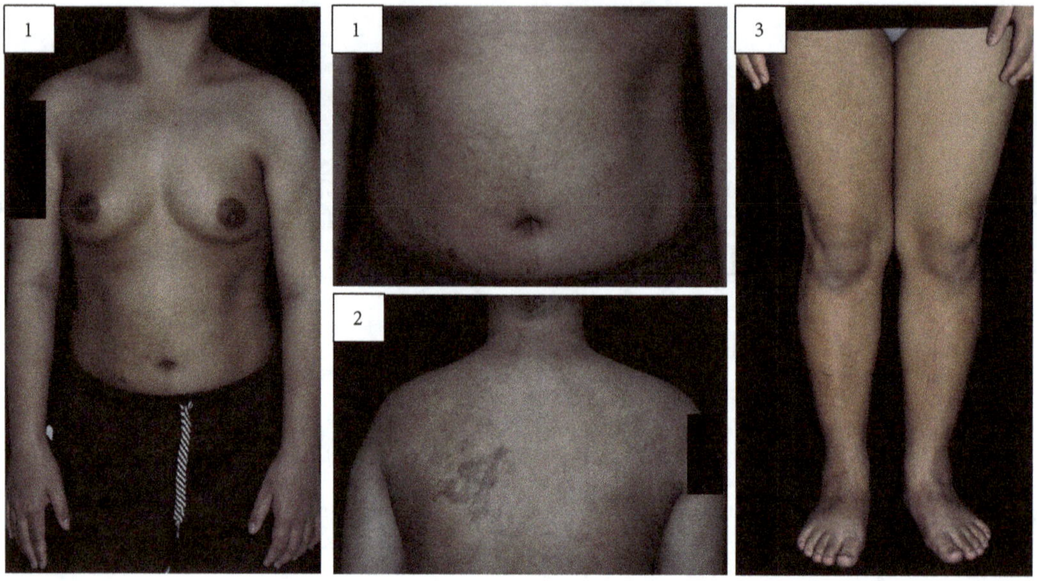

FIGURE 1: Multiple Becker nevi on (1) anterior trunk resembling a checkerboard mosaic pattern, (2) left upper back extending toward left shoulder, and (3) the whole right leg. Slight smaller left breast and right leg circumference are seen.

3. Discussion

Although most Becker nevi are found as isolated findings, some can be associated with abnormalities. Their precise etiopathogenesis still remains unclear. However, recent findings demonstrated that postzygotic lethal mutations in ACTB gene, a gene coding for beta-actin, may underlie the development of both Becker nevus and Becker nevus syndrome [2]. It has been hypothesized that in Becker nevus syndrome this sporadic mutation might occur during early developmental period, thus affecting multiple cell lineages compared with an isolated Becker nevus [2]. Androgen-dependent mechanism is another proposed pathogenesis of the disease according to its onset during puberty, the presence of hypertrichosis, and acneiform eruption [3], as well as the increase in androgen receptors restricted to the involved region [4].

According to a systematic literature review by Schneider et al., there is a regional correspondence between the skin manifestation of Becker nevus and the malformation, providing a clue that there might be a common mutation during embryogenesis. Breast hypoplasia, maxillofacial dysplasia, and lipodystrophy were reported to have the strongest regional correspondence [1]. In this patient, we present an interesting case of Becker nevus syndrome with checkerboard mosaic skin pattern with left breast hypoplasia and right leg lipodystrophy. Apparently, these two abnormalities are correlated with the sites of Becker nevi. Hence, this case is an excellent example showing the regional correspondence and raising awareness that Becker nevus may accompany some abnormalities, so careful examination should be performed.

Checkerboard or flag-like or block-like pattern is one of the archetypical patterns, which is characterized by alternating squares with a sharp midline separation. It can be found in either cases of cutaneous mosaicism or genetic chimerism. In case of mosaicism, if the mutation occurred early in embryogenesis, it is more likely that abnormal clone will be widely spread, contributing to a larger number of skin lesions and multiorgan involvement [5]. As a result, checkerboard skin pattern, which consists of multiple skin lesions, is sometimes reported to co-occur with extracutaneous abnormalities with frequent topographic correspondence between the skin lesions and the tissues involved. It is occasionally found in a number of different genetically determined syndromes [6]. Though multiple Becker nevi in one patient can be found from time to time, only few exhibit the real checkerboard configuration, emphasizing that checkerboard-like skin pattern is considered a rare condition among cases of Becker nevi or Becker nevus syndrome. Up to present, from our review, only three cases have been reported with multiple Becker nevi distributed in checkerboard configuration and none of them coexists with regional correspondence abnormalities like in our case.[7, 8]

The nature of Becker melanosis is benign; however, three reports have revealed that it might be associated with keratinocyte carcinomas such as basal cell carcinoma and Bowen disease. All of three cases developed cancerous lesions over the area of Becker nevus, which was a sun-protected and atypical site in a low-risk patient [9, 10]. Though it might be coincidental, awareness should be raised about long-term malignancy development in Becker nevus. We recommend a thorough and regular long-term follow-up in both cases of Becker nevus and Becker nevus syndrome. Especially in cases with leg dysplasia, long-term monitoring for joint deformities is warranted. Last but not least, from all the discussion so far, we would like to propose 3 more B's; Bowen disease, Basal cell carcinoma, and Beta-actin to the already well-known Becker, Breast, and Bone as an easy mnemonic for Becker nevus syndrome.

In conclusion, we present a case of Becker nevus syndrome which has very unique and interesting features. It is one of few cases that reveal a checkerboard mosaic pattern of

Becker nevi and apparently point up the correlation between sites of Becker nevi and abnormalities involved. Moreover, we strengthen the point that long-term follow-up should be kept in mind for upcoming associated abnormalities, complication, and malignancy.

References

[1] M. E. Schneider, E. Fritsche, U. Hug, and P. Giovanoli, "Becker nevus syndrome and ipsilateral breast hypoplasia: a systematic literature review," *European Journal of Plastic Surgery*, vol. 40, no. 6, pp. 489–498, 2017.

[2] E. D. Cai, B. K. Sun, A. Chiang et al., "Postzygotic mutations in beta-actin are associated with becker's nevus and becker's nevus syndrome," *Journal of Investigative Dermatology*, vol. 137, no. 8, pp. 1795–1798, 2017.

[3] J. Bolognia, J. Schaffer, and L. Cerroni, "Dermatology," in *Benign Melanocytic Neoplasm*, Chapter 112, pp. 1954–1988, Elsevier, China, 4th edition, 2017.

[4] H. Grande Sarpa, R. Harris, C. D. Hansen, K. P. Callis Duffin, S. R. Florell, and M. L. Hadley, "Androgen receptor expression patterns in Becker's nevi: An immunohistochemical study," *Journal of the American Academy of Dermatology*, vol. 59, no. 5, pp. 834–838, 2008.

[5] V. Molho-Pessach and J. V. Schaffer, "Blaschko lines and other patterns of cutaneous mosaicism," *Clinics in Dermatology*, vol. 29, no. 2, pp. 205–225, 2011.

[6] D. Torchia and R. Happle, "Segmental hypomelanosis and hypermelanosis arranged in a checkerboard pattern are distinct naevi: Flag-like hypomelanotic naevus and flag-like hypermelanotic naevus," *Journal of the European Academy of Dermatology and Venereology*, vol. 29, no. 11, pp. 2088–2099, 2015.

[7] K. Khaitan, Y. Manchanda, R. Mittal et al., "Multiple becker's naevi: a rare presentation," *Acta Dermato-Venereologica*, vol. 81, no. 5, pp. 374-375, 2001.

[8] F. Li, T. Wang, and L. Wang, "A rare case of multiple Becker's nevi without systemic involvement," *Indian Journal of Dermatology, Venereology and Leprology*, vol. 84, pp. 194–197, 2018.

[9] P. Sahu, S. Dayal, S. Kaur, and V. K. Jain, "Becker's nevus associated with basal cell carcinoma: An unusual presentation in a sun-protected area," *Anais Brasileiros de Dermatologia*, vol. 92, no. 1, pp. 145–147, 2017.

[10] M. Honda, T. Suzuki, K. Kudoh, and H. Tagami, "Bowen's disease developing within a Becker's melanosis (Becker's naevus)," *British Journal of Dermatology*, vol. 137, no. 4, pp. 659–661, 1997.

7

Giant Dermatofibroma: A Rare Presentation as a Large Scaly Plaque

T. Iqbal[1] and V. Mudaliar[2]

[1]Department of Dermatology, Leighton Hospital, Mid Cheshire Hospitals NHS Foundation Trust, Crewe, UK
[2]Department of Pathology, University Hospital of North Midlands NHS Trust, Stoke-on-Trent, UK

Correspondence should be addressed to T. Iqbal; tayaba.iqbal@mcht.nhs.uk

Academic Editor: Sergio A. Cuevas Covarrubias

A rare form of dermatofibroma (DF) is described in the literature as giant dermatofibroma. Due to the rarity and distinct presentation that can be confused with more sinister skin tumours, these can cause diagnostic uncertainty and require clinicopathologic correlation. Familiarity with this rare presentation of an otherwise common entity is required to prevent unnecessary clinical doubt and excessive interventions. We report a case of giant dermatofibroma on the leg of a 29-year-old healthy male that presented with a 7 cm, nonulcerated pink, brown plaque, adding to the limited literature of less than 30 known cases.

1. Introduction

A rare variant of this disease has been described as giant dermatofibroma with less than 30 reported cases. Dermatofibroma (DF), also known as fibrous histiocytoma, is a common benign lesion that is frequently encountered in clinical practice with easily recognisable appearance as pink, brown papules or nodules tethered to the skin causing dimple sign and central pallor with surrounding faint pigmentation on dermoscopy. These are slow growing and mostly solitary asymptomatic lesions up to 1.5 cm in diameter. Multiple lesions can be seen in cases of altered immunity [1].

Giant dermatofibromas are usually larger than 5 cm presenting as polypoidal or ulcerated plaques that have a benign course despite their concerning appearance. Most giant DFs reported hitherto have been found in adult patients over limbs and torso with the exceptions of a paediatric case in China and another case of an ulcerated lesion on the head and neck [2, 3]. Apart from two cases of nonulcerated plaques, all other known giant DFs have presented in the form of ulcerated and pedunculated lesions [2–5].

2. Case Report

We report the case of a 29-year-old male who presented with an asymptomatic, pink, brown, scaly plaque of an irregular shape and with some satellite lesions, measuring 7 cm on the right patellar region. This had gradually enlarged over many years. Dermoscopy showed nondiagnostic erythema and some glomerular vessels (Figure 1).

The patient was in good general health with no known systemic conditions or immunosuppression.

Histopathology was characteristic of typical DF, showing slightly acanthotic epidermis, and dermal cells with a histiocyte-like elongated appearance of myofibroblasts. There was no cytological atypia or mitotic activity. The lesion extended focally in the subcutis along the septa and was associated with hyalinised collagen and a small number of blood vessels (Figures 2 and 3).

The biopsy was repeated to ensure that histopathology was representative of the lesion, and showed similar results. Further mapping biopsies from the large lesion for an accurate clinicopathologic correlation also supported this finding, confirming the diagnosis of rare giant, atrophic

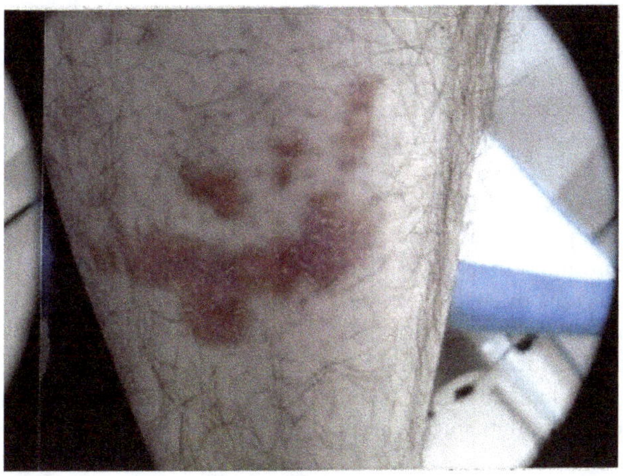

Figure 1: A 7 cm, irregular scaly pink, brown plaque of giant dermatofibroma with satellite lesions on the right shin of a young male. An asymptomatic and slow growing lesion which was nonulcerated.

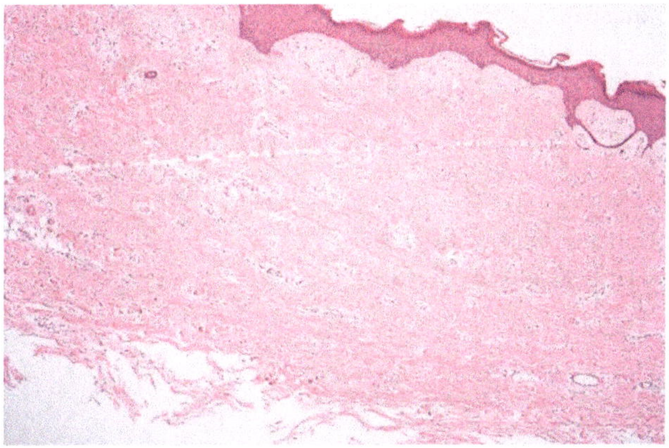

Figure 2: Histopathology of the large plaque with H&E stain at 40*x* magnification. Dermatofibroma with the overlying grenz zone and epidermal hyperplasia.

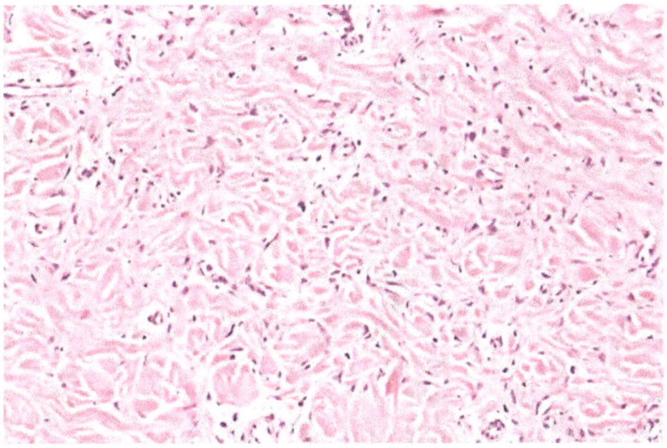

Figure 3: Histopathology H&E stain (magnification × 100). Weaving bland spindle cells around reticular collagen in the dermis.

fibrous histiocytoma. We did not find any features of dermatomyofibroma and dermatofibrosarcoma protuberans in histopathology.

Though a benign course was reported in the literature, the patient opted for wide local excision with grafting.

3. Discussion

Both neoplastic and reactive pathogeneses have been postulated in the formation of conventional DFs; however, even for giant DFs, no recurrences or metastases have been reported so far after surgical excision, giving these findings a good prognostic outlook. This is supported by this case report. One female patient reported in the literature had muscle ulceration and invasion and developed no metastasis in 5 years after wide resection with myocutaneous flap-plasty [5].

In many cases, giant DFs can mimic sinister lesions such as sarcomas, dermatofibrosarcoma protuberans, desmoplastic melanomas, and nonmelanoma skin cancers, but histopathology reveals storiform arrangement of benign spindle cells. Aneurysmal, heamosiderotic, and xanthomatous histologic variants have been described [2]. Immunostaining is positive for factor VIII A and negative for CD34. In our patient, histopathology showed benign spindle cells ruling out any sinister pathology.

To our knowledge, our report is the third case of a nonulcerated form of this rare entity and a significant addition to the limited literature on giant DFs [4]. Familiarity about this clinical entity among clinicians can lead to avoidance of unnecessary alarm among patients and doctors, as well as need for repeated biopsies and interventions that are prompted by diagnostic uncertainty.

Consent

Informed consent was obtained from the patient for publication of the case description and clinical and histological images.

References

[1] E. Calonje, "Soft-tissue tumours and tumour-like conditions," in *Rook's Textbook of Dermatology*, Wiley Blackwell, Hoboken, NJ, USA, 9th edition, 2016.

[2] T. Karlidag, E. Keles, I. Orhan, M. E. Kaplama, and B. Cobanoglu, "Giant ulcerative dermatofibroma," *Case Reports in Otolaryngology*, vol. 2013, Article ID 254787, 3 pages, 2013.

[3] M. S. Ng, A. Foong, and M. Koh, "Ulcerated giant dermatofibroma following routine childhood vaccination in a young boy," *Case Reports in Dermatol*, vol. 8, no. 2, pp. 210–217, 2016.

[4] L. J. Leow, P. A. Sinclair, and J. J. Horton, "Plaque-like dermatofibroma: a distinct and rare benign neoplasm?" *Australasian Journal of Dermatology*, vol. 49, no. 2, pp. 106–108, 2008.

[5] H. Kinoshita, T. Ishii, H. Kamoda et al., "Giant muscle invasive dermatofibroma clinically mimicking a malignant tumor," *Case Reports in Dermatology Medicine*, vol. 2019, Article ID 4503272, 4 pages, 2019.

8

Leukocytoclastic Vasculitis following the First Dose of the Elasomeran COVID-19 Vaccination

Jarett J. Casale, Mikél E. Muse, Tara J. Snow, Karen P. Gould, and Natalie D. Depcik-Smith

Campbell University at Sampson Regional Medical Center, Clinton 28328, NC, USA

Correspondence should be addressed to Tara J. Snow; tjsnow0505@email.campbell.edu

Academic Editor: Ravi Krishnan

Our case highlights leukocytoclastic vasculitis as a potential side effect of the elasomeran COVID-19 vaccine. As the elasomeran vaccine becomes more widely available to the public, cutaneous reactions should be noted and looked for as potential side effects of the vaccine. Our patient had a history of immune thrombocytopenic purpura, making this a potential predisposing condition to the development of vasculitis following elasomeran administration. The case of vasculitis in our patient, although diffuse in distribution, was self-resolving. Our patient was counseled of the potential risk of worsening reaction to the second dose of the vaccine and instructed to proceed at their own risk. He elected to receive the second vaccination dose without any further reaction or side effects. Primary teaching points from this case include the potential of developing leukocytoclastic vasculitis following the elasomeran vaccination. Patients who develop LCV following the first dose should be counseled of the risks associated with receiving the second dose, including progression to systemic organ involvement.

1. Introduction

Leukocytoclastic vasculitis refers to inflammation of small blood vessels resulting from immune-complex deposition within blood vessel walls leading to tissue destruction [1]. Infections and medications are the most common identifiable causes of leukocytoclastic vasculitis; however, up to 50% of cases are idiopathic in etiology [2]. The clinical course is often self-limiting and resolves with avoidance of the offending agent [1, 3]. Treatment is primarily supportive but may include systemic corticosteroids or other more potent immunosuppressive agents for severe cutaneous disease [2, 3].

We present a patient with leukocytoclastic vasculitis that developed 72 hours after administration of the first dose of the Spikevax (elasomeran) vaccination developed by Moderna. This vaccination is a two-part vaccination that utilizes mRNA technology to promote an immunological response to the spike protein of the Sars-CoV-2 virus. While the efficacy and safety of mRNA vaccination technology have been studied at length, the COVID-19 pandemic is the first time in which widespread utilization of this vaccine technology has been employed. This case highlights leukocytoclastic vasculitis as a potential rare side effect of the COVID-19 vaccination.

2. Case Synopsis

An 80-year-old male with a history of immune thrombocytopenic purpura (ITP) presented for evaluation of multiple small, red, violaceous petechiae involving the bilateral dorsal feet, legs, thighs, buttocks, and arms (Figures 1and 2) that appeared 72 hours after his first dose of the vaccine. The patient denied any recent illness, fever, weight changes, weakness, fatigue, shortness of breath, chest pain, myalgias, arthralgias, abdominal pain, chest pain, dyspnea, cough, neuropathy, or changes to his medications. Current medications include atorvastatin taken for 12 years, alprazolam as needed for 3 years with no recent increase in use, losartan taken for 8 years, carvedilol taken for 3 years, aspirin taken for 12 years, and fluticasone as needed for 5 years with no recent increase in use. A 4 mm punch biopsy was taken from the right thigh.

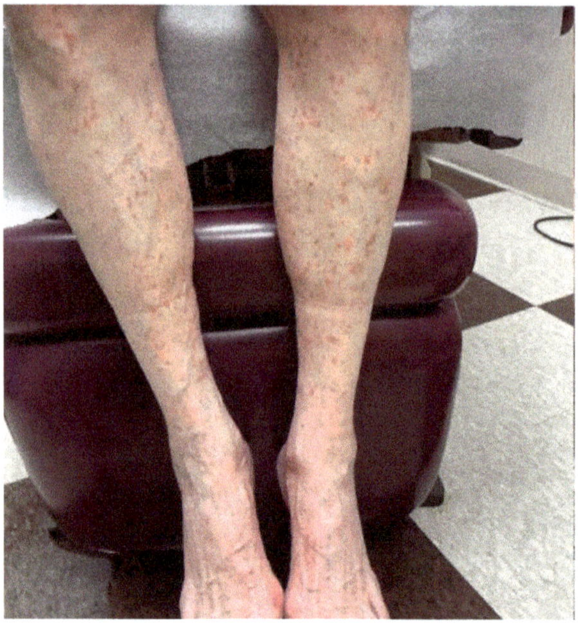

Figure 1: Image of the patient's bilateral lower legs demonstrating symmetrically distributed small, red, violaceous petechiae.

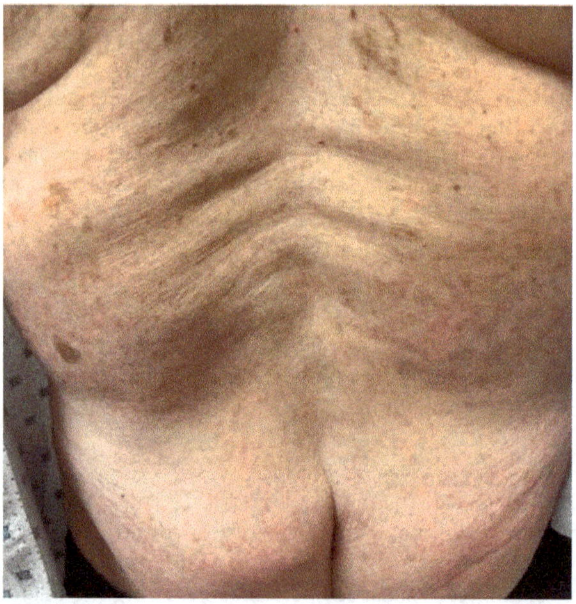

Figure 2: Image of the patient's back demonstrating symmetrically distributed small, red, violaceous petechiae.

Histology showed a perivascular lymphocytic infiltrate with extravasated red blood cells suggestive of vascular injury (Figures 3 and 4). Fibrinoid changes of the lumina and red cell extravasation without the involvement of deep vessels were observed. Pathology favored an early evolving leukocytoclastic vasculitis secondary to a vaccine reaction given the clinical history of the patient.

The patient was managed supportively and seen for follow-up 10 days after the initial biopsy was taken. Physical examination at that time revealed nearly complete resolution of the initial lesions. The patient was counseled of the

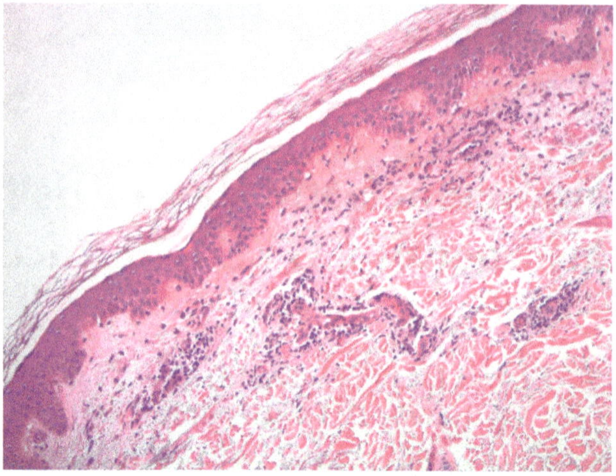

Figure 3: H&E (10x) shows a perivascular infiltrate with fibrinoid changes consistent with leukocytoclastic vasculitis.

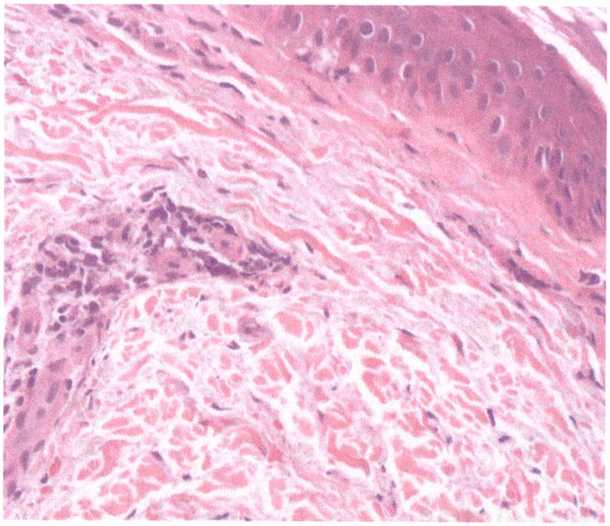

Figure 4: H&E (40x) shows early fibrinoid changes and scattered neutrophils consistent with leukocytoclastic vasculitis.

potential risks associated with receiving the second vaccine dose including worsening cutaneous reaction or potential for more severe systemic involvement and instructed to proceed at their own risk. The patient elected to receive the second dose of the elasomeran and denied any skin reactions.

3. Case Discussion

Leukocytoclastic vasculitis (LCV) is caused by the deposition of immune complexes within blood vessels leading to immune system activation and fibrinoid necrosis, resulting in characteristic vasculitic skin lesions [1]. The etiology of LCV is 45–55% idiopathic, 15–20% infectious, 15–20% autoimmune connective tissue disease or inflammatory disorders, 10–15% drug-induced hypersensitivity reactions, and 5% malignancy or lymphoproliferative disorders [2]. Although exceedingly rare, LCV has been reported as a side effect of the influenza vaccine [4]. The SARS-CoV-2 (COVID-19) pandemic has resulted in the United States Food and Drug Administration Emergency Use Authorization of two highly effective vaccinations from Moderna and Pfizer-BioNTech using mRNA vaccination technology [5].

Messenger RNA vaccine technology has been studied at length and offers strong safety advantages compared to traditional vaccine technology [6]. The primary advantage is due to the vaccine containing only genetic material needed for the expression of a selected encoded protein, rather than direct inoculation with a given antigen. In addition to mRNA, both the Moderna and Pfizer-BioNTech vaccines contain various other preservative compounds including the preservative propylene glycol. The elasomeran vaccine also contains the lipid compounds SM-102 (proprietary to Moderna), 1,2-distearoyl-sn-glycero-2-phosphocholine, cholesterol, inactive salts, and buffers such as tromethamine hydrochloride, acetic acid, and sodium acetate. We are uncertain which vaccine ingredient was the likely immune reactant leading to the development of LCV in our patient from the first dose. Previous studies of cutaneous reactions due to the elasomeran vaccine have found that the incidence of a delayed reaction after the first dose is more common on days 7 and 8, while a reaction with the 2nd dose is likely to be less severe and develop faster within 1–3 days, without severe adverse or allergic events [7]. Our patient did not report any symptoms following the second dose of the vaccine.

LCV presents clinically as symmetrically distributed palpable purpura or infiltrated erythema most commonly on the bilateral lower extremities [2, 3]. Deposition of immune complexes in LCV is predominantly limited to superficial postcapillary venules, leading to complement activation and neutrophil recruitment [2]. This results in fibrinoid necrosis of vessel walls, leading to edema of endothelial cells and red blood cell extravasation [1, 2]. Extravasation of red blood cells causes the characteristic macroscopic findings of inflammatory purpura, which can be further examined by diascopy. The lesions will often demonstrate a blanchable component due to underlying inflammation, and a nonblanchable component due to subcutaneous hemorrhage [2].

LCV is diagnosed by punch biopsy preferably within 18–48 hours of lesion onset. After this time frame, dissipation of immune complexes and recruitment of various mononuclear cells in addition to neutrophils makes the histopathological findings less specific for LCV [2]. In addition to H&E, a biopsy for direct immunofluorescence is often helpful to narrow the differential diagnosis by distinguishing among various immunoglobulin causes, such as IgA-associated Henoch–Schönlein purpura [3]. In cases of LCV with evidence of systemic involvement based on a thorough review of systems, laboratory testing is recommended and typically includes a CBC, LFTs, renal function tests, and urinalysis [1, 2].

Treatment for a primary episode of cutaneous vasculitis is aimed at avoidance of suspected triggers (in our patient, elasomeran vaccine), as well as supportive treatment such as leg elevation, antihistamines, and NSAIDs. For mild refractory LCV, antineutrophilic agents such as colchicine and dapsone are considered first-line agents [3]. Severe refractory LCV requires more potent systemic immunosuppressive agents such as mycophenolate mofetil, azathioprine, and tapering systemic corticosteroids [1–3]. In cases of vasculitis with extensive systemic involvement, a high risk of end-organ damage or death requires therapy with a combination of high potency corticosteroids and cyclophosphamide [3].

4. Conclusion

Our case highlights LCV as a potential novel side effect of the elasomeran vaccination. The case of LCV in our patient was self-limiting, however, the potential for a more severe immunological reaction with systemic involvement should be considered a possibility, and patients should be counseled of the risks associated with receiving the second dose of the elasomeran vaccine. In the case of our patient with a history of ITP, a predisposition for an amplified immunological response is considered as a potential confounding variable. Further research is required to isolate specific compounds within the vaccination associated with a high risk for an immunological reaction.

Consent

Patient written informed consent was obtained to publish case details.

References

[1] D. Baigrie, P. Bansal, A. Goyal, and J. S. Crane, "Leukocytoclastic vasculitis," in *StatPearls. Treasure Island (FL),* StatPearls Publishing, St. Petersburg, FL, USA, 2020.

[2] M. R. Goeser, V. Laniosz, and D. A. Wetter, "A practical approach to the diagnosis, evaluation, and management of cutaneous small-vessel vasculitis," *American Journal of Clinical Dermatology*, vol. 15, no. 4, pp. 299–306, 2014.

[3] K. R. Chen and J. A. Carlson, "Clinical approach to cutaneous vasculitis," *American Journal of Clinical Dermatology*, vol. 9, no. 2, pp. 71–92, 2008.

[4] A. E. Rosenblatt and S. L. Stein, "Cutaneous reactions to vaccinations," *Clinics in Dermatology*, vol. 33, no. 3, pp. 327–332, 2015.

[5] A. Banerji, P. G. Wickner, R. Saff et al., "mRNA vaccines to prevent COVID-19 disease and reported allergic reactions: current evidence and suggested approach," *Journal of Allergy and Clinical Immunology: In Practice*, vol. 9, 2021.

[6] T. Schlake, A. Thess, M. Fotin-Mleczek, and K. J. Kallen, "Developing mRNA-vaccine technologies," *RNA Biology*, vol. 9, no. 11, pp. 1319–1330, 2012.

[7] D. E. McMahon, E. Amerson, M. Rosenbach et al., "Cutaneous reactions reported after Moderna and Pfizer COVID-19 vaccination: a registry-based study of 414 cases," *Journal of the American Academy of Dermatology*, vol. 85, no. 1, pp. 46–55, 2021.

9

Coexistence of Neonatal Lupus Erythematous and Sturge–Weber Syndrome

Zahra Nikyar [1,2] Parvaneh Hatami [1] Zeinab Aryanian [1,3] Kambiz Kamyab Hesari [4] Azadeh Goodarzi [5] and Anahita Borzouei [6]

[1] *Autoimmune Bullous Diseases Research Center, Tehran University of Medical Sciences, Tehran, Iran*
[2] *Department of Dermatology, School of Medicine, Razi Hospital, Tehran University of Medical Sciences, Tehran, Iran*
[3] *Department of Dermatology, Babol University of Medical Sciences, Babol, Iran*
[4] *Department of Dermatopathology, School of Medicine Razi Hospital, Tehran University of Medical Sciences, Tehran, Iran*
[5] *Department of Dermatology, School of Medicine, Rasoul Akram Hospital, Iran University of Medical Sciences, Tehran, Iran*
[6] *Department of Dermatology, Mashhad University of Medical Sciences, Mashhad, Iran*

Correspondence should be addressed to Parvaneh Hatami; p_hatami2001@yahoo.com and Zeinab Aryanian; z_aryanian@yahoo.com

Academic Editor: Hristo Dobrev

Neonatal lupus erythematous (NLE) is a rare condition presented by lupus dermatitis shortly after birth or later following sun exposure. Sturge–Weber syndrome (SWS) is also an uncommon congenital condition characterized by extensive capillary malformation and ophthalmic and/or neurologic involvement. Here, we describe the first case of coexistence of NLE and SWS which posed a significant diagnostic challenge to clinicians.

1. Introduction

Neonatal lupus erythematous (NLE) is a rare condition produced by the transplacental passage of maternal autoantibodies [1]. NLE usually presented with lupus dermatitis including annular erythemato-squamous plaques developing shortly after birth or later following sun exposure [2].

The skin lesions often resolve spontaneously with or without leaving hypopigmented or hyperpigmented scar within the first year of life.

Sturge–Weber syndrome (SWS) is also an uncommon congenital condition characterized by extensive capillary malformation and ophthalmic and/or neurologic involvement [3].

Here, we describe a case that looks worthy of record since it presented with both NLE and SWS which has not been previously reported.

2. Case Report

A 3-month-old girl, born to nonconsanguineous parents, presented to our clinic with extensive port-wine stain on the left facial area since birth (Figure 1).

She was the full-term production of an uncomplicated pregnancy to a healthy mother without a history of abortion or any known medical condition.

On physical examination, the patient had a generally good condition. An extensive port-wine stain was noted distributing on V1, V2, and V3 areas on the left side of the face without involvement of mucosa. Multiple atrophic and hyperpigmented patches with telangiectasia on both sides of the face were seen which were more prominent on the forehead and temporal region and around the eyes. They presented since birth and were more obvious on the right side of the face due to presence of the port-wine stain on the

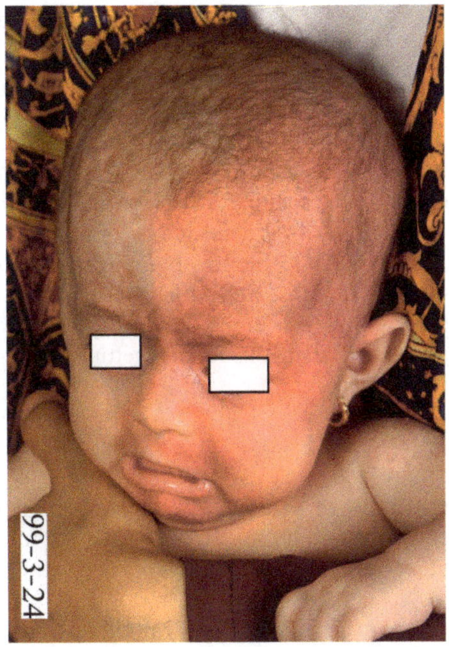

Figure 1: Extensive port-wine stain since birth.

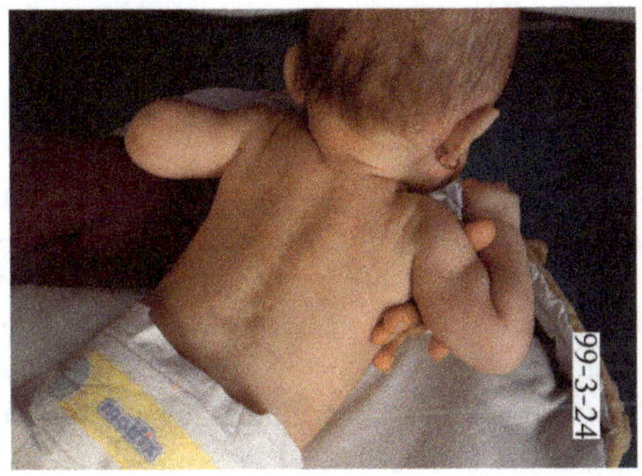

Figure 2: Multiple erythematous/hyperpigmented macules.

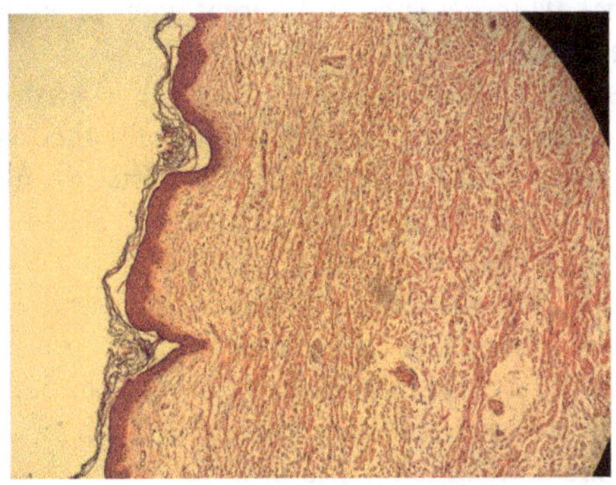

Figure 3: Dermal infiltration of spindle cells in a collagenous stroma containing abundant mucin intermixed with some mast cells.

other side. Multiple erythematous and/or hyperpigmented punched-out lesions, some with scaly appearance and/or atrophic surface, were noted on the trunk and proximal parts of extremities (Figure 2).

Initially, it was assumed to be a case of SWS and the patient was referred to the pediatric department for further ophthalmologic and neurologic examinations regarding presence of any abnormality in favor of SWS. No remarkable finding was noted in evaluations, except for bilateral benign horn cyst found in brain sonography.

However, we did not have any explanation for her atrophic punched-out lesions in the setting of SWS. Therefore, histiocytosis, mastocytosis, Goltz syndrome, and scar formation following maternal viral or parasitic infections during pregnancy including TORCH infections (toxoplasmosis, rubella, cytomegalovirus, and herpes simplex) were considered as the most relevant differential diagnoses, despite the absence of any applicable maternal history. A 4 mm punch biopsy was taken from one of the atrophic lesions of her trunk. Histopathologic assessment showed dermal infiltration of spindle cells in a collagenous stroma containing abundant mucin intermixed with some mast cells which was more compatible with "progressive mucinous histiocytosis" (Figures 3 and 4). "Cutaneous mucinosis of infancy" and "self-healing juvenile cutaneous mucinosis" were also suggested as differential diagnoses.

However, clinical manifestation of these disorders was quite different from that seen in our case.

Moreover, IHC study for CD 31, S100, C-kit, and lysozyme was performed which was not diagnostic for any of these diagnoses.

Unfortunately, we could not perform serologic evaluation for TORCH infections because of some financial issues.

Considering clinical appearance of the lesions including atrophy and telangiectasia and existence of abundant mucin in histopathologic assessment which has been reported as a rare finding in patients with lupus erythematosus [4], a diagnosis of NLE was suspected and relevant laboratory data were requested. Serologic examination of sera of the patient and her mother revealed the presence of anti-Ro/SS-A and anti-La/SS-B in high values in both and FANA positivity in her mother (titer: 1/3200).

Fortunately, any heart block or other cardiologic abnormalities were not found by the pediatric cardiologist, and other laboratory evaluations were within the normal range.

These data confirmed the diagnosis of NLE without internal involvement for our patient.

Considering the fact that extensive capillary malformation was previously reported as a rare manifestation of NLE [3] and also normal ophthalmologic and neurologic evaluations in our patient, the diagnosis of SWS seemed to be unlikely and port-wine stain was assumed to be an uncommon feature of her NLE.

Surprisingly, she developed an episode of nonfebrile tonic-clonic seizure about one month later. Hence, she was admitted and received phenytoin, phenobarbital, and Tegretol. Brain CT scan revealed mild subdural hematoma and streaky calcification compatible with leptomeningeal angiomatosis which, in context of having an extensive port-wine stain, returned us to the diagnosis of SWS. A secondary ophthalmologic consultation was requested in which glaucoma was noted in the left eye and the diagnosis was even more confirmed.

Then, the patient was discharged on phenobarbital 15 mg/BD and syrup Tegretol 60 mg/BD.

The patient remained seizure-free until the 10th month of her life when the second episode of tonic-clonic seizure happened, and her medication was changed to phenobarbital, clonazepam, and aspirin. A brain MRI was performed which revealed leptomeningeal enhancement and hypotrophy in the left cerebral hemisphere indicative of SWS.

Now, the child is 15 months old. No seizure occurred within the last 5 months. Her port-wine stain considerably improved following 4 sessions of PDL (pulsed-dye laser) therapy and other cutaneous lesions getting better spontaneously (Figures 5 and 6).

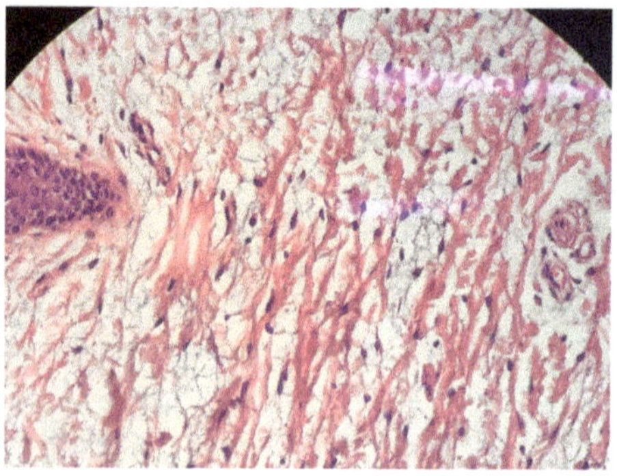

Figure 4: A magnified view of histopathological changes seen in the patient's tissue sample.

3. Discussion

We reported a case of NLE and SWS where both of them are considered as rare conditions. To the best of our knowledge, the coexistence of these disorders has not been reported until now.

NLE is an uncommon disorder caused by transplacental transfer of maternal anti-Ro and anti-La autoantibodies. The most common manifestation of NLE is cutaneous lesions developed in 50% of cases, and they usually appear in the first months of life [5] but can be noted since birth in a minority of cases, such as ours.

In our patient, most of the lesions presented as atrophic and telangiectatic macules on the scalp and trunk which is more likely representative of occurrence of inflammatory phase during pregnancy. This might explain the absence of distinct inflammatory features of LE on histopathologic evaluation. In fact, the absence of typical annular lesions of NLE, as well as unspecific histopathologic findings in this case, indicates the importance of having clinical suspicion for reaching correct diagnosis.

It is worthy to note that the presence of abundant mucin in histopathologic assessment might be a feature of NLE lesions [5] and should not mislead us to more common differential diagnoses such as different types of mucinosis in case of clinical suspicion to LE.

Widespread cutaneous lesions of NLE at birth are very rare and might be considered as a proof for the hypothesis that UV radiation, despite previous reports [6], might not have an essential role in the expression of intranuclear antigen and developing clinical lesions.

Another interesting feature of our case was the fact that her mother initially seemed to be healthy, but a more detailed history revealed that she had arthralgia and hence was referred to the rheumatology department where it turned out that she had some criteria of SLE.

SWS is also a rare syndrome characterized with facial angioma reaching territory V1, ophthalmologic anomaly (mostly congenital glaucoma), and neurological malformation, such as leptomeningeal angioma might lead to seizure or neurological deficit [2]. SWS is classified into 3 types: type 1 (complete or classic), type 2 (bisymptomatic), and type 3 (rough form) [7].

Our case was initially presented by facial port-wine stain which could be considered as an uncommon cutaneous presentation of NLE considering normal first ophthalmologic and neurologic evaluation. However, occurrence of subsequent seizure episodes and detecting glaucoma on further assessments confirmed the diagnosis of SWS with complete manifestation (type 1).

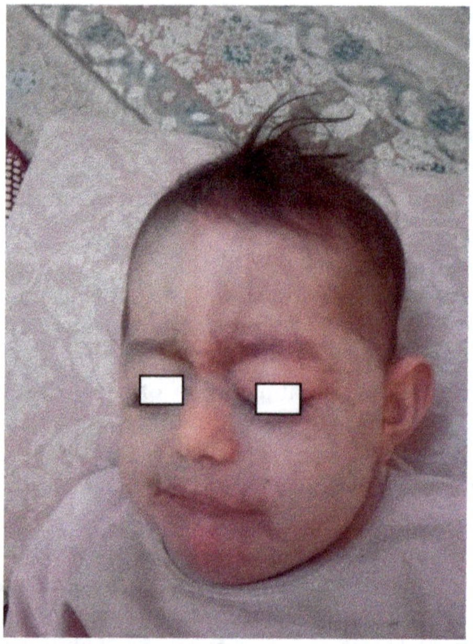

Figure 5: Remarkable resolution of port-wine stain following PDL therapy.

As mentioned above, nothing abnormal was found on the first ophthalmologic assessment of our patient which might be due to developing glaucoma later, during the course of the disease.

Even though the most common form of ocular complication in SWS is congenital glaucoma, it can also develop during childhood or even later in life [8] which shows the significance of careful ophthalmic follow-up of these patients.

In conclusion, we report an extraordinary case of NLE not only for having lesions since birth and with lack of maternal history which posed a significant diagnostic challenge but also for simultaneously having another rare condition (SWS) which made it even more challenging to diagnosis.

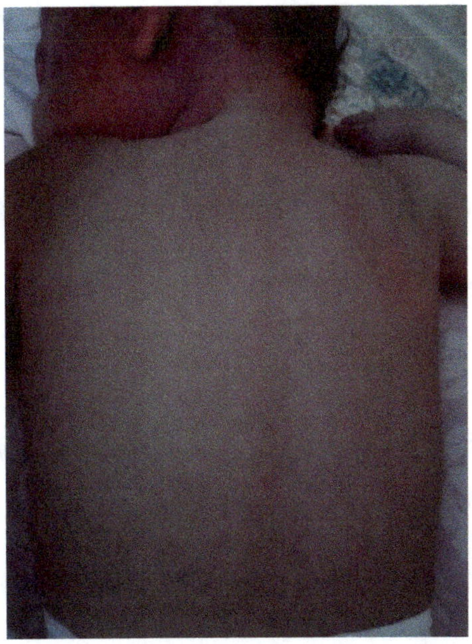

Figure 6: Spontaneous resolution of cutaneous lesions of NLE.

Making correct diagnosis in this case was important in several aspects: firstly, diagnosis of each of these disorders necessitates more systemic evaluations which led to detection of glaucoma in our case. Another important issue for patients with NLE is a relatively higher risk of developing other autoimmune disorders such as rheumatoid arthritis and Hashimoto thyroiditis during their childhood. Hence, they need long-term follow-up even though they experience spontaneous resolution of their extra cardiac manifestations [9].

Moreover, diagnosis of NLE in this case led to detection of SLE in her mother which was previously neglected. This also mandates strict follow-up of her mother during subsequent pregnancies due to higher risk of complete heart block in neonates which can be prevented by using IVIG and hydroxychloroquine early during pregnancy [10–14].

Therefore, careful examination and clinical suspicion besides appropriate paraclinical assessment are the key factors for correct diagnosis and management of patients.

Consent

The patient's parents provided written informed consent to publication of this case report and accompanying images.

Authors' Contributions

Conception or design of the work was carried out by Z. N. Data were collected by Z. A. Data analysis and interpretation were performed by K. K. and A. G. The article was drafted by P. H. and Z. A. Critical revision of the article was conducted by Z. N. and A. G. Final approval of the version to be published was given by P. H. and Z. N.

Acknowledgments

This study was performed at the Autoimmune Bullous Diseases Research Center, Razi Hospital, Tehran, Iran.

References

[1] T. Chaikul and S. Chaithirayanon, "Unusual skin manifestations in neonatal lupus erythematosus," *Medical Journal of the Medical Association of Thailand*, vol. 98, no. Suppl 10, pp. S147–S149, 2015.

[2] I. Niang, K. M. Ndiaye, A. M. Diop et al., "Sturge Weber syndrome, when brain CT is enough for diagnosis: about a case," *Pan African Medical Journal*, vol. 36, p. 308, 2020.

[3] F. Vílchez-Márquez, A. Martín-Fuentes, R. Conejero et al., "Neonatal lupus erythematosus mimicking extensive capillary malformation," *Pediatric Dermatology*, vol. 30, no. 4, pp. 495–497, 2013.

[4] Y. Yu, L. Du, J. Pan, J. Zheng, A. Chen, and L. Chen, "A 10-year retrospective study of neonatal lupus erythematous in China," *Asian Pacific Journal of Allergy and Immunology*, vol. 34, no. 2, pp. 174–178, 2016.

[5] V. Vega, M. Duque, D. Don-Pedro, and S. Bhatta, "A neonate with annular cutaneous lesions," *Cureus*, vol. 12, no. 7, Article ID e9138, 2020.

[6] S. Admani and A. C. Krakowski, "Neonatal lupus erythematosus presenting as atypical targetoid-like lesions involving genitals and soles of feet following brief sun exposure," *The Journal of clinical and aesthetic dermatology*, vol. 6, no. 5, pp. 19–23, 2013.

[7] L. Siri, L. Giordano, P. Accorsi et al., "Clinical features of Sturge-Weber syndrome without facial nevus: five novel cases," *European Journal of Paediatric Neurology*, vol. 17, no. 1, pp. 91–96, 2013.

[8] P. C. Luna, "Transplacentally acquired dermatoses," *Harper's Textbook of Pediatric Dermatology*, vol. Volume 1, Wiley, Hoboken, NJ, USA, Fourth Edition, Chapter 8, , pp. 93–100, 2019.

[9] M. Silverstein and J. Salvin, "Ocular manifestations of Sturge-Weber syndrome," *Current Opinion in Ophthalmology*, vol. 30, no. 5, pp. 301–305, 2019.

[10] A. Saxena, P. M. Izmirly, B. Mendez, J. P. Buyon, and D. M. Friedman, "Prevention and treatment in utero of autoimmune-associated congenital heart block," *Cardiology in Review*, vol. 22, no. 6, pp. 263–267, 2014.

[11] A. Brucato, R. Cimaz, R. Caporali, V. Ramoni, and J. Buyon, "Pregnancy outcomes in patients with autoimmune diseases and anti-Ro/SSA antibodies," *Clinical Reviews in Allergy and Immunology*, vol. 40, no. 1, pp. 27–41, 2011.

[12] P. M. Izmirly, M. Y. Kim, C. Llanos et al., "Evaluation of the risk of anti-SSA/Ro-SSB/La antibody-associated cardiac manifestations of neonatal lupus in fetuses of mothers with systemic lupus erythematosus exposed to hydroxychloroquine," *Annals of the Rheumatic Diseases*, vol. 69, no. 10, pp. 1827–1830, 2010.

[13] C. N. Pisoni, A. Brucato, A. Ruffatti et al., "Failure of intravenous immunoglobulin to prevent congenital heart block: findings of a multicenter, prospective, observational study," *Arthritis & Rheumatism*, vol. 62, no. 4, pp. 1147–1152, 2010.

[14] D. M. Friedman, C. Llanos, P. M. Izmirly et al., "Evaluation of fetuses in a study of intravenous immunoglobulin as preventive therapy for congenital heart block: results of a multicenter, prospective, open-label clinical trial," *Arthritis & Rheumatism*, vol. 62, no. 4, pp. 1138–1146, 2010.

10

Cryosurgery, Intralesional Methotrexate and Imiquimod for Keratoacanthoma: Tuning the Combination

Georgios Gaitanis and Ioannis D. Bassukas

Department of Skin and Venereal Diseases, Faculty of Medicine, School of Health Sciences, University of Ioannina, Ioannina, Greece

Correspondence should be addressed to Ioannis D. Bassukas; ibassuka@uoi.gr

Academic Editor: Ravi Krishnan

Keratoacanthomas (KA) are self-regressing, destructively expanding keratinocyte skin neoplasms typically characterized by sudden onset of explosive growth followed by complete involution. Cryosurgery, intralesional methotrexate and imiquimod have been used alone or in combination of two for the treatment of KA. Presently 3 patients (49, 60, and 65 years old; two females, one suspected with Ferguson-Smith syndrome), with 5 KA (6–24 mm maximal diameter) were treated with the combination of cryosurgery (liquid N_2, open spray, 2 cycles of 15 sec each) and intralesional methotrexate (2.5–30 mg cumulative dose) and subsequent daily application of imiquimod (14–35 days). Starting with 4 cryosurgery/intralesional methotrexate sessions and 5 weeks daily imiquimod, to document feasibility and efficacy we progressively reduced the intensity of the treatment to one cryosurgery/intralesional methotrexate (total dose: 5 mg) session and 14 days of daily imiquimod without compromising efficacy. KA stopped growing promptly with sustained clearance after 6–24 months follow up, implicating a huge potential of therapeutic synergy of the employed modalities in the management of KA. We suggest that, optimized, the present three modalities combination (one session mild cryosurgery/low dose, 5 mg intralesional methotrexate and 2 weeks once daily imiquimod) is a promising treatment for KA that merits evaluation in further studies.

1. Introduction

Keratoacanthoma (KA) is a distinct subset of self-regressing, locally invasive and destructively expanding keratinocyte skin neoplasms with squamous cell carcinoma micromorphology. KA are characterized by the sudden onset of an explosive, though limited growth phase followed by complete tumor tissue involution [1]. However, the evolution process of any particular KA is somehow unpredictable and few cases may acquire large dimensions that can eventually result in dysmorphic, potentially mutilating scars. This coupled with the possibility of missing a frank squamous cell carcinoma (SCC) prompts therapeutic intervention for all patients with this neoplasm [1]. Furthermore, multiple KA may appear in younger ages within the framework of syndromic KA forms, like the Ferguson-Smith syndrome. More recent interest for novel treatment modalities for KA has revived as KA emerges as an important toxicity event of the vemurafenib [2] and probably also of the pembrolizumab [3] treatment in patients with advanced malignant melanoma.

In the present retrospective study we describe the successful treatment of KA with the minimally invasive combination of concomitant sessions of cryosurgery and intralesional methotrexate and cycles of once-daily imiquimod application starting at the same evening of the cryosurgery-methotrexate treatment day. Initially, we evaluated the feasibility of the combination treatment protocol with an intensive plan of weekly repetitions of cryosurgery-methotrexate (moderate high dose) sessions during a 5-week once daily imiquimod application cycle. In the following, we optioned a step-wise up-down adaptation of the intensity of all three composing modalities, to optimize the feasibility-efficacy relationship of the proposed combination. Aim of this explorative study was to enhance the selectivity of the present triple combination modality for KA by (a) documenting feasibility and (b) adapting the intensity of all combined modalities to optimize efficacy.

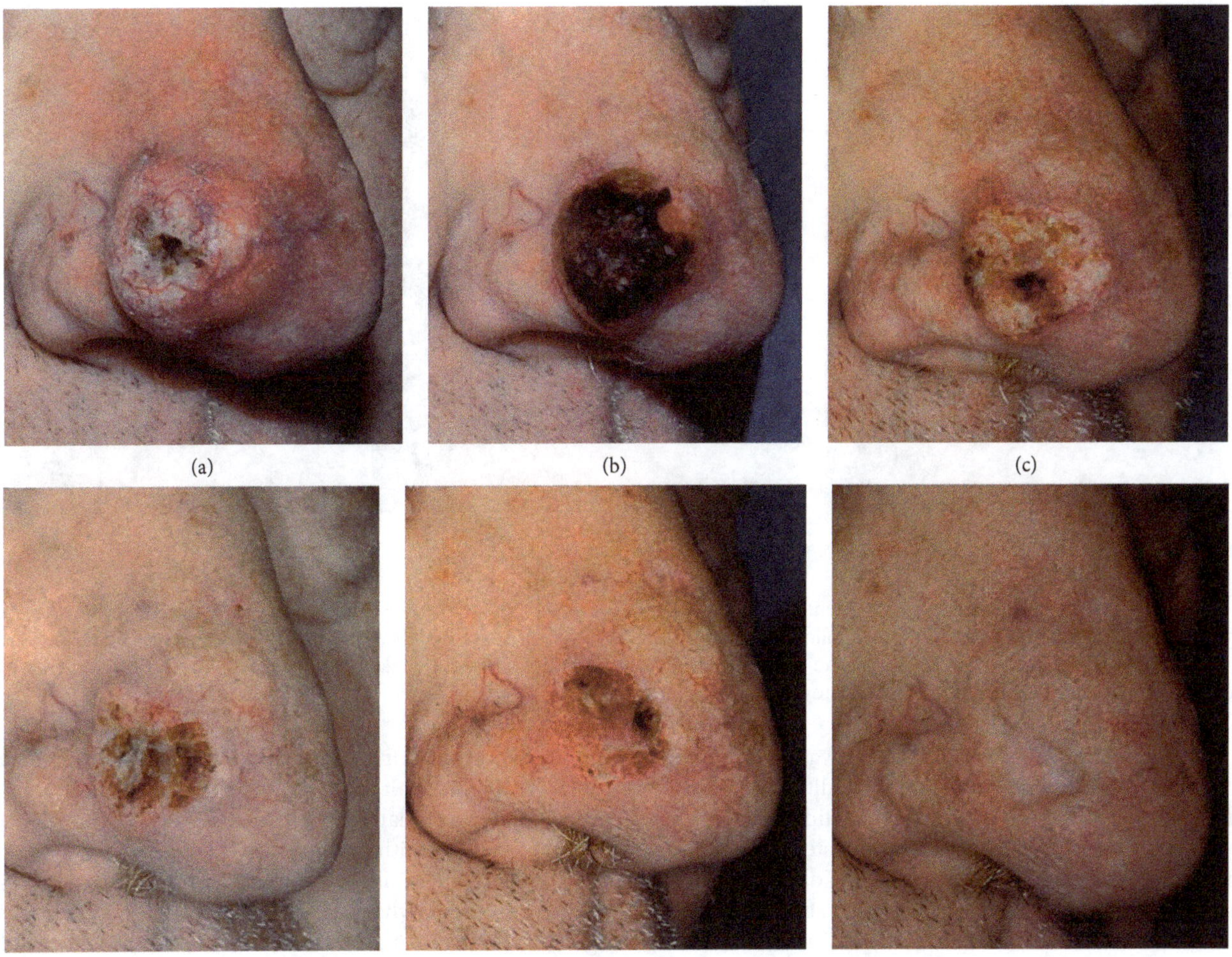

(a) (b) (c) (d) (e) (f)

FIGURE 1: Patient 1 with a 24 mm in maximal diameter keratoacanthoma. The patient was treated with weekly sessions of cryosurgery (liquid N_2, open spray, 2 cycles of 15 sec each), intralesional methotrexate (7.5 mg/weekly sessions) (Panels a–d) and daily application of imiquimod. Panel a: The tumor at baseline. Panels b–d: The tumor at weekly intervals at the days of cryosurgery and intralesional methotrexate. Panel e: Gradual tumor involution is achieved and the patient is treated with daily imiquimod for another week (35 days imiquimod in total). Panel f: The tumor has cleared and a deep scar has remained, representing the "tumor ghost", i.e., the area destroyed by the rapidly expanding keratoacanthoma. Photographs were acquired with modification of a previously used equipment [20] employing a Nikon D610 camera with a spatial resolution of 6016 × 4016 pixels. A 60 mm prime lens was adapted with a vertical polarized filter and a SIGMA EM-140 Macro ring flash with an additional vertical polarized filter. The photographs were taken with the axons of polarization of the two filters in vertical position to each other for cross-polarization to enhance the visualization of the vascular bed [21].

2. Case Reports

Single KA were biopsied prior to the intervention, while in the case of multiple KA treated in parallel, only one per treatment session was biopsied. Monitoring of methotrexate was performed according to corresponding treatment guidelines [4].

Patient 1 (Figure 1). A 65-year old man with unremarkable medical history presented with a rapidly enlarging tumor on the nose that within one month acquired 24 mm maximal diameter in size. Merging the clinical features and the findings of a punch biopsy we diagnosed KA. Once weekly cycles of concomitant cryosurgery (liquid N_2, open spray, 2 cycles of 15 sec each) and intralesional methotrexate (7.5 mg per session) were initiated in parallel to once daily 5% imiquimod cream application locally to the KA and a 0.5 cm wide skin rim around it for a total of 35 days. Four sessions of cryosurgery and intralesional methotrexate (total dose: 30 mg) were applied. The KA regressed rapidly, leaving a shallow scar corresponding approximately to the area destructed by the tumor during growth. The patient was relapse-free at the 24-month evaluation.

Patient 2. A 60-year old female presented with a KA of 2 weeks duration at the left mandible, 10 mm in maximal diameter. Biopsy, cryosurgery (liquid N_2, open spray, 2 cycles of 15 sec each) and intralesional methotrexate (5 mg) were provided in one session and once daily imiquimod application for 5 weeks was started. The lesion rapidly regressed and the patient is relapse free for 24 months, with a hypopigmented scar at the site of treatment.

Patient 3 (Figure 2). A 49-year old female with a history of 8 resected KA from the age of 28 presented with 2 new KA lesions, on the nose and the lower lip (8 mm and 6 mm in maximal diameters, respectively). Her medical history was otherwise unremarkable and in the family no KA cases could

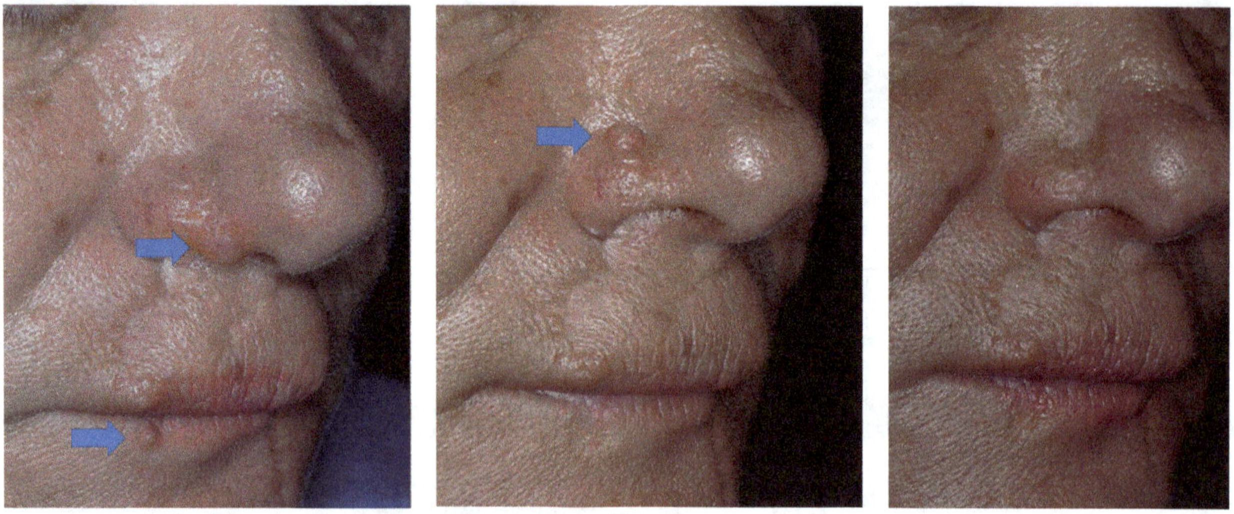

FIGURE 2: Patient 3. Panel a: The patient at presentation with two keratoacantoma lesions (arrays). Scars from previous surgeries for the same diagnosis are evident. Panel b: At 12 months follow-up the two lesions in complete remission with a swallow scar. Meanwhile a new lesion has appeared (arrow). Panel c: The patient at the 18 months follow-up. All photographs are taken with parallel polarization to increase the perception of skin relief [21]. For details of photography see Figure 1.

be recorded. Ferguson-Smith syndrome was suspected [1]; however, the patient did not consent for additional screening. The KA were treated with cryosurgery (liquid N_2, open spray, 2 cycles of 15 sec), intralesional methotrexate (2.5 mg/lesion) and daily application of imiquimod for 14 days. The shorter scheme was selected based on the observation that lesions rapidly involuted in the aforementioned Patients 1 and 2. At 12 months follow-up, a new lesion (8 mm maximal diameter) at the left side of the nose was treated likewise. All treated lesions regressed promptly and remained in complete remission, at 24 months follow-up, from her initial presentation.

3. Discussion

Experts still advocate surgery (conventional or Mohs'), if feasible, as the first line modality to manage KA [1]. As a main argument discussed in favor of this proposal is the traditionally quite subjective approach to the KA diagnosis [5], resulting in uncertainty to differentiate KA from SCC, at least in an appreciable subset of cases [1]. However, recent advances in the pathophysiology of KA clearly underline its unique nature, provide molecular evidence to differentiate it from SCC and have substantially sharpened our clinical-laboratory instruments to distinguish between the two conditions at the patient's level [6, 7]. Consequently, these latter developments call for reevaluation of the therapeutic priorities to approach the treatment of KA, by optimally addressing the benign biological behavior on one hand and the unpredictable tissue-destructive potential of this self-limited, skin growth on the other. Accordingly, in order to successfully substitute surgery as the mainstream modality, any proposed alternative modality should fulfill the same achievements, i.e., (a) abrupt growth stop as typical for surgical lesion removal, (b) sustained clearance of the treated lesion, and (c) minimal risk of KA induction in the surrounding skin areas by the therapeutic intervention itself. It is worth noting that, if effective, minimally invasive modalities are more efficacious in the management of patients with multiple KA lesions.

To date, the available nonsurgical modalities, employed alone, are of somewhat inferior effectiveness compared to surgery [1]. A way to improve effectiveness of these latter modalities is to evaluate rational combinations of them for synergy to enhance selectivity [8]. Herein we reported the preliminary results of an exploratory, minimally invasive approach to the treatment of KA with a fixed timing combination of three modalities, i.e., cryosurgery, intralesional methotrexate and imiquimod. All three are widely available modalities and were selected to be studied in a designed combination based on their accepted efficacy for KA, however, in adequately high treatment intensities, and also because they are not known to possess antagonistic therapeutic potential to each other. They have been applied with appreciable success either alone [9, 10] or in certain combinations of two [11] to treat KA. Our main aim was through a fixed combination to minimize the intensity of each consisting modality whereas optimizing the efficacy of the treatment. Intralesional MTX was collected as the backbone of the present combination, as it is the most preferable drug reported in the literature for the intralesional treatment of KA due to sufficient effectiveness (overall cure rate: 91%) [12], quite moderate costs per procedure and convenience of application (less pain compared e.g., to intralesional 5 fluorouracil) [13]. Mean total doses of 38.2 mg MTX in an average of 2.1 injections per lesion were needed to achieve above effectiveness levels [14]. The timing of the combination was designed to concentrate the intensity of the intervention in the very beginning of the treatment cycle, i.e., in a fashion mimicking as close as possibly the surgical excision. Due to its highest toxicity potential compared to the other two combination constituents (cryosurgery and topical imiquimod), our first priority was to enquire possible reduction of the MTX dose. Based on the encouraging feasibility and efficacy outcome, with the most intensive starting treatment scheme variation (Patient 1), we subsequently limited the applied methotrexate dose to a total of 5 mg and the cryosurgery sessions to a single one, whereas we retained the "typical" for "immunocryosurgery" 5-week imiquimod application period, as established in the treatment of basal cell carcinoma [15] (Patient 2). By the way, the total methotrexate dose applied to treat this latter lesion (Patient 2) is as low as those used for hypersensivity screening in candidates for methotrexate treatment initiation [4]. Based on the observation of optimal efficacy with this latter reduced scheme in Patient 2, in the last assessment step (Patient 3) we restricted the duration of imiquimod use from 5 to 2 weeks only once daily applications with very encouraging treatment outcome, however, in overall relatively smaller tumors. For comparison, according to literature data, generally 4–11 weeks of application are needed to obtain complete remission with topical imiquimod monotherapy [1]. Also Jeon et al. [16] based on their observation of the clinical course of KA resolution after 9 to 11 weeks of imiquimod treatment proposed that for remission treatment duration as short as 5 to maximal 8 weeks might be sufficient to clear KA. It is worth noting that for tumors <1 cm in maximal diameter (the first two neoplasms of Patient 3) a total methotrexate doses of 2.5 mg was adequate to achieve prompt remission with the present combination modality. However, since a 5 mg dose is generally regarded safe we suggest the slightly higher dose (5 mg MTX) to initiate this treatment combination for all KA. We have had the opportunity to evaluate this latter combination in the treatment of the 3rd KA of Patient 3 with an excellent feasibility and efficacy-outcome.

Resuming, we propose for a newly diagnosed KA, a treatment cycle starting with a moderate cryosurgery session (liquid N_2, open spray, 2 cycles of 15 sec) immediately followed by intralesional methotrexate (5 mg) in this order and already from the first therapy day once daily topical imiquimod (5% cream) for 2 weeks. This is a significantly shorter treatment duration compared to the approximately 8 weeks required for imiquimod alone treatment for KA [16, 17], which, if confirmed in larger studies, would mean a considerable improvement of feasibility and an indication in favor of synergistic effects in the framework of the combination. Yet, from our experience with large basal cell carcinoma ([18, 19] and unpublished data) we know that the combination of imiquimod and cryosurgery is optimized with biweekly cryosurgery session repetitions. We would like to suggest that for inadequately responding KA to a single treatment cycle repetitions of the above cycle could be enquired to improve overall treatment efficacy.

The main limitation of the present proposal is the fact that it is supported by the results of a relatively limited trial. KA is a challenging diagnosis for which no unique therapeutic proposal is accepted; yet all herein combined modalities have been used as single therapeutic modalities and proved efficacious at acceptable high rates. Moreover, our observations in the present case series indicate to a clinically significant synergy potential of the combined modalities. In conclusion, we propose a two-weekly triple modality combination module for the nonsurgical therapeutic approach to KA that combines safety and efficacy, can be repeated as required to improve efficiency and could be evaluated within appropriately designed clinical trials.

References

[1] B. Kwiek and R. A. Schwartz, "Keratoacanthoma: an update and review," *Journal of the American Academy of Dermatology*, vol. 74, no. 6, pp. 1220–1233, 2016.

[2] P. Chen, F. Chen, and B. Zhou, "Systematic review and meta-analysis of prevalence of dermatological toxicities associated with vemurafenib treatment in patients with melanoma," *Clinical and Experimental Dermatology*, vol. 44, no. 3, pp. 243–251, 2019.

[3] A. Freites-Martinez, B. Y. Kwong, K. E. Rieger, D. G. Coit, A. D. Colevas, and M. E. Lacouture, "Eruptive keratoacanthomas associated with pembrolizumab therapy," *JAMA Dermatology*, vol. 153, no. 7, pp. 694–697, 2017.

[4] R. B. Warren, S. C. Weatherhead, C. H. Smith et al., "British association of dermatologists' guidelines for the safe and effective prescribing of methotrexate for skin disease 2016," *British Journal of Dermatology*, vol. 175, no. 1, pp. 23–44, 2016.

[5] R. A. Carr and J. P. Houghton, "Histopathologists' approach to keratoacanthoma: a multisite survey of regional variation in Great Britain and Ireland," *Journal of Clinical Pathology*, vol. 67, no. 7, pp. 637–638, 2014.

[6] T. Takai, "Advances in histopathological diagnosis of keratoacanthoma," *Journal of Dermatology*, vol. 44, no. 3, pp. 304–314, 2017.

[7] T. Gleich, E. Chiticariu, M. Huber, and D. Hohl, "Keratoacanthoma: a distinct entity?" *Experimental Dermatology*, vol. 25, no. 2, pp. 85–91, 2016.

[8] J. Lehár, A. Krueger, S. W. Avery et al., "Synergistic drug combinations tend to improve therapeutically relevant selectivity," *Nature Biotechnology*, vol. 27, no. 7, pp. 659–666, 2009.

[9] I. Manousaridis and M. Leverkus, "Malignant epithelial tumors: part II. Therapy and prevention," *Journal of the German Society of Dermatology*, vol. 11, no. 1, pp. 9–27, 2013.

[10] N. M. Annest, M. J. VanBeek, C. J. Arpey, and D. C. Whitaker, "Intralesional methotrexate treatment for keratoacanthoma tumors: a retrospective study and review of the literature," *Journal of the American Academy of Dermatology*, vol. 56, no. 6, pp. 989–993, 2007.

[11] D. Panther, T. Nino, K. D. Macknet, and C. Macknet, "Eruptive keratoacanthomas as a complication of fractionated CO_2 laser resurfacing and combination therapy with imiquimod and intralesional methotrexate," *Dermatologic Surgery*, vol. 41, no. 1, pp. 172–175, 2015.

[12] K. Chitwood, J. Etzkorn, and G. Cohen, "Topical and intralesional treatment of nonmelanoma skin cancer: efficacy and cost comparisons," *Dermatologic Surgery*, vol. 39, no. 9, pp. 1306–1316, 2013.

[13] N. Kiss, P. Avci, A. Bánvölgyi et al., "Intralesional therapy for the treatment of keratoacanthoma," *Dermatologic Therapy*, vol. 32, no. 3, p. e12872, 2019.

[14] V. Della Valle and M. Milani, "Efficacy and safety of intralesional methotrexate in the treatment of a large keratoacanthoma of the dorsal hand in a 99-year-old woman," *Case Reports Dermatology*, vol. 10, no. 3, pp. 247–250, 2018.

[15] G. Gaitanis and I. D. Bassukas, "Immunocryosurgery for nonsuperficial basal cell carcinoma: a pro-spective, open-label phase III study for tumours ≤ 2 cm in diameter," *Acta Dermato Venereologica*, vol. 94, no. 1, pp. 38–44, 2014.

[16] H. C. Jeon, M. Choi, S. H. Paik, C. H. Ahn, H. S. Park, and K. H. Cho, "Treatment of keratoacanthoma with 5% imiquimod cream and review of the previous report," *Annals of Dermatology*, vol. 23, no. 3, pp. 357–361, 2011.

[17] V. Di Lernia, C. Ricci, and G. Albertini, "Spontaneous regression of keratoacanthoma can be promoted by topical treatment with imiquimod cream," *Journal of the European Academy of Dermatology and Venereology*, vol. 18, no. 5, pp. 626–629, 2004.

[18] G. Gaitanis and I. Bassukas, "Intralesional bevacizumab as in-add adjuvant to immunocryosurgery for locally advanced basal cell carcinoma," *Journal of the European Academy of Dermatology and Venereology*, vol. 28, no. 8, pp. 1117–1121, 2014.

[19] G. Gaitanis, M. Tronnier, A. Zioga, P. Spyridonos, and I. D. Bassukas, "A neglected basal cell carcinoma in a young patient: successful treatment with immunocryosurgery," *International Journal of Advances in Medicine*, vol. 2, no. 4, pp. 406–410, 2015.

[20] P. Spyridonos, G. Gaitanis, A. Likas, and I. D. Bassukas, "Automatic discrimination of actinic keratoses from clinical photographs," *Computers in Biology and Medicine*, vol. 88, pp. 50–59, 2017.

[21] J. A. Muccini, N. Kollias, S. B. Phillips et al., "Polarized light photography in the evaluation of photoaging," *Journal of the American Academy of Dermatology*, vol. 33, no. 5, pp. 765–769, 1995.

11

CD5-Positive Primary Cutaneous Diffuse Large B-Cell Lymphoma-Leg Type

Alexandra Papoudou-Bai,[1] Leonidas Marinos,[2] Amalia Vassou,[3] Eleni Kapsali,[3] and Panagiotis Kanavaros[4]

[1] *Department of Pathology, Faculty of Medicine, School of Health Sciences, University of Ioannina, Ioannina, Greece*
[2] *Department of Hematopathology, Evangelismos General Hospital, Athens, Greece*
[3] *Department of Hematology, Faculty of Medicine, School of Health Sciences, University of Ioannina, Ioannina, Greece*
[4] *Department of Anatomy-Histology-Embryology, Faculty of Medicine, School of Health Sciences, University of Ioannina, Ioannina, Greece*

Correspondence should be addressed to Alexandra Papoudou-Bai; apapoudoubai@gmail.com

Academic Editor: Jaime A. Tschen

Most primary cutaneous B-cell lymphomas (PCBCL) are CD5 negative, and only a few cases were found to express CD5. We report the first well-documented CD5+ primary cutaneous diffuse large B-cell lymphoma-leg type (PCDLBCL-LT). A 71-year-old woman with a history of Multiple Sclerosis was admitted because of a nodule at the left thigh. Histological examination of the skin biopsy disclosed a diffuse dermal infiltration by large lymphoid cells. Immunohistochemistry revealed that these large cells were positive for CD5, CD20, CD79a, MUM1/IRF4, Bcl6, Bcl2, and cytoplasmic IgM/λ, whereas CD3, CD56, CD23, CD21, CD10, CD30, cyclin D1, CD68, lysozyme, myeloperoxidase, and CD34 were not detected. Thus, the diagnosis of a CD5+ PCDLBCL-LT was made. Despite treatment, the patient died 11 months after initial diagnosis.

1. Introduction

Primary cutaneous B-cell lymphomas (PCBCL) are the second most common form of primary cutaneous lymphomas (PCL) and account for approximately 25%-30% of all PCL [1, 2]. Low-grade PCBCL, namely, the primary cutaneous follicle center lymphoma (PCFCL) and the primary cutaneous marginal zone lymphoma (PCMZL), represent the vast majority of PCBCL and display an indolent clinical course and a very good prognosis [1–5]. In contrast to PCMZL and PCFCL, primary cutaneous diffuse large B-cell lymphoma-leg type (PCDLBCL-LT) have an unfavorable prognosis [1–5]. PCDLBCL-LT typically presents as nodules or tumors in one or two legs and approximately 10-15% of patients present with lesions outside the lower extremities [1–5]. The large neoplastic B-cells typically express CD20, CD79a, PAX5, MUM1/IRF4, Bcl2, and FOXP1 whereas BCL6 may be present or undetectable [1–5]. Interestingly, PCDLBCL-LT seems to be a "cutaneous counterpart" of activated B-cell-like nodal DLBCL with a similar cytogenetic and immunohistochemical profile [1–7]. Most PCDLBCL are CD5 negative and, to the best of our knowledge, only 5 cases of this tumor were found to express CD5 [1, 8–12]. We report the first well-documented CD5+ PCDLBCL-LT occurring in a 71-year-old woman with a history of Multiple Sclerosis.

2. Case Presentation

The patient was a 71-year-old woman with a history of Multiple Sclerosis during the past 12 years receiving dimethyl fumarate and baclofen. She also had hypertension and hyperlipidemia. She noticed a nodule at her left thigh, thought initially to be a mosquito bite. As the nodule grew bigger, a biopsy was performed. Histological examination demonstrated a diffuse dermal infiltration by large lymphoid cells (Figure 1(a)). Immunohistochemistry revealed that these large cells were positive for CD5, CD20, CD79a, MUM1/IRF4, Bcl6, Bcl2, and cytoplasmic IgM/λ whereas

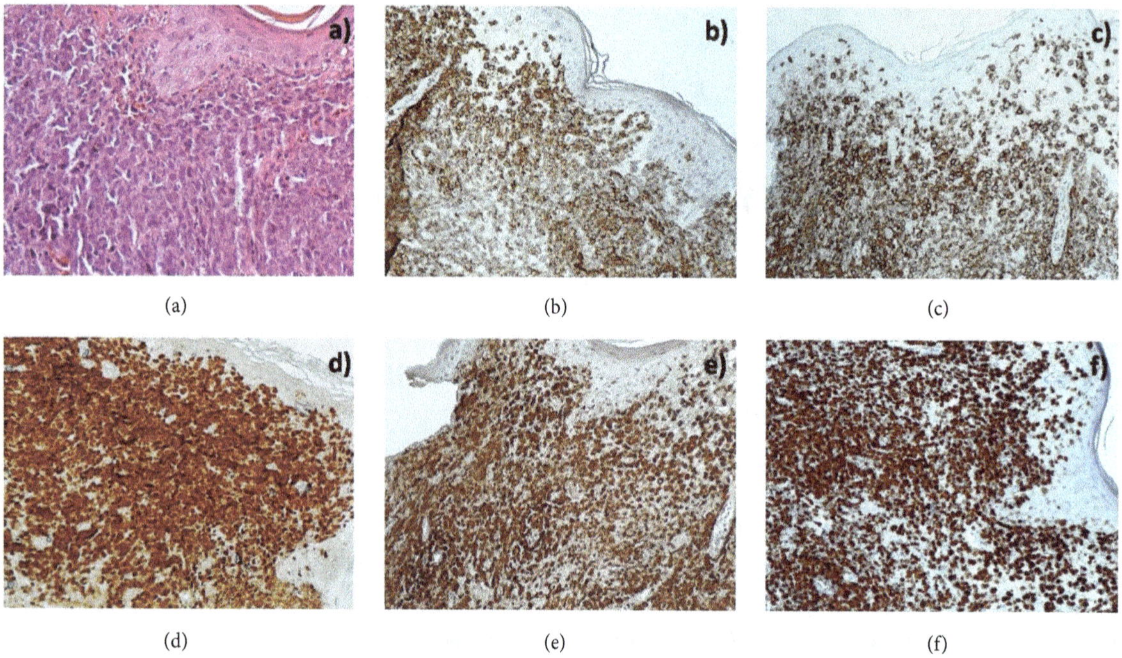

FIGURE 1: (a) Diffuse infiltration of the dermis by large lymphoid tumor cells with variable proportions of centroblasts and immunoblast-like cells (Hematoxylin-Eosin: magnification X400), (b–e) Positive immunostaining of large tumor cells for CD20, CD5, MUM1, and Bcl2, respectively (magnification X200) and (f) Ki67 immunostaining in approximately 90% of large tumor cells.

CD3, CD56, CD23, CD21, CD10, CD30, cyclin D1, CD68, lysozyme, myeloperoxidase, and CD34 were not detected (Figures 1(b)–1(e)). MYC immunopositivity was observed in 20% of tumor cells but our case was considered as MYC negative since the threshold for MYC immunohistochemical positivity in DLBCL is immunostaining of >40% of tumor cells [13]. Ki-67 immunostaining was detected in approximately 90% of large tumor cells (Figure 1(f)). Thus, the diagnosis of PCDLBCL-LT was made on the basis of clinical, histological, and immunohistochemical findings. The patient underwent Computed Tomography (CT) scans of thorax and abdomen and a bone marrow biopsy with no abnormal findings. She had four cycles of R-CHOP, with main side effect profound neutropenia. Ten months after the initial diagnosis she experienced right hemiplegia and entered the Neurology Department since worsening of Multiple Sclerosis was the primary diagnosis. A CT scan of the brain revealed lesions on basal ganglia and a biopsy was performed. On the basis of histological and immunohistochemical findings localization of DLBCL in Central Nervous system (CNS) was diagnosed. The patient was admitted to the Hematology Department and started treatment with methotrexate 3,5 mg/m^2. After the first cycle, she experienced an episode of hematuria and urinary infection with Enterococcus faecalis. After completing the antibiotic treatment, a second methotrexate treatment was given followed by a third cycle on schedule. Ten days after the last treatment, the patient had epileptic seizures and was transferred to the Intensive Care Unit where she died five days later because of progressive disease.

3. Discussion

In the present report, the diagnosis of PCDLBCL-LT was established on the basis of clinical, histological, and immunohistochemical findings. The most relevant differential diagnosis of PCDLBCL-LT is PCFCL with diffuse growth pattern that is based on morphology (centroblast- and immunoblast-like cells for PCDLBCL-LT vs centrocyte-like cells for PCFCL) and the immunophenotype (PCDLBCL-LT display strong positivity for Bcl-2, MUM1/IRF4 and cytoplasmic IgM, whereas MUM1/IRF4 and cytoplasmic IgM are undetectable in PCFCL and most of PCFCL are negative for Bcl-2) [1, 3, 4]. Notably, it was emphasized that any PCDLBCL with positivity for both Bcl2 and MUM1/IRF4 should be designated as leg-type, regardless of anatomical localization [4]. A diagnostic challenge may also result from CD30 expression in large B-cell lymphoma resembling anaplastic large T-cell lymphoma, but expression of CD20 and absence of T-cell markers lead to the diagnosis [1].

Interestingly, our case is CD5+ whereas most PCDLBCL-LT are CD5 negative [1, 3, 4]. To the best of our knowledge, only five cases of CD5+ PCLBL have been reported so far [8–12]. However, it was not possible to establish the diagnosis of PCDLBCL-LT in these 5 previous cases since immunostaining results for both MUM1/IRF4 and Bcl2 were not reported in any case [8–12]. Therefore, our case is the first well-documented CD5+ PCDLBCL-LT.

Notably, all previously reported cases of CD5+ PCLBL responded well to chemotherapy [8–12]. However, our patient died 11 months after diagnosis although she was treated with R-CHOP and methotrexate. Thus, further studies with additional cases are required to determine if there are prognostic differences between CD5-positive and CD5-negative PCDLBCL-LT.

It is noteworthy that our patient had a history of Multiple Sclerosis and a previously reported patient had a history of Rheumatoid arthritis [9]. This observation raises the possibility that the pathogenesis of CD5+ PCLBL might be related to autoimmunity [14, 15]. In this regard, it is noteworthy that CD5 is a negative regulator of T-cell Receptor (TCR) and B-cell Receptor (BCR) signalling and using animal models evidence was provided that increased expression of CD5 on either T cells or B cells protects against autoimmunity as a consequence of an increase of the threshold needed for TCR- or a BCR-mediated activation following antigen recognition [14]. Of potential interest is also the finding that a significantly increased percentage of CD19+CD5+ cells has been detected by two-colour fluorescence analysis in patients with progressive Multiple Sclerosis [16]. Further studies are required to gain insight into the putative role of the autoimmunity in the pathogenesis of CD5+ PCLBL.

In conclusion, we present the first well-documented CD5-positive PCDLBCL-LT occurring in a 71-year-old woman with a history of Multiple Sclerosis. Despite treatment with R-CHOP and methotrexate, the patient died 11 months after diagnosis.

References

[1] W. Kempf, D. V. Kazakov, and C. Mitteldorf, "Cutaneous lymphomas: An update. Part 2: B-cell lymphomas and related conditions," *American Journal of Dermatopathology*, vol. 36, no. 3, pp. 197–210, 2014.

[2] J. P. Nicolay and M. Wobser, "Cutaneous B-cell lymphomas - pathogenesis, diagnostic workup, and therapy," *JDDG: Journal der Deutschen Dermatologischen Gesellschaft*, vol. 14, no. 12, pp. 1207–1224, 2016.

[3] R. Willemze, E. S. Jaffe, G. Burg et al., "WHO-EORTC classification for cutaneous lymphomas," *Blood*, vol. 105, no. 10, pp. 3768–3785, 2005.

[4] A. L. Suárez, C. Querfeld, S. Horwitz, M. Pulitzer, A. Moskowitz, and P. L. Myskowski, "Primary cutaneous B-cell lymphomas," *Journal of the American Academy of Dermatology*, vol. 69, no. 3, pp. 343.e1–343.e11, 2013.

[5] M. Paulli, M. Lucioni, A. Maffi, G. A. Croci, M. Nicola, and E. Berti, "Primary cutaneous diffuse large B-cell lymphoma (PCDLBCL), leg-type and other: An update on morphology and treatment," *Giornale Italiano di Dermatologia e Venereologia*, vol. 147, no. 6, pp. 589–601, 2012.

[6] J. J. Hoefnagel, M. M. S. Mulder, E. Dreef et al., "Expression of B-cell transcription factors in primary cutaneous B-cell lymphoma," *Modern Pathology*, vol. 19, no. 9, pp. 1270–1276, 2006.

[7] A. Pham-Ledard, M. Prochazkova-Carlotti, L. Andrique et al., "Multiple genetic alterations in primary cutaneous large B-cell lymphoma, leg type support a common lymphomagenesis with activated B-cell-like diffuse large B-cell lymphoma," *Modern Pathology*, vol. 27, no. 3, pp. 402–411, 2014.

[8] M. Tanaka, R. Ichinohasama, M. Iwasaki, M. Sato, and H. Tagami, "Primary cutaneous B-cell lymphomas in Japan: A report of three cases and a comparison of Japanese and white patients," *Journal of the American Academy of Dermatology*, vol. 31, no. 1, pp. 54–60, 1994.

[9] T. Takahashi, Y. Kazama, H. Shimizu, M. Yoshimoto, M. Tsujisaki, and K. Imai, "De novo CD5-positive diffuse large B cell lymphoma solely presenting as multiple subcutaneous nodules," *Acta Haematologica*, vol. 107, no. 4, pp. 230–233, 2002.

[10] T. A. Hembury, B. Lee, R. D. Gascoyne et al., "Primary cutaneous diffuse large B-cell lymphoma: A clinicopathologic study of 15 cases," *American Journal of Clinical Pathology*, vol. 117, no. 4, pp. 574–580, 2002.

[11] H. Goto, M. Nishio, T. Endo et al., "Effective in vivo purging with rituximab and autologous peripheral blood stem cell transplantation in a woman with CD5 positive primary cutaneous diffuse large B-cell lymphoma," *European Journal of Haematology*, vol. 74, no. 6, pp. 526–528, 2005.

[12] J.-L. Dargent, L. Lespagnard, F. Feoli, L. Debusscher, M. Greuse, and D. Bron, "De novo CD5-positive diffuse large B-cell lymphoma of the skin arising in chronic limb lymphedema," *Leukemia & Lymphoma*, vol. 46, no. 5, pp. 775–780, 2005.

[13] A. Valera, S. Epistolio, L. Colomo et al., "Definition of MYC genetic heteroclonality in diffuse large B-cell lymphoma with 8q24 rearrangement and its impact on protein expression," *Modern Pathology*, vol. 29, no. 8, pp. 844–852, 2016.

[14] A. Dalloul, "CD5: A safeguard against autoimmunity and a shield for cancer cells," *Autoimmunity Reviews*, vol. 8, no. 4, pp. 349–353, 2009.

[15] Y. Baglaenko, K. P. Manion, N.-H. Chang, C. Loh, G. Lajoie, and J. E. Wither, "Suppression of autoimmunity by CD5(+) IL-10-producing B cells in lupus-prone mice," *Genes & Immunity*, vol. 16, no. 5, pp. 311–320, 2015.

[16] P. Bongioanni, C. Fioretti, R. Vanacore et al., "Lymphocyte subsets in multiple sclerosis A study with two-colour fluorescence analysis," *Journal of the Neurological Sciences*, vol. 139, no. 1, pp. 71–77, 1996.

12

Successful Treatment of Plaque Psoriasis with Allogeneic Gingival Mesenchymal Stem Cells: A Case Study

Sebo Gene Wang,[1] Nicholas C. Hsu,[1] Sebo Michelle Wang,[2] and Fu Nan Wang[1,3]

[1] *Top IVF USA, Hacienda Heights, CA, USA*
[2] *Loma Linda University School of Medicine, Loma Linda, CA, USA*
[3] *Stem Cell Life Science Corp., New Taipei City, Taiwan*

Correspondence should be addressed to Fu Nan Wang; funanwangmd@yahoo.com

Academic Editor: Alireza Firooz

Plaque psoriasis is the most common type of psoriasis that manifests as red scaly patches with white scales affecting body areas including scalp, elbows, knees, trunk, and buttocks. Although many treatment options are available including novel biologics, no cure is available. Mesenchymal stem cells (MSCs) have been safely used to treat a variety of human diseases. Allogeneic MSCs possess unique characteristics including hypoimmunogenicity, immunomodulatory, and anti-inflammatory properties, and they are currently being explored for potential therapeutic use for many systemic inflammatory diseases. The human gingival tissue is an easily accessible and obtainable source for the isolation of MSCs. MSCs from adult human gingiva are of fetal-like phenotype, multipotent, and easy to isolate and expand *in vitro*. Herein, we report a case of a 19-year-old man with a 5-year history of severe plaque psoriasis refractory to multiple topical and systemic therapies who was treated with allogeneic human gingival MSCs. Complete regression was achieved after 5 infusions with no adverse reaction occurred. The patient has been followed for three years and has remained disease free.

1. Introduction

Plaque psoriasis, the most common variant of psoriasis, makes up approximately 85 to 90 percent of all psoriasis cases [1]. This form of psoriasis typically presents with raised red scaly patches covered with white scales. These lesions/plaques most commonly occur on scalp, extensor surfaces of the elbows and knees, trunk, and buttocks, though it can appear on any location [2]. Psoriasis is associated with several other serious health conditions, such as diabetes, cardiovascular disease, lymphoma, and depression [2–4]. The etiology of psoriasis included genetic and environmental factors, yet it is complex and not well understood. Population and genetic studies have revealed a strong hereditary component, and the mode of inheritance is multifactorial [5–7]. Many environmental, physiologic, and psychological factors including infections, skin trauma, alcohol, tobacco, obesity, medications, and stress are known to trigger psoriasis and/or exacerbate existing condition [8]. Treatment options are diverse and range from topical medications including salicylic acid, coal tar, anthralin, corticosteroids, vitamin D3 analogs, calcineurin inhibitors, and tazarotene for mild disease, UV light therapy for moderate disease, and systemic agents such as methotrexate, oral retinoids, cyclosporine, and biologics for more severe disease [9]. Although these conventional therapies are effective for symptom control, there is no permanent cure for psoriasis [2, 9].

Present in virtually all tissues, mesenchymal stem cells (MSCs) are multipotent adult stem cells that possess the ability of self-renewal and multilineage differentiation [10–12]. MSCs can be readily isolated and expanded in vitro [13, 14] and, thus, hold great therapeutic potential in both autologous and allogeneic settings. Although autologous transplantation is a safe therapeutic option in the context of immunogenicity, the quantity, quality, and proliferation

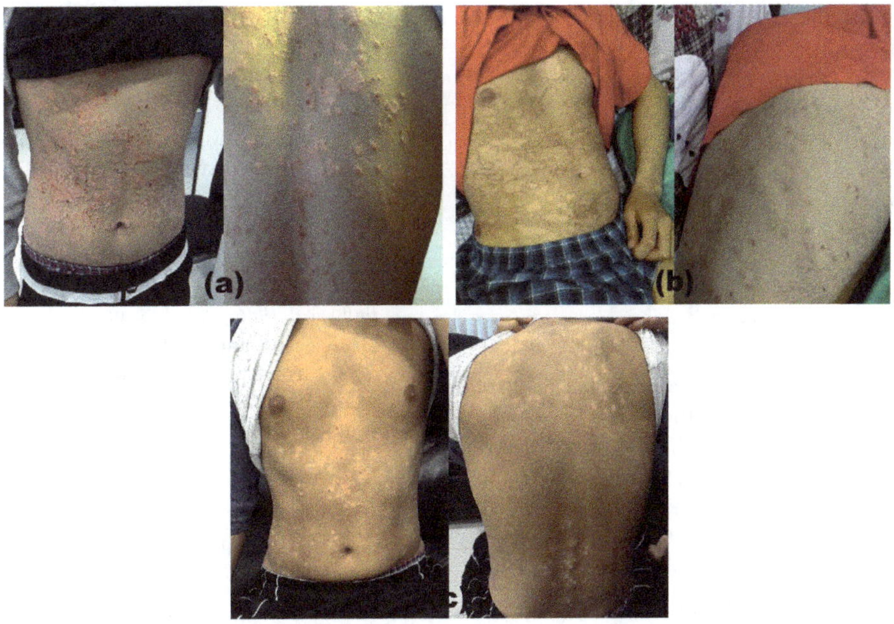

Figure 1: The effects of G-MSC infusions on a 19-year-old man with a 5-year history of severe plaque psoriasis. (a) Baseline/preinfusion images showing demarcated, round, erythematous plaques on upper chest and abdomen. (b) Gradual clearing of plaques after two successive weekly administrations of MSCs. (c) Lesions fully cleared after three more MSC infusions.

capability of MSCs were often reduced due to age and existing diseases of the patients [15–20]. MSCs are inherently hypoimmunogenic due to low-level major histocompatibility complex (MHC) class I expression and the lack of expression of MHC class II and co-stimulatory molecules [21, 22]. These unique immunosuppressive properties render them safe for allogeneic use [23–25]. The gingiva, composed of epithelium and connective tissues, is a unique biological barrier of the human periodontium. One of the gingiva's distinct characteristics is its fast wound healing ability following injury with little or no scarring [26]. Readily accessible and only minimally invasive procedure is needed for sampling, and this tissue represents an ideal source of multipotent postnatal stem cells for cell-based therapy in regenerative medicine. Here, we report a case of severe plaque psoriasis successfully treated with allogeneic gingiva-derived (G-) MSCs.

2. Case Report

A 19-year-old male college student presented with a 5-year history of severe plaque psoriasis. Physical examination revealed demarcated, round, erythematous plaques with overlying thick white scales distributed throughout his body (Figure 1(a)). The patient experienced itching often and described the intensity as unbearable. This disease had not only taken a toll on the patient physically, but he also suffered from depression and had suicidal thoughts. The patient had received several systemic treatments including methotrexate, acitretin, cyclosporine, and etanercept but with limited response. Because of the severity of the disease and lack of treatment response to prior systemic therapies, allogeneic MSC-based therapy was offered as an option based on earlier reports of success. The patient and the family were well informed regarding the experimental nature of MSC-based therapy. Written informed consent for treatment and data publication was obtained from the patient. The patient had not received phototherapy or other treatments during and after the MSC-based therapy.

Isolation and expansion of MSCs were performed according to the method previously described by Mitrano et al. [27]. Briefly, a biopsy of gingival connective tissue was obtained from a healthy adult donor. The tissue was minced for explant culture. The resulting cells were harvested and expanded in vitro for 3 to 4 weeks. Afterwards, the cells were aliquoted and cryopreserved. On days of treatment, the MSCs were thawed and made ready for administration. MSCs were suspended in 5 mL of normal saline prior to bolus injection. The patient received two successive weekly administrations of MSCs (3×10^6/Kg/infusion). Gradual clearing of plaques was observed, and no adverse effect was reported by patient (Figure 1(b)). Five weeks later, we gave the patient three more weekly MSC infusions. A week after the last injection, his psoriatic lesions fully cleared (Figure 1(c)). The patient has been free of psoriasis for 3 years now.

3. Discussion

With roughly 2% of population affected, psoriasis is a major public health burden worldwide [28]. Patients with psoriasis frequently experience comorbidities and are at higher risk for depression and suicide [2–4]. Although an array of treatment options exists, an effective and durable therapy has yet been developed. Psoriasis is an immune-mediated chronic systemic inflammatory disease. Because MSCs exert potent anti-inflammatory and immunomodulatory effects and possess important immunoevasive properties, there has been growing interest in the use of these cells as therapeutics for psoriasis [29–31]. G-MSCs form adult gingival mucosa which are of fetal-like phenotype and multipotent and possess strong immunomodulatory properties [32]. G-MSCs have notably several advantages as a candidate cell source over other MSCs. These cells are homogeneous and proliferate faster than other mesenchymal stem cells. G-MSCs also display stable morphology, maintain normal karyotype and telomerase activity at high passages [33]. Moreover, G-MSCs cells are abundant and easily accessible and can been effectively isolated and expanded *in vitro* for clinical use. To the best of our knowledge, this is the first study to report the safety and the effects of repeated administration of G-MSCs in a patient with psoriasis. The patient has been monitored for three years and has remained relapse free. This novel treatment vastly improved the quality of life and the psychological well-being of the patient. The findings of this study were in agreement with previous reports with regards to safety and feasibility of MSC infusions in patients with severe psoriasis [30, 31]. Therapeutic application of MSCs may be potentially superior to conventional clinical treatment modalities for severe psoriasis. Further studies that involved a larger sample size are needed to optimize key components of MSC therapies such as infusion frequency, method, and dosage.

Consent

The patient and the volunteer consented to participate in this study and have their data published.

References

[1] C. E. Griffiths and J. N. Barker, "Pathogenesis and clinical features of psoriasis," *The Lancet*, vol. 370, no. 9583, pp. 263–271, 2007.
[2] A. Menter, A. Gottlieb, S. R. Feldman et al., "Guidelines of care for the management of psoriasis and psoriatic arthritis," *Journal of the American Academy of Dermatology*, vol. 58, no. 5, pp. 826–850, 2008.
[3] A. B. Kimball, D. Gladman, J. M. Gelfand et al., "National Psoriasis Foundation clinical consensus on psoriasis comorbidities and recommendations for screening," *Journal of the American Academy of Dermatology*, vol. 58, no. 6, pp. 1031–1042, 2008.
[4] S. K. Kurd, A. B. Troxel, P. Crits-Christoph, and J. M. Gelfand, "The risk of depression, anxiety, and suicidality in patients with psoriasis: a population-based cohort study," *Archives of Dermatology*, vol. 146, no. 8, pp. 891–895, 2010.
[5] R. G. Langley, G. G. Krueger, and C. E. Griffiths, "Psoriasis: epidemiology, clinical features, and quality of life," *Annals of the Rheumatic Diseases*, vol. 64, no. 2, pp. ii18–ii23, 2005.
[6] F. Capon, R. C. Trembath, and J. N. Barker, "An update on the genetics of psoriasis," *Dermatologic Clinics*, vol. 22, no. 4, pp. 339–347, 2004.
[7] F. O. Nestle, D. H. Kaplan, and J. Barker, "Psoriasis," *New England Journal of Medicine*, vol. 361, no. 5, pp. 496–509, 2009.
[8] V. Chandran and S. P. Raychaudhuri, "Geoepidemiology and environmental factors of psoriasis and psoriatic arthritis," *Journal of Autoimmunity*, vol. 34, no. 3, pp. J314–J321, 2010.
[9] A. Menter and C. E. Griffiths, "Current and future management of psoriasis," *The Lancet*, vol. 370, no. 9583, pp. 272–284, 2007.
[10] D. J. Prockop, "Marrow stromal cells as stem cells for nonhematopoietic tissues," *Science*, vol. 276, no. 5309, pp. 71–74, 1997.
[11] F. Granero-Molto, J. A. Weis, L. Longobardi, and A. Spagnoli, "Role of mesenchymal stem cells in regenerative medicine: application to bone and cartilage repair," *Expert Opinion on Biological Therapy*, vol. 8, no. 3, pp. 255–268, 2008.
[12] H. K. Salem and C. Thiemermann, "Mesenchymal stromal cells: current understanding and clinical status," *Stem Cells*, vol. 28, no. 3, pp. 585–596, 2010.
[13] P. Bianco, P. G. Robey, and P. J. Simmons, "Mesenchymal stem cells: revisiting history, concepts, and assays," *Cell Stem Cell*, vol. 2, no. 4, pp. 313–319, 2008.
[14] M. F. Pittenger, A. M. Mackay, S. C. Beck et al., "Multilineage potential of adult human mesenchymal stem cells," *Science*, vol. 284, no. 5411, pp. 143–147, 1999.
[15] F. Cianfarani, G. Toietta, G. Di Rocco, E. Cesareo, G. Zambruno, and T. Odorisio, "Diabetes impairs adipose tissue-derived stem cell function and efficiency in promoting wound healing," *Wound Repair and Regeneration*, vol. 21, no. 4, pp. 545–553, 2013.
[16] Y. Sun, W. Deng, L. Geng et al., "Mesenchymal stem cells from patients with rheumatoid arthritis display impaired function in inhibiting Th17 cells," *Journal of Immunology Research*, vol. 2015, Article ID 284215, 13 pages, 2015.
[17] Y. Nie, C. Lau, A. Lie, G. Chan, and M. Mok, "Defective phenotype of mesenchymal stem cells in patients with systemic lupus erythematosus," *Lupus*, vol. 19, no. 7, pp. 850–859, 2010.
[18] E. U. Alt, C. Senst, S. N. Murthy et al., "Aging alters tissue resident mesenchymal stem cell properties," *Stem Cell Research*, vol. 8, no. 2, pp. 215–225, 2012.
[19] O. S. Beane, V. C. Fonseca, L. L. Cooper, G. Koren, and E. M. Darling, "Impact of aging on the regenerative properties of bone marrow-, muscle-, and adipose-derived mesenchymal stem/stromal cells," *PLoS One*, vol. 9, no. 12, Article ID e115963, 2014.
[20] A. Hermann, C. List, H.-J. Habisch et al., "Age-dependent neuroectodermal differentiation capacity of human mesenchymal stromal cells: limitations for autologous cell replacement strategies," *Cytotherapy*, vol. 12, no. 1, pp. 17–30, 2010.
[21] R. E. B. Fitzsimmons, M. S. Mazurek, A. Soos, and C. A. Simmons, "Mesenchymal stromal/stem cells in regenerative medicine and tissue engineering," *Stem Cells International*, vol. 2018, Article ID 8031718, 16 pages, 2018.
[22] B. Lukomska, L. Stanaszek, E. Zuba-Surma, P. Legosz, S. Sarzynska, and K. Drela, "Challenges and controversies in human mesenchymal stem cell therapy," *Stem Cells International*, vol. 2019, Article ID 9628536, 10 pages, 2019.
[23] M. M. Lalu, L. McIntyre, C. Pugliese et al., "Safety of cell therapy with mesenchymal stromal cells (SafeCell): a systematic review and meta-analysis of clinical trials," *PLoS One*, vol. 7, no. 10, Article ID e47559, 2012.
[24] A. A. Oliva, L. McClain-Moss, A. Pena, A. Drouillard, and J. M. Hare, "Allogeneic mesenchymal stem cell therapy: a regenerative medicine approach to geroscience," *Aging Medicine*, vol. 2, no. 3, pp. 142–146, 2019.

[25] J. Zhang, X. Huang, H. Wang et al., "The challenges and promises of allogeneic mesenchymal stem cells for use as a cell-based therapy," *Stem Cell Research & Therapy*, vol. 6, p. 234, 2015.
[26] H. Larjava, C. Wiebe, C. Gallant-Behm, D. A. Hart, J. Heino, and L. Häkkinen, "Exploring scarless healing of oral soft tissues," *Journal (Canadian Dental Association)*, vol. 77, no. 77, p. b18, 2011.
[27] T. I. Mitrano, M. S. Grob, F. Carrión et al., "Culture and characterization of mesenchymal stem cells from human gingival tissue," *Journal of Periodontology*, vol. 81, no. 6, pp. 917–925, 2010.
[28] E. Christophers, "Psoriasis-epidemiology and clinical spectrum," *Clinical and Experimental Dermatology*, vol. 26, no. 4, pp. 314–320, 2001.
[29] Y. S. Lee, S. K. Sah, J. H. Lee, K.-W. Seo, K.-S. Kang, and T.-Y. Kim, "Human umbilical cord blood-derived mesenchymal stem cells ameliorate psoriasis-like skin inflammation in mice," *Biochemistry and Biophysics Reports*, vol. 9, pp. 281–288, 2017.
[30] H. Chen, J.-W. Niu, H.-M. Ning et al., "Treatment of psoriasis with mesenchymal stem cells," *The American Journal of Medicine*, vol. 129, no. 3, pp. e13–e14, 2016.
[31] K. Comella, M. Parlo, R. Daly, and K. Dominessy, "First-in-man intravenous implantation of stromal vascular fraction in psoriasis: a case study," *International Medical Case Reports Journal*, vol. 11, pp. 59–64, 2018.
[32] M. E. Grawish, "Gingival-derived mesenchymal stem cells: an endless resource for regenerative dentistry," *World Journal of Stem Cells*, vol. 10, no. 9, pp. 116–118, 2018.
[33] G. B. Tomar, R. K. Srivastava, N. Gupta et al., "Human gingiva-derived mesenchymal stem cells are superior to bone marrow-derived mesenchymal stem cells for cell therapy in regenerative medicine," *Biochemical and Biophysical Research Communications*, vol. 393, no. 3, pp. 377–383, 2010.

13

Avelumab-Induced Scleroderma in a Patient with Metastatic Squamous Cell Carcinoma of the Lung

Jeffrey L. Dobrzynski,[1] Blake E. Vest,[2] and Brian L. Swick[2]

[1]*University of Iowa Roy J. and Lucille A. Carver College of Medicine, 375 Newton Rd, Iowa City, IA 52242, USA*
[2]*University of Iowa Hospitals and Clinics, Dermatology, 200 Hawkins Drive, Iowa City, IA 52242, USA*

Correspondence should be addressed to Jeffrey L. Dobrzynski; jeffrey-dobrzynski@uiowa.edu

Academic Editor: Ioannis D. Bassukas

Immune checkpoint inhibitors are associated with a spectrum of cutaneous immune-related adverse events. While maculopapular eruptions are the most common cutaneous adverse event, scleroderma can rarely develop. Herein, we report a case of new-onset scleroderma associated with avelumab treatment in the setting of metastatic squamous cell carcinoma of the lung. The pathophysiology of immune checkpoint inhibitor-induced scleroderma is not completely understood. A proposed mechanism is discussed along with the clinical presentation of symptoms and associated therapeutic response in cancer treatment. This case contributes to the few existing reports of immune checkpoint inhibitor-induced scleroderma to better understand the implications in the management of cutaneous immune-related adverse events.

1. Introduction

Immune checkpoint inhibitors (ICIs) are immunotherapy agents effective in treating a variety of cancers [1]. ICIs utilize antibodies that target immune checkpoint proteins such as the CTLA-4 receptor, PD-1 receptor, or PD-1 ligand. These checkpoint proteins function to downregulate the immune system. By blocking these targets, ICIs act to increase immune system activity and increase antitumor immunity. Despite their efficacy in treating advanced cancers, ICIs are associated with a spectrum of immune-related adverse events (irAEs) [1–3]. Of these, cutaneous immune-related adverse events (cirAEs) are the most common, affecting 20% to 40% of all patients treated with ICIs [4]. Although maculopapular eruptions occur most frequently, rarely scleroderma can develop [3]. Here we report a case of scleroderma induced by the PD-L1 inhibitor, avelumab.

2. Case Report

A 67-year-old female with metastatic squamous cell carcinoma of the lung on avelumab and utomilumab for almost 3 years presented with a 2-month history of a worsening rash. The rash started as rough spots on the volar wrists and posterior knees that progressed into diffuse areas of loose, sagging skin involving the trunk, extremities, and intertriginous areas (Figure 1). Immunotherapy was withheld due to the development of skin lesions.

Punch biopsies of the calf and thigh both showed thickened dermal collagen bundles, eccrine gland entrapment, and sparse, plasma cell-rich, chronic inflammation along the dermal-subcutaneous junction (Figure 2). Elastichrome stain exhibited normal elastin fibers. Serologic testing revealed elevated ANA of 1:320 with a coarse speckled pattern, but negative Scl-70, centromere, SM/RNP, RNA polymerase III, and PM-Scl-100 antibodies. These findings were consistent with a diagnosis of avelumab-induced scleroderma.

The patient was treated with methotrexate 17.5 mg weekly and a prednisone taper, starting at 60 mg daily and decreasing by 5 mg every week. The patient had neither improvement nor worsening on a one-month follow-up. Two months after discontinuation of immunotherapy, a new lesion of the left upper lobe of the lung was identified on

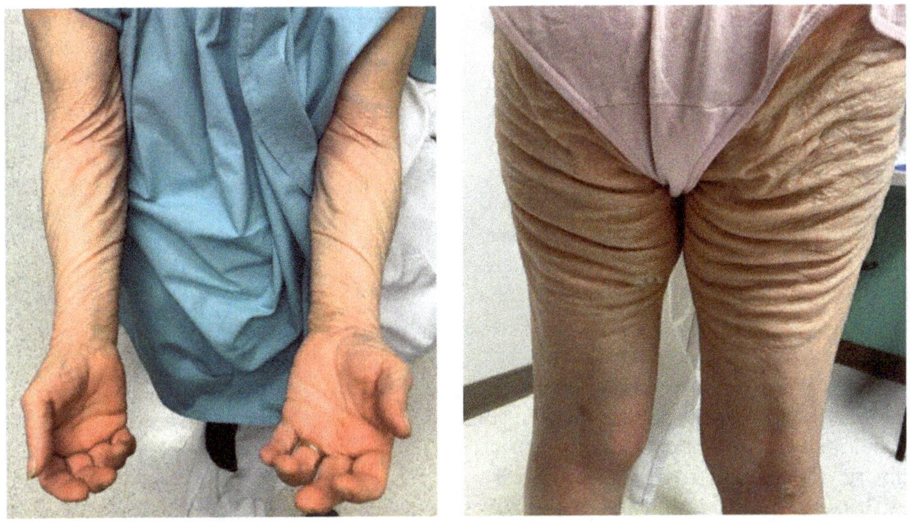

(a) (b)

FIGURE 1: Clinical photographs show areas of diffuse indurated, sagging skin, with decreased elasticity and fine scaling. (a) Ventral forearms and wrists. (b) Posterior thighs.

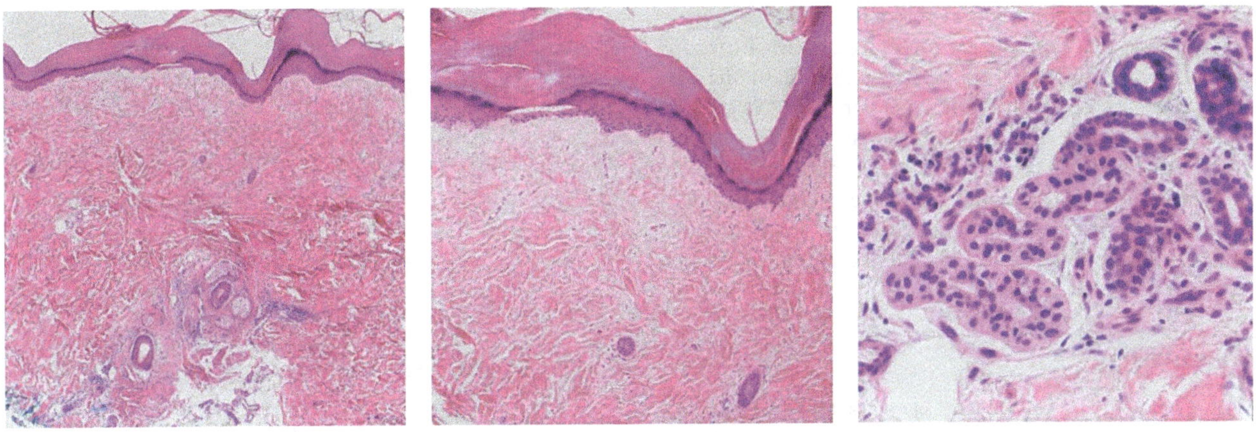

(a) (b) (c)

FIGURE 2: Punch biopsy showed thickened dermal collagen bundles, eccrine gland entrapment, and sparse plasma cells in the deep reticular dermis. (hematoxylin-eosin stain, original magnifications (a) ×40, (b) ×100, and (c) ×200).

chest CT, and the biopsy demonstrated small cell carcinoma. A new primary lesion was favored over the transformation of her original malignancy.

3. Discussion

Interaction between PD-L1 and the PD-1 receptor plays a key role in dermal thickening and the development of skin sclerosis and fibrosis in patients with scleroderma [5]. Although the pathophysiology is not completely understood, it is proposed that PD-1/PD-L1 inhibitor-induced scleroderma may result due to the development of Th1, Th2, and Th17 cells that induce profibrotic type 2 macrophages causing fibroblast activation and fibrosis [5].

A recent review of ICI-induced scleroderma found only 35 reported cases of ICI-induced scleroderma, with 30 cases caused by the PD-1 inhibitors pembrolizumab or nivolumab, three caused by the CTLA-4 inhibitor ipilimumab, and 2 caused by the PD-L1 inhibitors atezolizumab and durvalumab [5]. ICI-induced scleroderma may result in atypical presentations depending on the specific medication being used. Nivolumab seems to cause localized symptoms compared to pembrolizumab, which more often causes generalized skin thickening [5]. As opposed to the shiny, taught skin that spreads distally from the trunk seen in typical systemic scleroderma, our patient developed more distal extremity followed by truncal skin thickening with a wrinkled appearance, further demonstrating the variability in the clinical presentation of scleroderma induced by different ICIs. Additionally, drug-induced scleroderma lacks Raynaud's phenomenon and the internal organ involvement seen in systemic sclerosis [6].

Utomilumab is a fully human immunoglobulin G2 monoclonal antibody agonist of the T-cell costimulatory receptor 4-1BB/CD137. This agent is under investigation for the treatment of solid organ and hematologic malignancies. Overall, it has a favorable safety profile with no dose-limiting toxicities reported in a phase Ib trial [7]. Although less likely, the contribution of utomilumab to this patient's cutaneous adverse event cannot be completely excluded. Applying the WHO-UMC causality criteria, there is a probable/likely degree of association between avelumab and scleroderma observed in this case [8].

Multiple studies have shown that the development of irAEs is associated with increased therapeutic response in cancer treatment [9]. Two months after discontinuation of avelumab our patient had stable to improved cancer burden; however, she developed a new primary tumor diagnosed as small cell carcinoma of the lung. This was treated with stereotactic body radiation therapy and a follow-up CT of the chest, abdomen, and pelvis showed no residual or new tumors in the lungs. The patient's scleroderma was initially stable after the discontinuation of immunotherapy and initiation of methotrexate and prednisone. However, she developed a progression of scleroderma on the bilateral ankles after tapering off prednisone. These symptoms stabilized after restarting prednisone. Although high-dose systemic corticosteroids are often avoided when treating systemic sclerosis due to the risk of renal crisis, this along with methotrexate are mainstay treatments for the isolated skin findings without internal organ involvement seen in drug-induced scleroderma [6]. This case of avelumab-induced scleroderma contributes to the few existing reports of ICI-induced scleroderma to better understand the implications in the management of both cirAEs and the underlying malignancy.

References

[1] M. A. Postow, R. Sidlow, and M. D. Hellmann, "Immune-related adverse events associated with immune checkpoint blockade," *New England Journal of Medicine*, vol. 378, no. 2, pp. 158–168, 2018.

[2] I. Puzanov, A. Diab, K. Abdallah et al., "Managing toxicities associated with immune checkpoint inhibitors: consensus recommendations from the society for immunotherapy of cancer (SITC) toxicity management working group," *Journal for ImmunoTherapy of Cancer*, vol. 5, no. 1, p. 95, 2017.

[3] A. N. Geisler, G. S. Phillips, D. M. Barrios et al., "Immune checkpoint inhibitor-related dermatologic adverse events," *Journal of the American Academy of Dermatology*, vol. 83, no. 5, pp. 1255–1268, 2020.

[4] K. Tang, J. Seo, B. C. Tiu et al., "Association of cutaneous immune-related adverse events with increased survival in patients treated with anti-programmed cell death 1 and anti-programmed cell death ligand 1 therapy," *JAMA Dermatology*, vol. 158, no. 2, pp. 189–193, 2022.

[5] B. Terrier, S. Humbert, L. H. Preta et al., "Risk of scleroderma according to the type of immune checkpoint inhibitors," *Autoimmunity Reviews*, vol. 19, no. 8, Article ID 102596, 2020.

[6] Y. Hamaguchi, "Drug-induced scleroderma-like lesion," *Allergology International*, vol. 71, no. 2, pp. 163–168, 2022.

[7] E. E. W. Cohen, M. J. Pishvaian, D. R. Shepard et al., "A phase Ib study of utomilumab (PF-05082566) in combination with mogamulizumab in patients with advanced solid tumors," *Journal for ImmunoTherapy of Cancer*, vol. 7, no. 1, p. 342, 2019.

[8] S. Parida, "Clinical causality assessment for adverse drug reactions," *Indian Journal of Anaesthesia*, vol. 57, no. 3, pp. 325-326, 2013.

[9] A. Cortellini, S. Buti, V. Agostinelli, and M. Bersanelli, "A systematic review on the emerging association between the occurrence of immune-related adverse events and clinical outcomes with checkpoint inhibitors in advanced cancer patients," *Seminars in Oncology*, vol. 46, no. 4-5, pp. 362–371, 2019.

14

A Case of Psoriasis Vulgaris Treated with Brodalumab in a Hemodialysis Patient with End-Stage Renal Disease due to Diabetic Nephropathy

Masafumi Ishibashi and Rie Shiiyama

Department of Dermatology, Nippon Kokan Hospital, Kawasaki, Japan

Correspondence should be addressed to Masafumi Ishibashi; m_ishibashi@1997.jukuin.keio.ac.jp

Academic Editor: Ioannis D. Bassukas

Psoriasis vulgaris is not frequently seen in patients on hemodialysis. However, these patients have limited treatment for psoriasis due to concerns about complications. We report the case of a psoriatic patient with end-stage renal disease on hemodialysis, safely treated with brodalumab. A 60-year-old man who presented with a 20-year history of recalcitrant severe psoriasis. He had diabetes from 40 years ago, and hemodialysis was initiated due to the progression of renal dysfunction two months ago. He was treated with brodalumab, and skin lesions improved markedly. He began to have a chronic cough four months after starting brodalumab. CT showed diffuse ground-glass shadow and pleural effusion in both lungs. Transbronchial lung biopsy showed no findings suggestive of interstitial pneumonia. In bronchoalveolar lavage fluid, mycobacteria and fungi were not identified. The T-SPOT.TB test was negative. It was considered to be a symptom of overflow due to excessive fluid volume based on insufficient dietary management. Brodalumab was continued, and respiratory symptoms improved with proper weight setting and adequate dietary control. No recurrence of rash has been seen 12 months after the initiation of brodalumab. There were no serious adverse events.

1. Introduction

There have been several case reports of safe and effective biological treatment for psoriasis patients undergoing hemodialysis, with many cases treated with ustekinumab or adalimumab [1–3]. Recently, there was a report of a psoriasis patient on hemodialysis treated with anti-IL-17A antibody [4, 5].

2. Case Presentation

A 60-year-old man was diagnosed with psoriasis 20 years ago for a widespread rash on the trunk. He was diagnosed with diabetes in his twenties and hypertension in his thirties but was untreated. He developed a necrotizing soft tissue infection of the thigh 12 years ago, and diabetes treatment was started. He was treated with cyclosporine 10 years ago at another hospital; this was discontinued due to renal dysfunction. Renal function gradually declined, and hemodialysis was introduced 2 months ago. During his visit to our department, psoriatic plaques were seen on his scalp, face, trunk, and limbs (Figures 1(a) and 1(b)). He had a Psoriasis Area and Severity Index (PASI) score of 39.6. In clinical examination, blood urea nitrogen was 48 mg/dL, serum creatinine was 11.57 mg/dL, and C-reactive protein was normal. Serum 1, 3-beta-D-glucan was negative. The T-SPOT.TB test was negative. He had no history of interstitial pneumonia and no specific findings on chest computed tomography (CT). He had received hemodialysis for diabetic nephropathy. He previously suffered from necrotizing soft tissue infection and had a high risk of developing infection. Although his skin lesion was severe, his adherence to the treatment was poor. Rapid onset of efficacy was considered to be important for treatment adherence. Treatment with brodalumab was initiated in terms of the efficacy and safety. After 4 weeks, the generalized rash was mainly pigmented; 100% improvement in the PASI score was achieved at 12 weeks (Figures 2(a) and 2(b)). He began

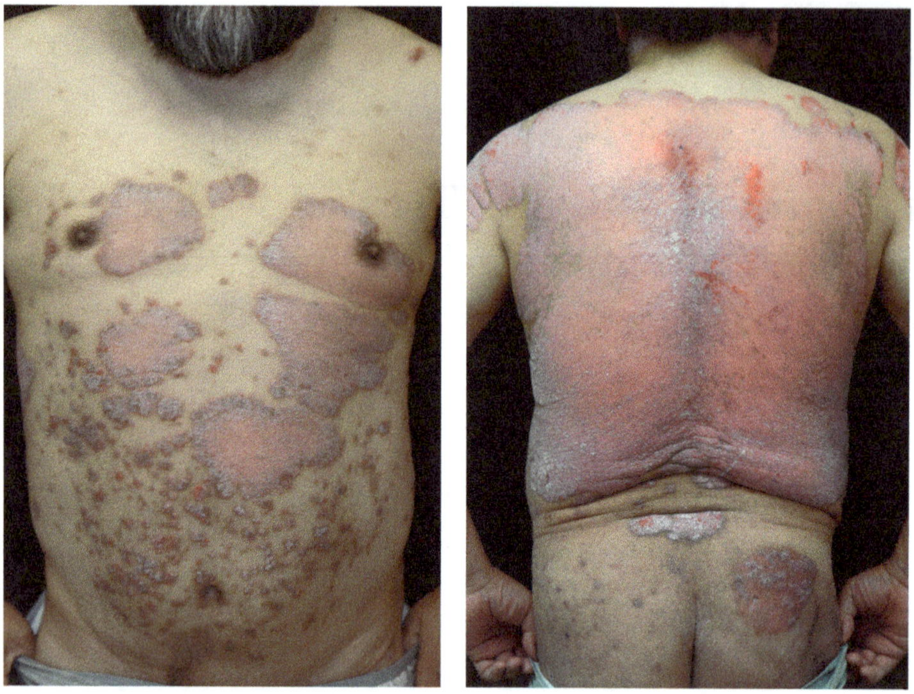

(a) (b)

Figure 1: (a, b) Scaling erythematous plaques on the trunk before brodalumab treatment.

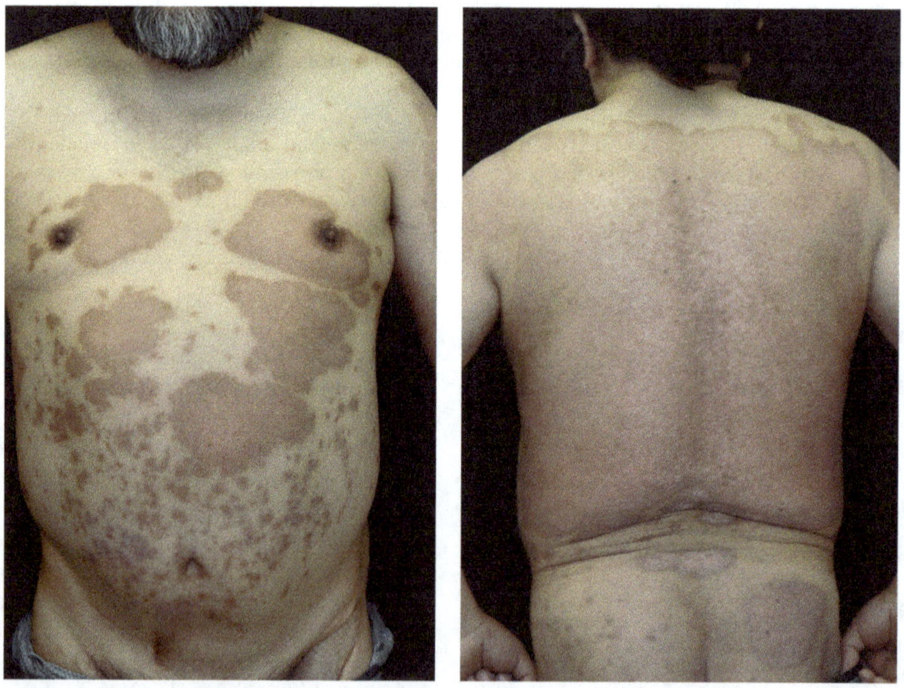

(a) (b)

Figure 2: (a, b) Almost complete clearance of psoriatic lesions at 12 weeks after the start of brodalumab treatment.

to have a chronic cough four months after the start of the biologic treatment. He ceased his dermatology visit and had not been given brodalumab for a month. Coughing continued, and CT showed diffuse ground-glass opacities and pleural effusions in both lungs (Figure 3(a)). Transbronchial lung biopsy showed no findings suggestive of interstitial pneumonia. Grocott staining was negative in bronchoalveolar lavage fluid (BALF), as were acid-fast bacilli and fungal cultures. *Mycobacterium tuberculosis*, *Mycobacterium avium*, and *Mycobacterium intracellulare* were not identified

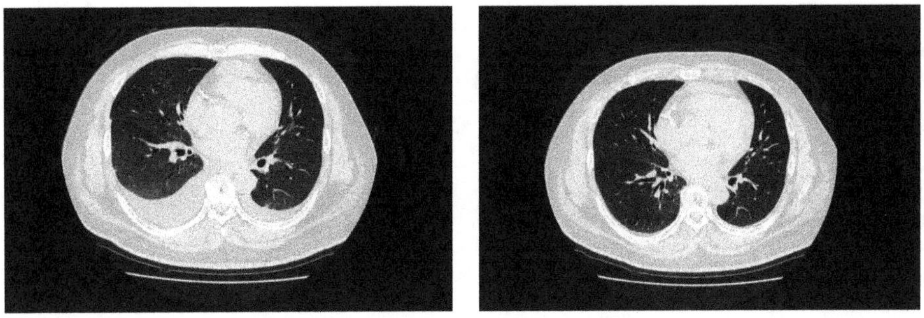

(a) (b)

FIGURE 3: (a) Chest CT four months after brodalumab initiation, which showed bilateral ground-glass opacities and pleural effusions. (b) Seven months after brodalumab initiation, bilateral ground-glass opacities and pleural effusions improved.

by polymerase chain reaction in BALF. The T-SPOT.TB test was also negative. It was considered to be a symptom of overflow due to excessive fluid volume because of insufficient dietary management. Brodalumab was continued, and respiratory symptoms improved with proper weight setting and adequate dietary control. Chest CT showed improved pleural effusion and opacity (Figure 3(b)). No recurrence of rash has been seen twelve months after the initiation of brodalumab. There were no serious adverse events.

3. Discussion

Chronic kidney disease (CKD) is significantly associated with uncontrolled diabetes and hypertension. Some skin conditions are associated with CKD and end-stage renal failure (ESRD). Meanwhile, severe psoriasis is a risk factor for CKD and ESRD [6, 7]. Two cohort studies in Taiwan showed psoriasis was associated with nearly a 2- and 3-fold increased risk of CKD and ESRD, respectively. Serious infections increase among patients with psoriasis, and psoriasis is an independent risk factor for serious infections, according to studies from the Netherlands and the United States [8, 9]. Furthermore, the severity of psoriasis is suggested to be a predictor for the risk of severe infection [10], as with diabetes. With regard to the risk of infection among patients treated with biologics, respiratory and skin infections can occur under tumor necrosis factor α antagonist administration [11], and infliximab increases the risk of serious infections in psoriasis patients compared to nonbiological systemic therapies [12]. During anti-IL-17 therapy, the incidence of *Candida* infection increases only marginally, but no basis for an increased incidence of tuberculosis is found. A meta-analysis showed that there was no significant difference in the incidence of serious adverse events among patients treated with Th17 inhibitors versus placebo [13]. Respiratory diseases to be differentiated when using biologics are bacterial pneumonia, mycobacterial infection, pneumocystis pneumonia, and drug-induced interstitial pneumonia. Since hemodialysis patients are immunocompromised, regular monitoring of infections such as tuberculosis is necessary in those treated with IL-17 inhibitors, as with other biologics. Brodalumab is a highly efficacious therapy for psoriasis and may have the fastest onset of action of any biologic therapy currently available [14]. To our knowledge, this is the first reported case of psoriasis patients undergoing dialysis treated with brodalumab. It is suggested that brodalumab is useful for the treatment of severe psoriasis in patients undergoing hemodialysis, but more cases need to be reported for a better understanding.

References

[1] Y. Kusakari, K. Yamasaki, T. Takahashi et al., "Successful adalimumab treatment of a psoriasis vulgaris patient with hemodialysis for renal failure: a case report and a review of the previous reports on biologic treatments for psoriasis patients with hemodialysis for renal failure," *The Journal of Dermatology*, vol. 42, no. 7, pp. 727–730, 2015.

[2] Y. Umezawa, M. Hayashi, S. Kikuchi et al., "Ustekinumab treatment in patients with psoriasis undergoing hemodialysis," *The Journal of Dermatology*, vol. 42, no. 7, pp. 731–734, 2015.

[3] K. Nimmannitya, C. Tateishi, Y. Mizukami et al., "Successful treatment with ustekinumab of psoriasis vulgaris in a patient undergoing hemodialysis," *The Journal of Dermatology*, vol. 43, no. 1, pp. 92–94, 2016.

[4] Y. Koike, Y. Fujiki, M. Higuchi, R. Fukuchi, S. Kuwatsuka, and H. Murota, "An interleukin-17 inhibitor successfully treated a complicated psoriasis and psoriatic arthritis patient with hepatitis B virus infection and end-stage kidney disease on hemodialysis," *JAAD Case Reports*, vol. 5, no. 2, pp. 150–152, 2019.

[5] D. Ikuma, M. Oguro, J. Hoshino et al., "Efficacy of secukinumab for plaque psoriasis in a patient on hemodialysis," *CEN Case Reports*, vol. 9, no. 1, pp. 55–58, 2019.

[6] C.-C. Chi, J. Wang, Y.-F. Chen, S.-H. Wang, F.-L. Chen, and T.-H. Tung, "Risk of incident chronic kidney disease and end-stage renal disease in patients with psoriasis: a nationwide population-based cohort study," *Journal of Dermatological Science*, vol. 78, no. 3, pp. 232–238, 2015.

[7] S. Yu, H.-P. Tu, C.-L. Yu, C.-H. Lee, and C.-H. Hong, "Is psoriasis an independent risk factor of renal disease? A nationwide retrospective cohort study from 1996 to 2010," *Dermatologica Sinica*, vol. 35, no. 2, pp. 78–84, 2017.

[8] M. Wakkee, E. de Vries, P. van den Haak, and T. Nijsten, "Increased risk of infectious disease requiring hospitalization among patients with psoriasis: a population-based cohort,"

Journal of the American Academy of Dermatology, vol. 65, no. 6, pp. 1135–1144, 2011.

[9] D. Y. Hsu, K. Gordon, and J. I. Silverberg, "Serious infections in hospitalized patients with psoriasis in the United States," *Journal of the American Academy of Dermatology*, vol. 75, no. 2, pp. 287–296, 2016.

[10] J. Takeshita, D. B. Shin, A. Ogdie, and J. M. Gelfand, "Risk of serious infection, opportunistic infection, and herpes zoster among patients with psoriasis in the United Kingdom," *Journal of Investigative Dermatology*, vol. 138, no. 8, pp. 1726–1735, 2018.

[11] W. G. Dixon, K. Watson, M. Lunt et al., "Rates of serious infection, including site-specific and bacterial intracellular infection, in rheumatoid arthritis patients receiving anti-tumor necrosis factor therapy: results from the British Society for Rheumatology Biologics Register," *Arthritis & Rheumatism*, vol. 54, no. 8, pp. 2368–2376, 2006.

[12] Z. Z. N. Yiu, D. M. Ashcroft, I. Evans et al., "Infliximab is associated with an increased risk of serious infection in patients with psoriasis in the U.K. and Republic of Ireland: results from the British Association of Dermatologists Biologic Interventions Register (BADBIR)," *British Journal of Dermatology*, vol. 180, no. 2, pp. 329–337, 2019.

[13] G. S. Naik, W. K. Ming, I. M. Magodoro et al., "Th17 inhibitors in active psoriatic arthritis: a systematic review and meta-analysis of randomized controlled clinical trials," *Dermatology*, vol. 233, no. 5, pp. 366–377, 2017.

[14] K. A. Papp and M. G. Lebwohl, "Onset of action of biologics in patients with moderate-to-severe psoriasis," *Journal of Drugs in Dermatology*, vol. 17, no. 3, pp. 247–250, 2017.

15

Interstitial Mycosis Fungoides: An Unusual Mimic of Interstitial Granuloma Annulare Not to Miss

Neha Singh,[1] Kiley K. Fagan,[2] and Douglas J. Grider[2,3]

[1]*Virginia Tech Carilion School of Medicine, Roanoke, VA, USA*
[2]*Section of Dermatology, Department of Internal Medicine, Virginia Tech Carilion School of Medicine, Roanoke, VA, USA*
[3]*Department of Basic Science Education, Virginia Tech Carilion School of Medicine, Roanoke, VA, USA*

Correspondence should be addressed to Kiley K. Fagan; kkfagan@carilionclinic.org

Academic Editor: Henry Wong

Interstitial mycosis fungoides is a rare histopathologic variant of mycosis fungoides that may resemble interstitial granuloma annulare, inflammatory morphea, and interstitial granulomatous dermatitis. Reported is a case of a 62-year-old African American female who presented with an asymptomatic, progressive rash of the left underarm and abdomen with histologic features suggestive of granuloma annulare. Biopsies revealed an interstitial pattern of cells in the dermis with prominent small aggregates of atypical lymphocytes, a few atypical lymphocytes in the lower epidermis, and a mild increase in dermal mucin. Immunohistochemistry staining revealed the atypical lymphocytes to be positive for CD3 and CD8 and negative for CD4 and CD7, an aberrant immunoprofile. Mixed in the dermis with the atypical lymphoid cells were a few CD68 positive histiocytes and S100 protein positive dermal dendritic cells. T-cell receptor beta gene rearrangement studies showed nearly the same clonal peaks for TCRB rearrangement in two biopsy specimens from separate sites, all supporting a diagnosis of interstitial mycosis fungoides. The patient is undergoing treatment with full body narrowband UVB (nbUVB) phototherapy with notable improvement in skin discoloration and resolution of several abdominal lesions. A diagnosis of interstitial mycosis fungoides is challenging to make based on clinical features alone and is often clinically misdiagnosed. Awareness of histopathologic features is critical to make an accurate diagnosis and thus patient management.

1. Introduction

Interstitial mycosis fungoides (IMF), first described by Shapiro and Pinto in 1994, is a rare histopathologic variant of mycosis fungoides (MF) that often presents with erythematous patches and/or plaques of the trunk and proximal limbs. IMF shares many clinical and histological features with interstitial granuloma annulare, inflammatory morphea, and interstitial granulomatous dermatitis, which make it challenging to accurately diagnose. There are several key histopathologic features to make a diagnosis of IMF that have been described in the literature and are emphasized in this report.

1.1. Case Report. A 62-year-old African American female presented to the dermatology clinic for a rash present for the past 5 years. It started under her left underarm, and then, she developed various patches on her abdomen that have since grown, covering less than 10% of the body surface area. The rash was asymptomatic but cosmetically bothersome to her. A physical exam revealed a large well-demarcated hyperpigmented thin plaque with a rim of annular erythema extending from the left axilla to the medial upper arm, suggestive of uncertain etiology (Figure 1). Various subtle hyperpigmented ill-defined patches with a wrinkled appearance were present on the lateral right abdomen (Figure 2). The patient had no lymphadenopathy.

Three punch biopsies were obtained from the axilla and abdomen, all of which revealed an interstitial pattern of cells in the dermis with prominent small aggregates of mildly enlarged atypical lymphocytes and a few histiocytes associated with a mild increase in dermal mucin (Figures 3(a)–3(c) and 4). There were a few atypical lymphocytes noted in the lower portion of the overlying epidermis. No dermal wiry collagen was present.

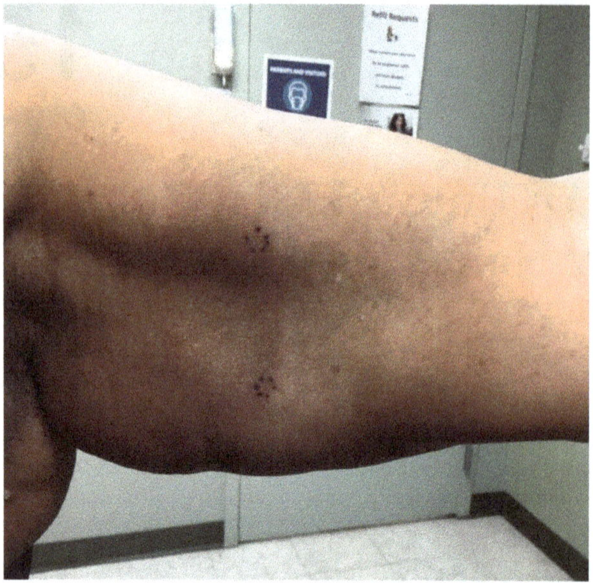

FIGURE 1: An ill-defined hyperpigmented patch with a wrinkled surface.

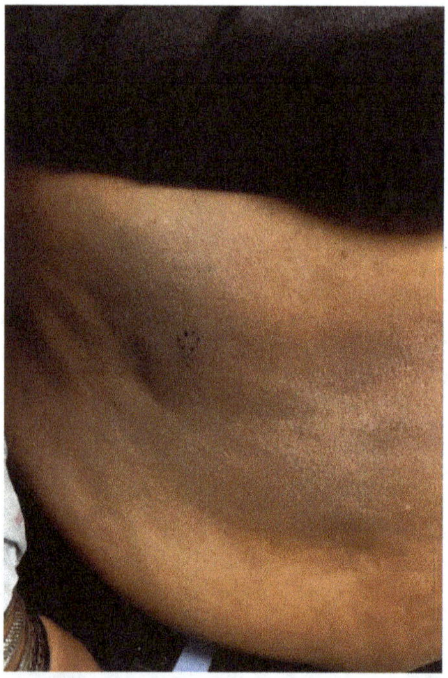

FIGURE 2: A large, slightly scaling, hyperpigmented patch on the right abdomen.

Ancillary immunohistochemistry demonstrated that the atypical lymphocytes in the dermis stained positive for CD3 and CD8 (Figure 5) and negative for CD4 and CD7 (Figure 6), an aberrant immunoprofile. There were insignificant numbers of CD20 positive B lymphocytes. CD68 stained a few intermixed dermal histiocytes (Figure 7), and S100 protein stained dermal dendritic cells as well as marked Langerhans cells in the overlying epidermis (Figure 8), producing a pattern mimicking interstitial granuloma annulare. T-cell receptor beta (TCRB) gene rearrangement studies showed nearly the same clonal peaks for TCRB rearrangement in biopsies from the left axilla (270, 305) and right abdomen (277, 305).

The patient is currently undergoing treatment with full body narrowband UVB (nbUVB) phototherapy with sessions 2–3 days per week. After 37 sessions, she has shown an improvement in the discoloration of the skin lesion in the left axilla and almost complete resolution of abdominal lesions. She has also been applying hydrocortisone 2.5% cream once daily to these areas.

2. Discussion

IMF is a rare histopathologic variant of MF that may resemble interstitial granuloma annulare (IGA), inflammatory morphea, and interstitial granulomatous dermatitis (IGD), and interstitial granulomatous drug reaction [1–7]. Histopathologically, this patient's lesions raised suspicion for granuloma annulare.

The concept of IMF was initially described by Shapiro and Pinto in 1994 and was later reintroduced by Ackerman in 1997 [8, 9]. Shapiro and Pinto reported on the presence of interstitial dermal infiltrates as one of the rare histopathologic patterns of MF and addressed their resemblance to granuloma annulare, while few case series and reports of IMF have been published to date, and they have been observed in both early and advanced stages [1, 9–12]. In the largest published case series to date by Reggiani et al, IMF was found to be a true histopathologic variant of MF with an otherwise conventional clinical presentation [2]. Affected individuals usually display erythematous patches and/or plaques, but macules and nodules have also been described [1, 2]. The disease typically affects the trunk and proximal limbs [1, 2].

Some data suggest IMF may be a transient histopathologic variant of otherwise conventional MF, in which interstitial patterns do not represent the only manifestation of the disease seen in different biopsies taken over time [2, 11]. An interstitial pattern representing the sole histopathologic presentation has been reported in only 2 cases [2]. Histology of IMF reveals prominent, linear aggregates of dermal interstitial infiltrates of small-to-medium sized lymphocytes intermixed with a few histiocytes [2, 12]. Lesion biopsies also show collections of lymphocytes splaying collagen bundles, involving mainly the dermis [1, 2]. In some cases, dermal mucin deposition or follicular mucinosis can be seen [1, 13]. A coarse pattern of fibrosis to the papillary dermis with a lichenoid infiltrate can also be seen in IMF [1].

IMF can also share many similar histopathologic features with MF, including epidermotropism, band-like papillary dermal infiltrates, and clonal T-cell proliferation [2]. Immunohistochemical staining reveals predominantly CD3 positive T cells in the epidermis and dermis with intermixed CD68 positive histiocytes and S100 protein dermal dendritic cells. In a series of 21 patients with IMF, a CD8 positive phenotype was found in 9 of 18 tested cases [2].

The histopathologic patterns detailed above aid in differentiating IMF from other differential diagnoses. In contrast to interstitial granuloma annulare and interstitial

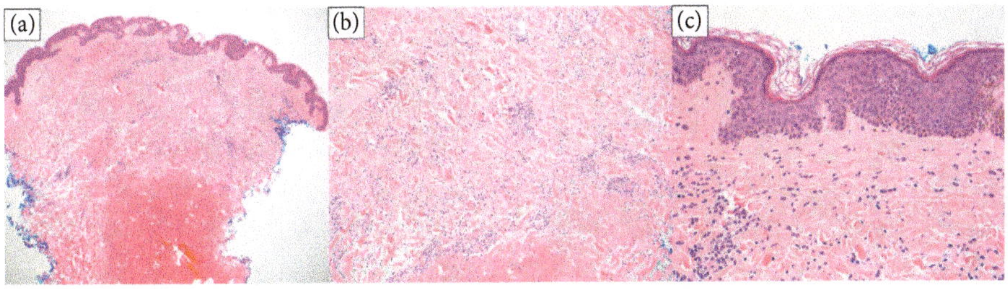

FIGURE 3: a–c) Lymphocytes, some larger and atypical, in the interstitial pattern in the dermis (hematoxylin & eosin, 4×, 10×, and 20× magnification).

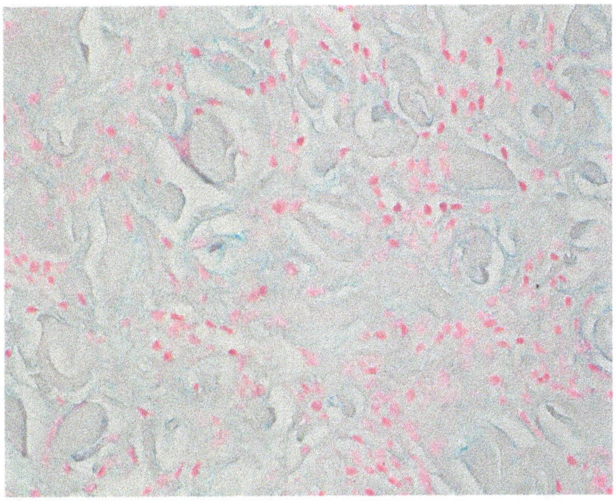

FIGURE 4: Increased dermal mucin between mononuclear cells (colloidal iron with digestion, 40× magnification).

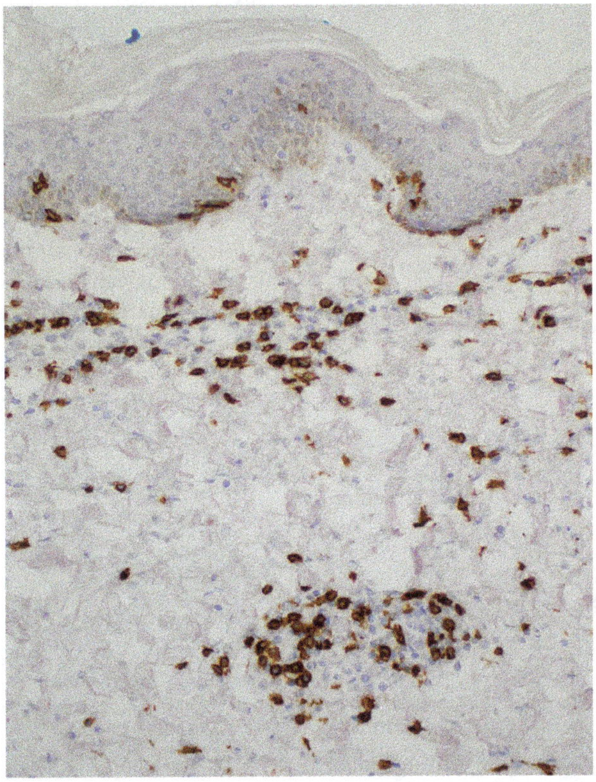

FIGURE 5: Atypical, enlarged interstitial lymphocytes with positive staining for CD8 in the biopsy from the L axilla (CD8 immunostain, 20× magnification).

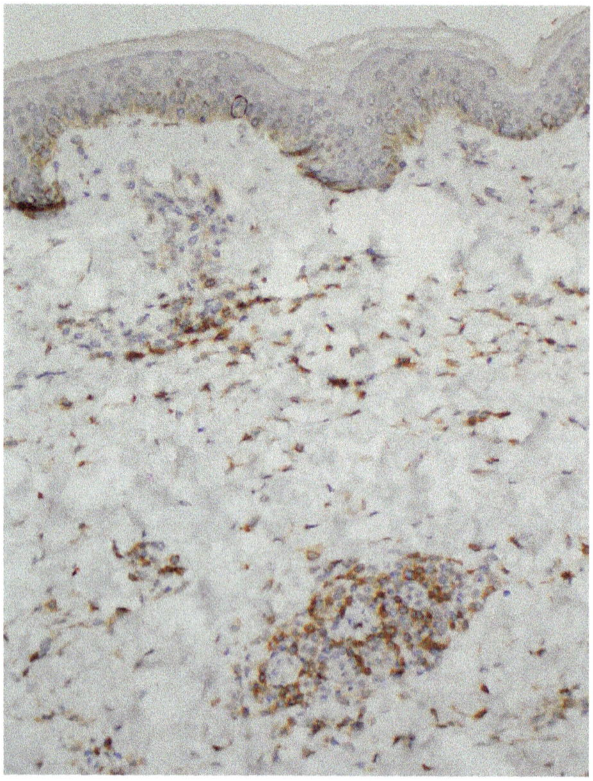

Figure 6: CD4 staining of lymphocytes is decreased in number in the biopsy from the L axilla when compared to CD8 (CD4 immunostain, 20× magnification).

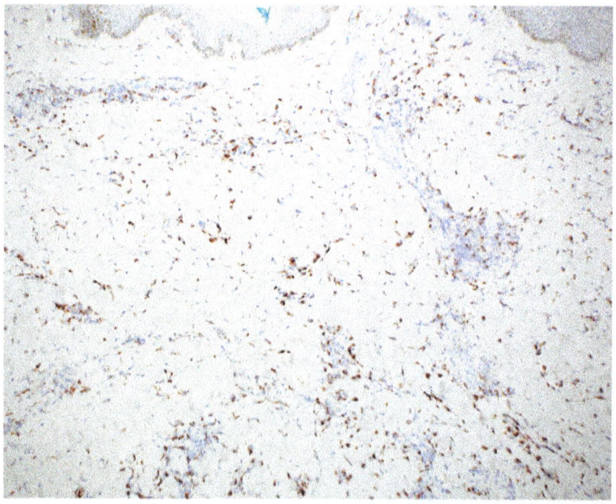

Figure 7: CD68 staining of dermal histiocytes (CD68 immunostain, 10× magnification).

granulomatous dermatitis in which CD68 positive histiocytes predominate, IMF usually presents with a predominance of CD3 positive atypical lymphocytes. In addition, these lymphocytes localize to the superficial dermis compared to the deeper dermis seen in interstitial granuloma annulare [1, 8, 10, 12, 14]. IMF can also be distinguished from inflammatory morphea based on the absence of plasma cells, lymphocytes, and histiocytes aggregating along the dermal-subcutaneous junction and absence of sclerosis [15].

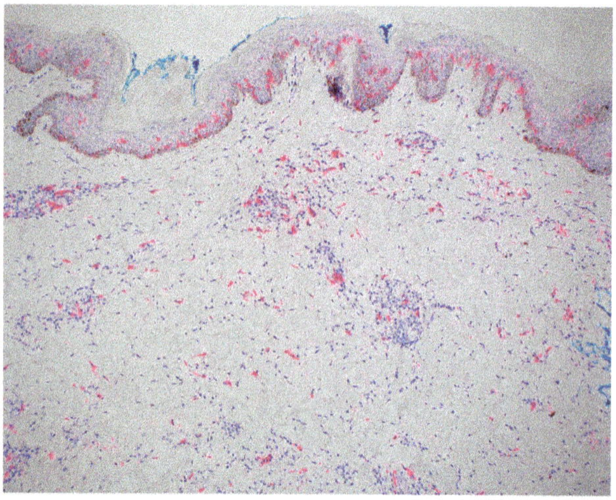

Figure 8: S100 protein staining dermal dendritic cells and Langerhans cells in the epidermis (S100 protein immunostain, 10× magnification).

Inflammatory morphea also shows superficial and deep, moderately dense interstitial, periadnexal, and perivascular infiltrates of lymphocytes between dermal collagen [1]. Plasma cells are also observed along the dermal-subcutaneous junction.

Based on these nuanced findings, histopathologic evaluation with particular focus on dermal interstitial lymphohistiocytic infiltrates and proper clinicopathologic correlation are necessary for an accurate diagnosis of IMF. This emphasizes the importance of performing a punch biopsy over a superficial shave biopsy, as sufficient depth of the dermis is critical in establishing the diagnosis of IMF [16].

3. Conclusion

IMF is a rare histopathologic variant of MF. Clinically and histopathologically, IMF may resemble interstitial granuloma annulare, inflammatory morphea, and interstitial granulomatous dermatitis. Although the clinical behavior, prognosis, and treatment for IMF are similar to classic MF, it is still important for dermatologists and dermatopathologists to be aware of IMF and its mimics because it is easy to misdiagnose.

References

[1] L. D. Su, Y. H. Kim, P. E. LeBoit, S. M. Swetter, and S. Kohler, "Interstitial mycosis fungoides, a variant of mycosis fungoides resembling granuloma annulare and inflammatory morphea," *Journal of Cutaneous Pathology*, vol. 29, no. 3, pp. 135–141, 2002.

[2] C. Reggiani, C. Massone, R. Fink-Puches, C. Cota, and L. Cerroni, "Interstitial mycosis fungoides: a clinicopathologic study of 21 patients," *The American Journal of Surgical Pathology*, vol. 40, no. 10, pp. 1360–1367, 2016.

[3] K. Mizuno, A. Suzuki, N. Kato, T. Isei, and H. Okamoto, "CD8-positive granulomatous mycosis fungoides mimicking generalized granuloma annulare," *Journal of Dermatology*, vol. 39, no. 12, pp. 1068-1069, 2012.
[4] T. Jouary, M. Beylot-Barry, B. Vergier, J. Paroissien, M. Doutre, and C. Beylot, "Mycosis fungoides mimicking granuloma annulare," *British Journal of Dermatology*, vol. 146, no. 6, pp. 1102-1103, 2002.
[5] U. Khanna and J. P. North, "Patch-type granuloma annulare: an institution-based study of 23 cases," *Journal of Cutaneous Pathology*, vol. 47, no. 9, pp. 785–793, 2020.
[6] W. Kempf, S. Ostheeren-Michaelis, M. Paulli et al., "Granulomatous mycosis fungoides and granulomatous slack skin: a multicenter study of the cutaneous lymphoma histopathology task force group of the European organization for research and treatment of cancer (EORTC)," *Archives of Dermatology*, vol. 144, no. 12, pp. 1609–1617, 2008.
[7] J. Y. Li, M. P. Pulitzer, P. L. Myskowski et al., "A case-control study of clinicopathologic features, prognosis, and therapeutic responses in patients with granulomatous mycosis fungoides," *Journal of the American Academy of Dermatology*, vol. 69, no. 3, pp. 366–374.e4, 2013.
[8] P. E. Shapiro and F. J. Pinto, "The histologic spectrum of mycosis fungoides/Sezary syndrome (cutaneous T-cell lymphoma). A review of 222 biopsies, including newly described patterns and the earliest pathologic changes," *The American Journal of Surgical Pathology*, vol. 18, no. 7, pp. 645–667, 1994.
[9] A. M. Freedman and A. B. Ackerman, "What is the clue and what is the diagnosis?" *Dermatopathol Pract & Concept*, vol. 3, pp. 171–174, 1997.
[10] G. Ferrara, G. Crisman, I. Zalaudek, G. Argenziano, and C. M. Stefanato, "Free-floating collagen fibers in interstitial mycosis fungoides," *The American Journal of Dermatopathology*, vol. 32, no. 4, pp. 352–356, 2010.
[11] M. T. Paoletti, F. Comoz, A. Dompmartin-Blanchere, M. Bagot, and N. Ortonne, "Interstitial mycosis fungoid: a rare variant of mycosis fungoids. Two cases," *Annales de Pathologie*, vol. 31, no. 1, pp. 36–40, 2011.
[12] M. Di Leonardo, "Pattern analysis: interstitial type of granuloma annulare vs interstitial type of mycosis fungoides vs interstitial granulomatous dermatitis with arthritis," *Dermatopathol Pract & Concept*, vol. 4, pp. 320-321, 1998.
[13] P. Gerami and J. Guitart, "The spectrum of histopathologic and immunohistochemical findings in folliculotropic mycosis fungoides," *The American Journal of Surgical Pathology*, vol. 31, no. 9, pp. 1430–1438, 2007.
[14] A. B. Ackerman, *Histologic Diagnosis of Inflammatory Skin Diseases*, Williams & Wilkins, Philadelphia, PA, USA, 1997.
[15] C. Jaworsky, "Connective tissue disorders," *Lever's Histopathology of the Skin*, p. 274, Lippincott-Rven, Philadelphia, PA, USA, 1997.
[16] P. E. Shapiro and P. E. LeBoit, "Interstitial mycosis fungoides: setting the record straight," *The American Journal of Surgical Pathology*, vol. 41, no. 2, pp. 282-283, 2017.

16

Reactive Eccrine Syringofibroadenoma on the Heel, Clinically Mimicking Squamous Cell Carcinoma

Yuri Sugita, Teruhiko Makino, Kotaro Matsui, and Tadamichi Shimizu

Department of Dermatology, Graduate School of Medicine and Pharmaceutical Sciences, University of Toyama, Toyama 930-0194, Japan

Correspondence should be addressed to Tadamichi Shimizu; shimizut@med.u-toyama.ac.jp

Academic Editor: Soner Uzun

The authors present a case of eccrine syringofibroadenoma that clinically mimicked squamous cell carcinoma and briefly comment on the current knowledge about its clinical and histopathological features and therapeutic options.

1. Introduction

Eccrine syringofibroadenoma (ESFA) is a rare benign skin disease that originates from the eccrine ducts. First described by Mascaro in 1963 [1], ESFA is histologically characterized by anastomosing strands of epithelial cells embedded in a fibro-vascular stroma. However, despite its distinct histological manifestation, the clinical appearance of ESFA is nonspecific and variable. We herein report a case of reactive ESFA with hyperkeratosis and hematomas on the heel, clinically mimicking squamous cell carcinoma.

2. Case Presentation

A 90-year-old Japanese woman presented with a 4-year history of hyperkeratotic lesions on her left heel that had not been improved by topical treatment with salicylic acid petrolatum ointment or 10% urea cream. There was no history of trauma, but she gradually found it hard to walk because of her left heel pain. The patient had been taking clopidogrel, aspirin, azosemide, metformin hydrochloride, and alogliptin benzoate for the treatment of chronic heart failure, angina, and diabetes mellitus, and all of these symptoms had been well controlled. At the first visit, a clinical examination revealed an erythematous plaque with multiple brown macules, ulcer, and hyperkeratosis (Figure 1).

Dermoscopy demonstrated glomerular vessels with regular arrangement in the ulcer area (Figure 2(a)) and red-black homogeneous areas in the erythematous area (Figure 2(b)). She had no particular family history. Although we recommended that she undergo a skin biopsy to diagnose the skin lesion, the patient and her family expressed a strong desire to treat the lesion through a single surgical operation because she was at an advanced age, and the possibility of squamous cell carcinoma could not be completely excluded. Therefore, the skin lesion was totally excised.

The histopathological examination revealed hyperkeratosis and thin anastomosing strands of cuboidal cells extending from the epidermis to the upper dermis (Figure 3(a)). Small ductal structures and cystic changes were observed within the interconnected strands of cells. Hematomas were found in the intracorneal region and upper dermis (Figure 3(b)). No mitotic or dysplastic cells were observed. The cells of the ductal and cystic structures were positive for carcinoembryonic antigen (CEA) (Figures 3(c) and 3(d)). Based on these findings, the lesion was diagnosed as a reactive ESFA.

3. Discussion

ESFA is commonly classified into five subtypes: (i) solitary ESFA, (ii) multiple ESFA associated with hidrotic ectodermal dysplasia (Schöpf syndrome), (iii) multiple ESFA without associated cutaneous findings (eccrine syringofibroadenomatosis), (iv) non-familial unilateral linear ESFA (nevoid ES), and (v) reactive ESFA associated with an inflammatory or neoplastic process [2–4]. The present patient was diagnosed with reactive

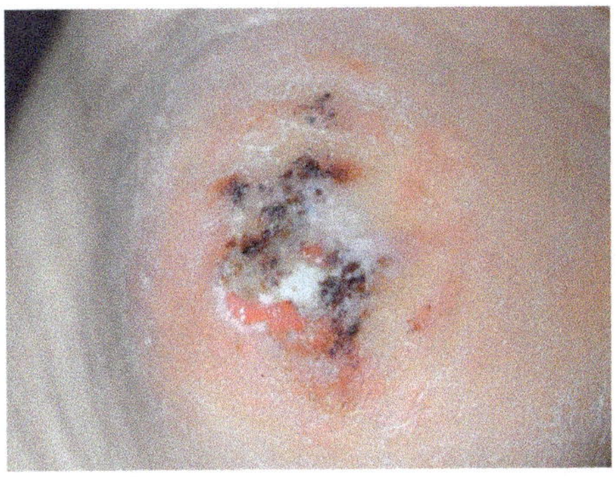

FIGURE 1: Clinical findings of the patient. Erythema plaque with multiple brown macules, ulcer, and hyperkeratinization on the left heel.

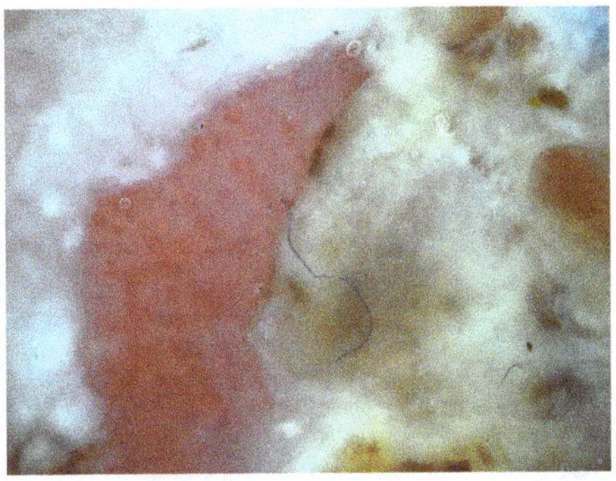

(a)

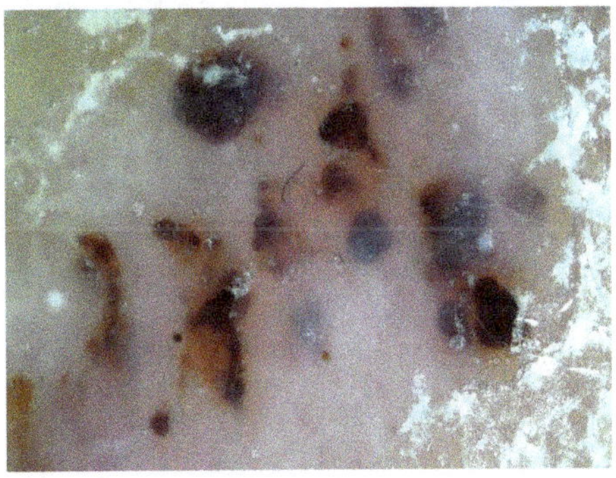

(b)

FIGURE 2: (a) Dermoscopy of the ulcer lesion. Glomerular vessels with regular arrangement in the ulcer area. (b) Dermoscopy of the erythematous plaque. There were features of intracorneal hemorrhaging.

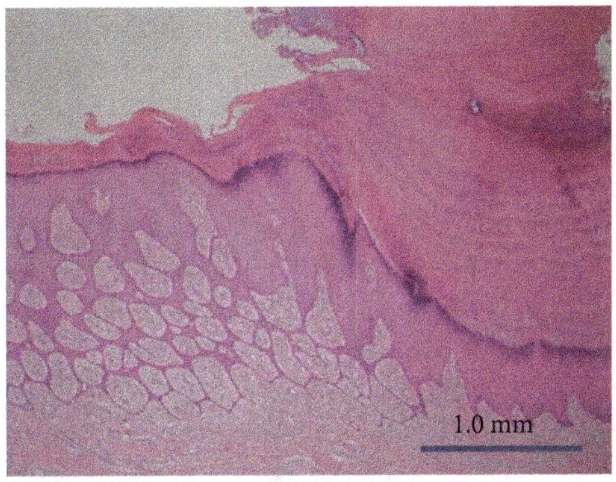

(a)

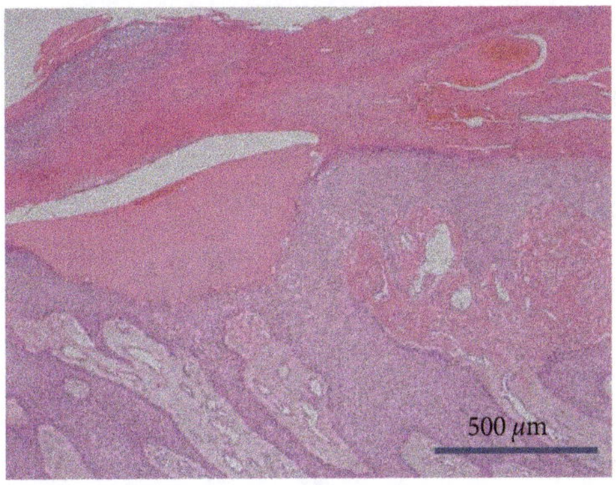

(b)

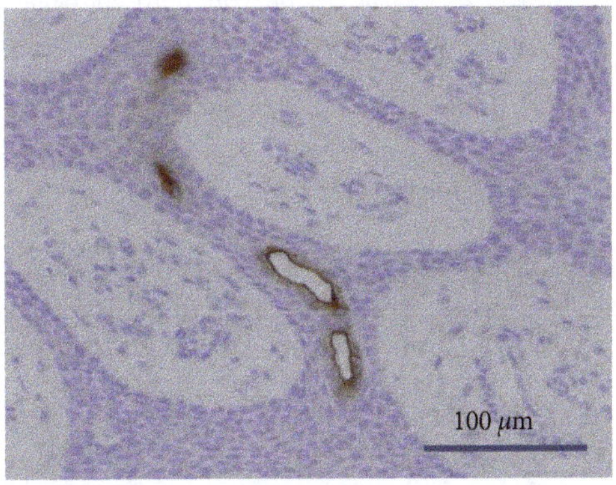

(c)

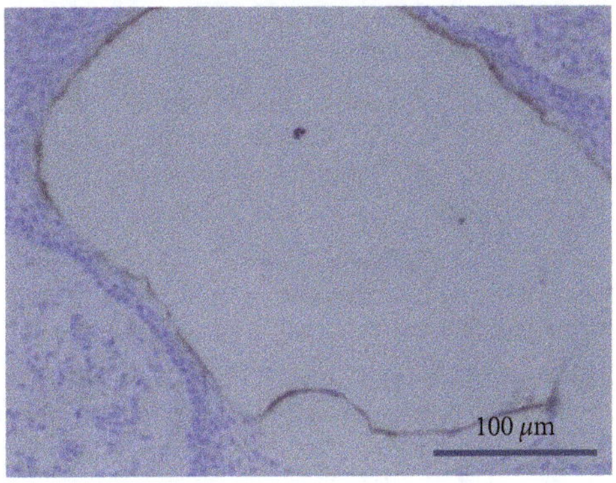

(d)

FIGURE 3: (a) Hyperkeratosis with thin anastomosing strands of cuboidal cells extending from the epidermis to the upper dermis (H&E stain, original magnification × 2). (b) Hematomas in the intracorneal region and upper dermis (H&E stain, original magnification × 4). (c) The cells of the ductal and cystic structures (d) were positive for CEA (original magnification × 20).

ESFA based on the characteristic histological and immunohistochemical findings.

Reactive ESFA is associated with tissue remodeling and has been found together with erosive palmoplantar lichen planus [3], bullous pemphigoid [5], burn scar [6], lepromatous leprosy [7], diabetes mellitus with polyneuropathy and chronic ulcers [8], nevus sebaceous, or squamous cell carcinoma [9]. In the present patient, both chronic stimulation and repetitive ulceration may have been associated with the development of reactive ESFA. The lesion in the present patient demonstrated unique findings, such as hyperkeratosis, ulceration, and hematomas. Although ESFA is well known to show a varied clinical appearance, no findings similar to ours have yet been reported. In addition, the clinical appearance in this case suggested the possibility of squamous cell carcinoma. Repetitive bleeding, which was enhanced by aspirin, may modify the clinical appearance.

In some subtypes of ESFA, malignant transformation into syringofibrocarcinoma or eccrine porocarcinoma has occasionally been observed [10]. However, reactive ESFA usually shows no malignant transformation; surgical excision may therefore be unnecessary for treating reactive ESFA, although the skin lesion in the present patient was totally excised. Reactive ESFA showing atypical findings may clinically resemble squamous cell carcinoma; therefore, physicians should consider reactive ESFA as a disease that should be distinguished from skin malignancy.

Consent

The examination of the patient was conducted according to ICMJE guidelines.

References

[1] J. M. Mascaro, "Considerations on fibro-epithelial tumors: exocrine syringofibroadenoma," *Annals of Dermatology and Syphiligraphy*, vol. 90, pp. 143–153, 1963.

[2] T. M. Starink, "Eccrine syringofibroadenoma: multiple lesions representing a new cutaneous marker of the Schöpf syndrome, and solitary nonhereditary tumors," *Journal of the American Academy of Dermatology*, vol. 36, no. 4, pp. 569–576, 1997.

[3] L. E. French, E. Masgrau, P. Chavaz, and J. H. Saurat, "Eccrine syringofibroadenoma in a patient with erosive palmoplantar lichen planus," *Dermatology*, vol. 195, no. 4, pp. 309–310, 1997.

[4] L. E. French, "Reactive eccrine syringofibroadenoma: an emerging subtype," *Dermatology*, vol. 195, no. 4, pp. 399–401, 1997.

[5] K. Nomura and I. Hashimoto, "Eccrine syringofibroadenomatosis in two patient with bullous pemphigoid," *Dermatology*, vol. 195, no. 4, pp. 395–398, 1997.

[6] E. Ichikawa, Y. Fujisawa, Y. Tateishi, S. Imakado, and F. Otsuka, "Eccrine syringofibroadenoma in a patient with a burn scar ulcer," *British Journal of Dermatology*, vol. 143, no. 3, pp. 591–594, 2000.

[7] H. L. Tey, W. S. Chong, and S. N. Wong, "Leprosy-associated eccrine syringofibroadenoma of Mascaro," *Clinical and Experimental Dermatology*, vol. 32, pp. 533–535, 2007.

[8] S. Thirawut, R. Salinee, and V. Vasanop, "Reactive eccrine syringofibroadenoma associated with neuropathy, venous stasis, and diabetic foot ulcer," *Case Reports in Dermatology*, vol. 8, no. 2, pp. 124–129, 2016.

[9] C. R. Schadt and A. S. Boyd, "Eccrine syringofibroadenoma with coexistent squamous cell carcinoma," *Journal of Cutaneous Pathology*, vol. 34, no. 1, pp. 71–74, 2007.

[10] T. Bjarke, A. Ternesten-Bratel, M. Hedblad, and A. Rausing, "Carcinoma and eccrine syringofibroadenoma: a report of five cases," *Journal of Cutaneous Pathology*, vol. 30, no. 6, pp. 382–392, 2003.

17

Mixed Cutaneous Infection Caused by Leishmania and Dermatophytes: A Rare Coincidence or Immunological Fact

Amresh Kumar Singh[1] **Ankur Kumar**[1] **Jayesh Pandey**[1] **Vivek Gaur**[1] **Pratima Tripathi**[1] **and Indra Prasad Adhikari**[2]

[1]*Department of Microbiology, Baba Raghav Das Medical College, Gorakhpur, Uttar Pradesh 273013, India*
[2]*Department of Biochemistry, Baba Raghav Das Medical College, Gorakhpur, Uttar Pradesh 273013, India*

Correspondence should be addressed to Amresh Kumar Singh; amresh.sgpgi@gmail.com

Academic Editor: Sergio A. Cuevas Covarrubias

Leishmaniasis was first described in 1824, in the Jessore district of Bengal (now Bangladesh) and more prevalent in Bihar, Uttar Pradesh, Jharkhand, and West Bengal. The disease is associated with depressed cellular immunity. Tinea is a fungal infection of the skin, which can become more extensively pathogenic particularly in patients with depressed cell-mediated immunity. Regulatory T cells and Th17 cells have been shown to be responsible for post-kala-azar dermal leishmaniasis (PKDL). We present a rare case of a 52-year-old house wife with a history of recurrent itching, depigmentation of the skin of extremities, and loss of appetite for 2-3 months followed by progressive spread of such lesion all over the body in an apparently healthy female. On examination, there were many hypopigmented scaly lesions mainly over the extensor aspect of the body. Skin lesions were characteristics of tinea infection with or without PKDL. A diagnosis of PKDL with tinea was made based on the history of kala-azar and on the skin slit smear for amastigote forms, *rK39* test, and KOH mount. Routine blood investigations showed negative serology for HIV and lower normal CD4+T counts. The patient was advised for treatment on systemic antifungal therapy with antihistaminics and later with miltefosine. We have highlighted that PKDL, although uncommon, is a distinct manifestation of VL. In our case study, we also tried to find the reason of coinfection; this was probably due to the depressed cellular immunity, skin abruptions, and acquired dermatophytic infection which is prevalent and associated with lower CD4+ T cell count.

1. Introduction

Visceral leishmaniasis (kala-azar) is a slowly progressing indigenous, neglected, and endemic disease caused by a protozoan parasite of the genus *Leishmania*. Leishmaniasis is a parasitic disorder transmitted by the bite of an infected female sandfly in developing countries, named *Phlebotomus* as per the National Vector Borne Disease Control Programme (NVBDCP) Govt of India and Lainson R. [1, 2]. The disease is transmitted by sandflies, which inoculate flagellated promastigotes into the skin of the host [3]. In human beings, leishmaniasis presents in four different clinical forms with different clinical manifestations: visceral leishmaniasis, or kala-azar; cutaneous leishmaniasis; mucocutaneous leishmaniasis; and diffuse cutaneous leishmaniasis [4].

Post-kala-azar dermal leishmaniasis (PKDL) is a late (usually posttreatment) complication of visceral leishmaniasis (VL) caused by *Leishmania donovani*. VL is one of the major neglected tropical diseases as per the World Health Organization (WHO), and it is especially prevalent among the poorest communities in endemic areas [5]. PKDL is a non-life-threatening cutaneous form characterized by a variety of skin manifestations, from hypopigmented macules to papular or nodular lesions. PKDL is generally linked to a previously occurring VL, and the lesions tend to appear 2-3 years after the completion of treatment in the Indian subcontinent [6]. The risk of developing PKDL seems to be associated with incomplete sodium stibogluconate (SSG) treatment [7]. However, PKDL has also been reported in patients treated with other antileishmanial drugs (i.e., miltefosine, amphotericin B, and paromomycin) and in individuals with no history of VL [6, 8, 9]. PKDL cases are relevant in the transmission of *L. donovani,* because they can act as reservoirs. However, except for cosmetic considerations, PKDL does not cause any physical limitation, and thus, patients do not tend to seek medical care for it. Active case detection is required to ensure adequate identification and treatment of patients [10].

PKDL is more prevalent in East Africa, where up to 50% of VL cases develop PKDL, whereas, on the Indian subcontinent, only 5%–18% of cases develop this cutaneous form [6]. However, the number of studies estimating the prevalence of PKDL in the Indian subcontinent is limited. A recent study showed that 2.4% of treated VL patients developed PKDL in Nepal but the exact prevalence is not known [7]. The PKDL incidence has been rising, and the estimated PKDL prevalence was 6.2/10,000 in Bangladesh [10, 11]. In India, to our knowledge, only one study was conducted in Uttar Pradesh and reported a PKDL prevalence of 48.2/10,000 in 1987 [12]. Therefore, the actual prevalence of confirmed PKDL cases was 1.8/10,000. Even if the incidence of PKDL seems to be decreasing in India according to surveillance data, there are no recent studies assessing the burden of PKDL in endemic areas [13].

Tinea corporis is a fungal infection that affects superficial layers of the skin caused by dermatophytes. It is defined based on the site of the lesions that may involve the trunk, neck, arms, legs, and groin. These include the scalp (tinea capitis), the face (tinea faciei), groin (tinea cruris), hands (tinea manuum), and feet (tinea pedis) [14]. Tinea corporis is common worldwide, and its prevalence is increasing day by day. Dermatophytes are the most prevalent causative agents of superficial fungal infections. There are many predisposing factors for rising prevalence: excessive heat, high relative humidity, and tight-fitted clothing [15]. Tinea can become more extensively pathogenic, particularly in patients with depressed cell-mediated immunity. T cell responses have been identified, such as regulatory T cells and Th17 cells that have been shown to be implicated in various forms of leishmaniasis as well as post-kala-azar dermal leishmaniasis (PKDL). The immunocompromised patients also have an increased prevalence of Majocchi granuloma, a type of tinea corporis folliculitis that invades the deep dermal layers [16].

Here, we are presenting a unique interesting case of mixed infection caused by *Leishmania* spp. and *Trichophyton rubrum* presenting with skin lesions.

2. Case Report

A 64-year-old female patient residing at Jagdishpur village, Deoria district, UP, India, a housewife, was referred from the District Government Hospital, Deoria, for diagnosis and management of "post-kala-azar dermal leishmaniasis." The patient was attending our hospital in December 2020 complaining of recurrent itching, depigmentation of the skin of extremities, and loss of appetite for 2-3 months followed by a progressive spread of such lesion all over the body. Hypopigmented rashes were present all over the body for two months. The patient was apparently fine 2 years earlier when she started complaining of malaise, rashes, and loss of appetite on and off. She took local symptomatic treatment (paracetamol for malaise and multivitamins with unknown ointment) for about one month but did not get any relief and gradually started developing progressive itching lesions from the extremities to the anterior abdominal wall. After history taking, she has mentioned that she was diagnosed as a case of visceral leishmaniasis in 2017 based on history, epidemiology, visceromegaly, and *rk39* test. For that, she has completed treatment as per the guideline and she cured clinically.

On examination, multiple hypopigmented, multiple circular, or ovoid in appearance lesions are present. These annular lesions demonstrate sharp marginations with raised erythematous scaly edges at a few places. In some of these lesions, the degree of inflammation was variable as seen in Figures 1(b) and 1(c). The lesions spread centrifugally, leaving a central clearing and mild residual scaling; this appears as a "ring" shape so, named as "ringworm." Since this case was referred from the periphery for evaluation of PKDL, we evaluated as per this case the need and suspicion.

Thus, in lieu of suspicion for tinea and PKDL, we have planned to do a first skin scraping and then skin slit biopsy and serological test for leishmaniasis. The diagnosis of tinea corporis with PKDL was made based on a clinical thorough history and physical examination. However, testing was to be done to confirm the diagnosis.

2.1. Skin Scraping. A skin scraping was examined under a microscope with a potassium hydroxide (KOH) preparation which revealed hyaline, septate, and branching long narrow hyphae with occasional arthroconidia suggestive of dermatophytic infection as seen in Figures 2(b) and 2(c). This finding was supportive for the diagnosis of extensive dermatophytosis based on the extent of lesions. However, up to 15% of cases may yield false negatives when only using KOH preparations for diagnosis [17].

2.2. Fungal Culture. Therefore, another method for confirmation which is a fungal culture has been placed. Fungal cultures are important to diagnose genus and species but take time for definitive identification. The culture was done using skin scraping samples in Sabouraud dextrose agar (SDA). Cultures showed growth of the fungal pathogen in about five days. The colony was mostly flat to slightly raised, white to cream, suede-like to downy, with yellow-brown to wine-red reverse. The most common isolation medium used for fungal cultures is SDA (1% glucose, 4% mycological peptone agar, water). Identification was done by examining the morphology, pigmentations, and surface topography of the culture as a *Trichophyton rubrum* as seen in Figures 1(a) and 1(b) [18].

2.3. Lacto Phenol Cotton Blue-Stained Microscopy. Most cultures show scanty to moderate numbers of slender clavate to pyriform microconidia under lactophenol cotton blue-stained wet smear made after teasing of fungal growth.

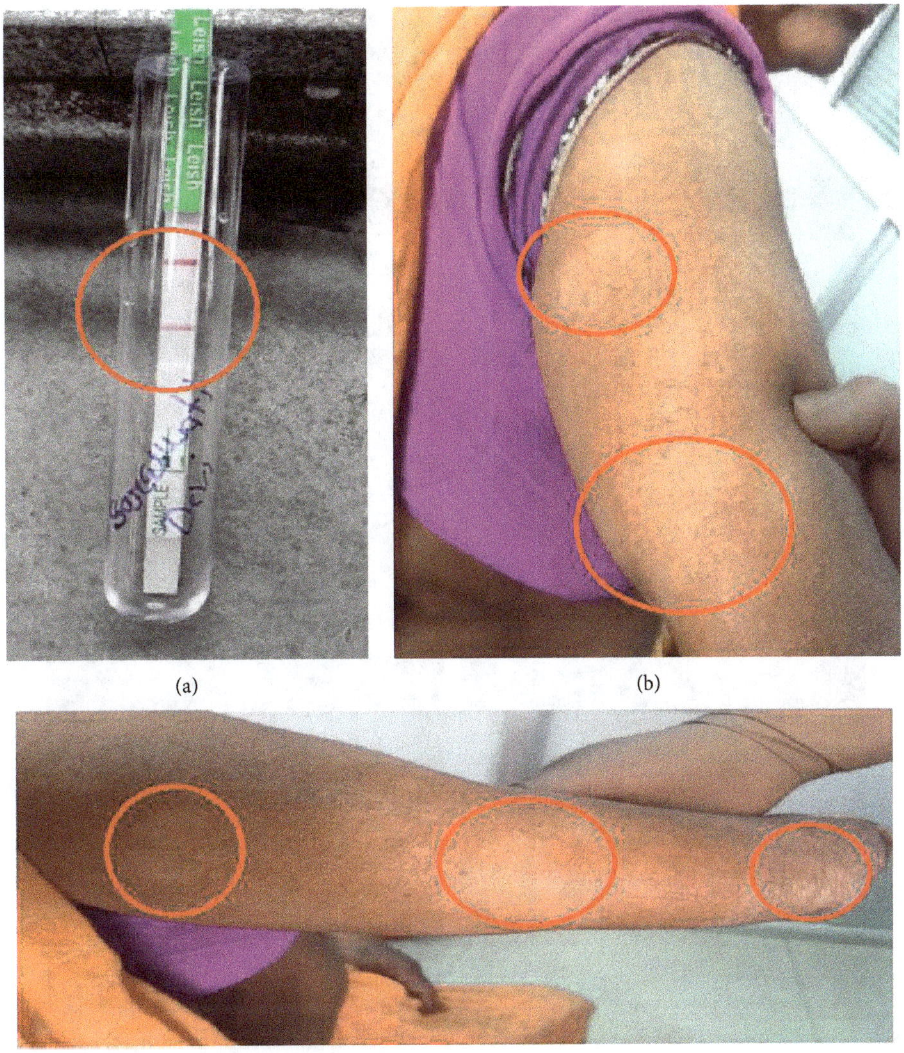

(a) (b) (c)

FIGURE 1: a) rK39 rapid card test (positive result). (b) and (c) Multiple hypopigmented lesions in the extensor aspect of upper limbs.

Macroconidia are usually absent, but when present, they are smooth, thin-walled, multiseptate, slender, and cylindrical to cigar-shaped as seen in Figures 1(c), 3(a), and 3(b). The shape of microconidia varies from slender clavate to pyriform; the numbers of macroconidia range from none to scanty to many and may or may not have terminal projections.

2.4. Biochemical Test for Identification. Based on the battery of different morphological tests and biochemical tests like hydrolysis of urea (urease test) in broth and on urea agar slants and Petri plates incubated at 22°C, 28°C, and 37°C, *in vitro* hair perforation (blond child, sheep, and goat hair), pigment production on cornmeal dextrose agar (CMDA), and the genus and species level identification by biochemical tests like urease test as *T. rubrum* [19] were performed.

2.5. rK39 Rapid Immune-Chromatographic Test (ICT). The *rK39* strip is a nitrocellulose strip impregnated with recombinant rK39 antigen and a commercially available test to diagnose *Leishmania* spp. infection (InBios International, Seattle, Washington, USA). One drop of serum from peripheral blood was applied at the base of nitrocellulose strips. After being air-dried, 2-3 drops of the test buffer (phosphate-buffered saline plus bovine serum albumin) were added, and the strip was placed upright for one minute. The appearance of a lower red band (control) indicates the proper functioning of the test, while the appearance of an upper red band indicates the presence of anti-rK39 IgG signifying a positive *rK39* test as seen in Figure 2(a) [20].

2.6. Skin Slit Smear. Collection of skin slit smear samples was performed using a sterile surgical blade, by a trained pathologist of our institute after taking proper consent. The important steps of this procedure were explained in detail. Local anesthesia (Xylocaine 1%) was given underneath the skin lesion at 3-4 places after sensitivity testing. Multiple imprint smears of the inner surface of the biopsy specimen were prepared immediately on three

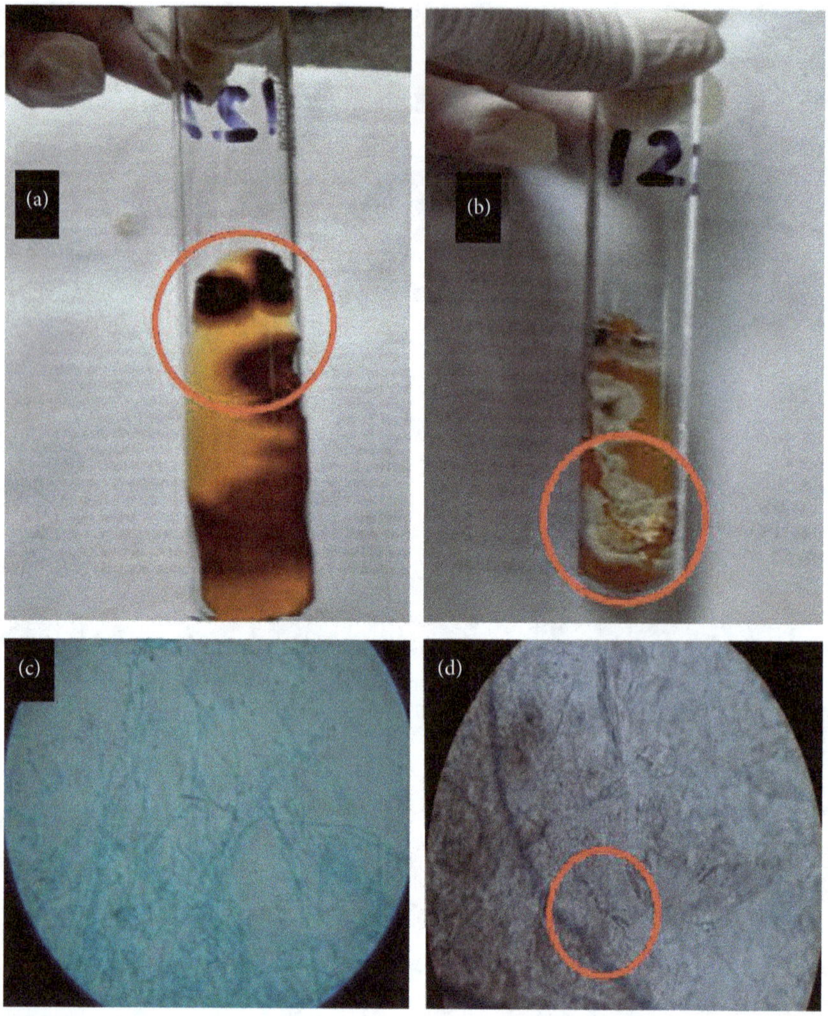

Figure 2: (a) Reverse side of fungal growth (*T. rubrum*) in SDA media. (b) Obverse side of fungal growth. (c) Lactophenol cotton blue (LCB) wet mount examination of fungal growth under high power microscopy (40X). (d) KOH mount examination of skin scarping under high power microscopy (40X).

clean grease-free glass slides and fixed with methanol before staining.

2.7. Giemsa-Stained Microscopy. Giemsa-stained imprint smears were examined microscopically by two laboratory personnel for demonstration of Leishmania parasites (amastigote form), and the findings were confirmed by the pathologist. The histiocytes showed numerous intracytoplasmic amastigote forms of *Leishmania* spp. after Giemsa stain as shown in Figure 4 [21].

2.8. PCR Test for Leishmania spp. The skin specimen was cut from the filter paper with a disposable sterile scalpel and incubated in 250 μl cell lysis buffer. DNA was extracted from the lysates with phenol-chloroform, and the pellets were air-dried. After being dissolved in 50 μl Tris-EDTA buffer, the DNA was kept at 4°C until analyzed by PCR. The kinetoplast DNA (kDNA) PCR showed a positive result, correctly diagnosing as a confirmed positive sample. The kDNA PCR is considered to be the most sensitive method for diagnosing leishmaniasis.

2.9. Other Laboratory Findings. The routine laboratory investigations revealed anemia (HB: 8.1G/dl), mild thrombocytopenia (PLT: 0.9 lacs/cumm), and leukopenia (total leukocyte counts: 3300/cumm) with relative eosinophilia (E: 08%). In routine serology, HIV was negative, C-reactive protein was normal, CD4+T count was 670/cumm (lower side of normal range), and the ESR was peaked at 22 mm. The finding of chest X-ray was normal. Ultrasonography was performed to know the visceromegaly and it showed no evidence of visceromegaly.

2.10. Treatment Plan of PKDL with Tinea Infection. Based on laboratory findings, in this particular case, the first antifungal therapy with oral terbinafine with antihistaminics was started for two weeks, and after proper clinical cure, miltefosine will be given at the dose of 150 mg/day for 60 days [22]. Now, the patient has improved a lot, as far as

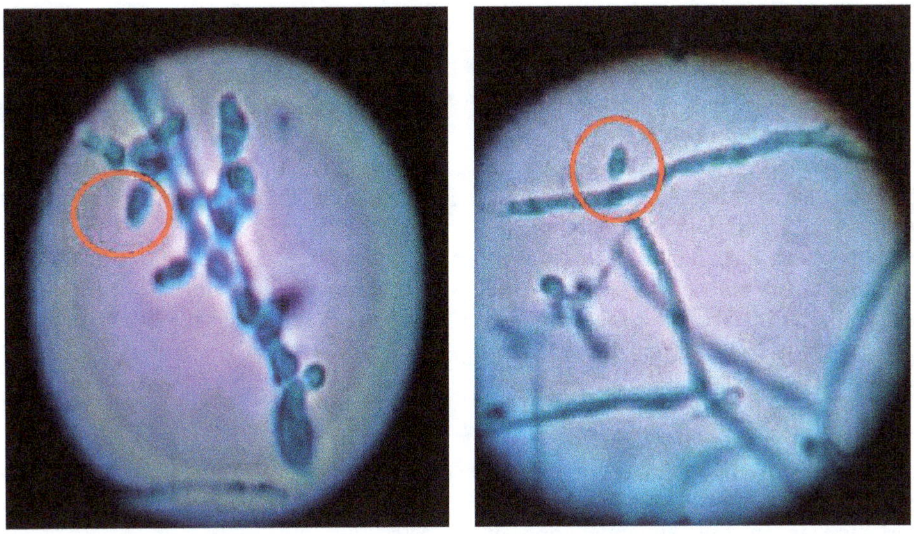

(a) (b)

Figure 3: Lactophenol cotton blue mounted examination under 100X shows moderate numbers of slender clavate to pyriform microconidia suggestive of *T. rubrum*.

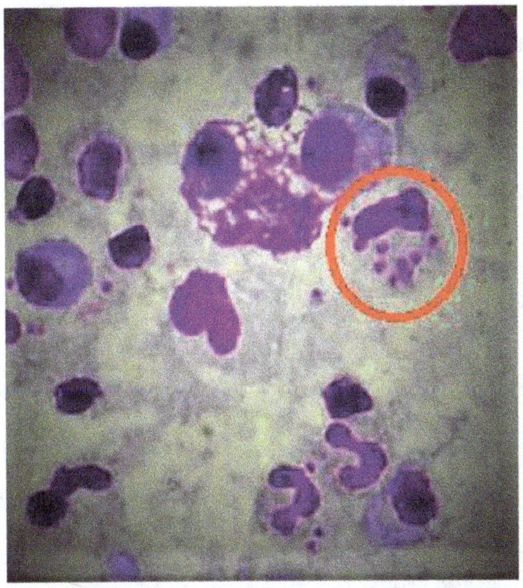

Figure 4: Giemsa-stained smear shows the typical presence of amastigote forms of *Leishmania* spp.

hypopigmented lesions were improved, but currently, the patient is on miltefosine as per standard dose. We have called the patient, after the completion of antileishmanial therapy for microbiological assessment for a complete parasitic cure.

2.11. Differential Diagnosis. In this case, skin lesions were evaluated clinically, and the differential diagnosis may mimic the appearance of tinea corporis with or without PKDL. Cases that are refractory to unknown antifungal ointment and treatment should warrant further investigation to rule out other skin lesions. Other common differential diagnoses include PKDL, erythema annulare, centrifugum, nummular eczema, tinea versicolor, contact dermatitis, cutaneous candidiasis, subacute cutaneous lupus erythematosus, pityriasis rosea, atopic dermatitis, seborrheic dermatitis, and psoriasis.

3. Discussion

Tinea is a fungal infection of the skin, which can become more extensively pathogenic particularly in patients with depressed cell-mediated immunity. Visceral leishmaniasis is also associated with depressed cellular immunity [23]. This may be the reason for the mixed infection caused by *T. rubrum* and *Leishmania* spp. Immune responses in leishmaniasis are often described in terms of (T helper) Th1 and Th2 cellular immune responses [24]. In addition, other T cell responses have been identified, such as regulatory T cells and Th17 cells that have been shown to be implicated in various forms of leishmaniasis as reported by Zijlstra [25]. After treatment with antileishmanial drugs, the immune response changes to a predominantly Th1 response characterized by the presence of IL-12 production and INF-γ production by T cells. Macrophage activation with the subsequent killing of parasites is a key factor in disease control [26]. PKDL is characterized by an intermediate position between a Th1 and Th2 response, and this transition stage may govern the typical clinical features. As a result of antileishmanial treatment of leishmaniasis, the PKDL patient was no longer systemically ill and has no fever, and the liver and spleen are normal, as seen in this case. Only the amastigote forms of parasites persist that may have been there since VL [27].

The immune response to dermatophytes ranges from a nonspecific host reaction to a humoral and cell-mediated immune response. The currently accepted fact is that a cell-mediated immune response is responsible for dermatophytosis control. On the other hand, some individuals develop a chronic or recurrent infection mediated by the downregulation of cell-mediated immune response.

Understanding the nature and function of the immune response to dermatophytes is a unique challenge that might lead to novel approaches in the research of treatment and immunological prophylaxis for dermatophytosis as shown by Almeida [28].

Although, *Trichophyton rubrum* was found in 20% of cases of dermatophytic infection in this geographical region in a previous study conducted for etiology of dermatophytes [29]. The *Trichophyton* spp. was also subjected to a urease test for the differential identification of *T. mentagrophytes* (showing a positive result) and *T. rubrum* (having a negative result) as in this case [19, 29]. *Trichophyton rubrum* is an anthropophilic fungus that has become the most widely distributed dermatophyte. Therefore, coinfection must be seriously considered, especially in patients who are supposed to be immunocompromised. Any hypopigmented patches and cutaneous papular polymorphic skin lesions must be investigated by the clinician in this endemic zone of leishmaniasis and some degree of dermatophytes; hence, for effective control of VL and to interrupt the transmission of kala-azar infection, its reservoir host PKDL needs to be detected early and treated adequately in the eastern part of Uttar Pradesh which is closely connected with the endemic zone of the Bihar state of India [30].

While reporting this case, we have highlighted the fact that PKDL, although uncommon, is a distinct manifestation of VL. Accurate early identification and management of these cases are crucial in eliminating a potential source of disease in the future. In our case study, we also tried to find the source of coinfection; this was probably due to the patient primarily suffering from PKDL and skin abruption, an acquired dermatophytic infection which was prevalent in this geographical region, and other factors (mainly immunological) as in this case because of lower CD4+T cell count also contribute to acquiring such mixed cutaneous infection. This may be because of the fact that these cases belong to rural areas and the majority of the patients consulted first with traditional healers or quack practitioners before being referred to a higher medical health facility. The patient was living in a house made up of stone and mud in an endemic area of eastern UP. Further, they also had a cattle shed in their yard all with conditions favorable for sand fly breeding as reported previously [31]. Even though kala-azar is endemic in the eastern UP and adjoining north-western part of Bihar, this patient was remained undiagnosed for a considerable period of time. Moreover, other risk factors which include lower socioeconomic status, lack of awareness about vector-borne or zoophilic infections, and mismanagement are the major causes that contribute to the high prevalence of these infections [32].

Limitations of this case report are the following. All immunological parameters were not analyzed to know the level of depressed cellular immunity except CD4+T cell count. Second, we have not analyzed the follow-up response of this case as this particular patient was first advised of oral antifungal therapy with antihistaminics and later planned for treatment with an antileishmanial drug.

Moving forward, this report will be useful to physicians as well as health policymakers on how to identify and diagnose such coinfection of dermatophyte with or without a history of VL. The technique used to identify and diagnose the suspected cases was easy to perform at any basic laboratory or clinical setup for early diagnosis and it also helps the clinician for the management of mixed PKDL and dermatophytic infections. As a final note, this case was rare and unique while considering cutaneous infection etiology could be mixed with PKDL and dermatophytes in India; therefore, clinicians as well as microbiologists should consider this approach during diagnosis and treatment management of the unusual cases of PKDL.

Consent

Written informed consent was obtained before collecting the different clinical samples.

Acknowledgments

The authors are highly thankful for the study subject to provide her consent to participate in this study. The authors would like to thank Dr. Gyan Chand, Program Officer (VL), PATH Organization for Neglected Tropical Disease, UP, for providing support in the diagnosis and management of this case. The authors would like to thank their laboratory technicians (Mr. Akhilanand Rai and Mr. Jagmohan Prasad) and microbiologists for their support.

References

[1] Extent of Problem of Kala-Azar in India, National Vector Borne Disease Control Programme (NVBDCP), MOHFW, https://nvbdcp.gov.in/index4.php?lang=1&level=0&linkid=534&lid=3742.

[2] R. Lainson, "The American leishmaniases: some observations on their ecology and epidemiology," *Transactions of the Royal Society of Tropical Medicine and Hygiene*, vol. 77, no. 5, pp. 569–596, 1983.

[3] P. Desjeux, "Human leishmaniasis: epidemiology and public health aspects," *World Health Statistics Quarterly*, vol. 45, no. 2-3, pp. 267–275, 1992.

[4] M. Pourahmad, F. Hooshmand, and M. Rahiminejad, "Cutaneous leishmaniasis associated with visceral leishmaniasis in a case of acquired immunodeficiency syndrome," *International Journal of Dermatology*, vol. 48, no. 1, pp. 59–61, 2003.

[5] M. Boelaert, F. Meheus, A. Sanchez et al., "The poorest of the poor: a poverty appraisal of households affected by visceral leishmaniasis in Bihar, India," *Tropical Medicine & International Health*, vol. 14, no. 6, pp. 639–644, 2009.

[6] E. Zijlstra, A. Musa, E. Khalil, I. El Hassan, and A. El-Hassan, "Post-kala-azar dermal leishmaniasis," *The Lancet Infectious Diseases*, vol. 3, no. 2, pp. 87–98, 2003.

[7] S. Uranw, B. Ostyn, A. Rijal et al., "Post-kala-azar dermal leishmaniasis in Nepal: a retrospective cohort study (2000-2010)," *PLoS Neglected Tropical Diseases*, vol. 5, no. 12, p. e1433, 2011.

[8] V. N. R. Das, P. Das, R. K. Topno et al., "Development of post-kala-azar dermal leishmaniasis (PKDL) in miltefosine-treated

visceral leishmaniasis," *The American Journal of Tropical Medicine and Hygiene*, vol. 80, no. 3, pp. 336–338, 2009.

[9] K. Pandey, V. N. R. Das, D. Singh et al., "Post-kala-azar dermal leishmaniasis in a patient treated with injectable paromomycin for visceral leishmaniasis in India," *Journal of Clinical Microbiology*, vol. 50, no. 4, pp. 1478-1479, 2012.

[10] D. Mondal, K. N. Nasrin, M. M. Huda et al., "Enhanced case detection and improved diagnosis of PKDL in a kala-azar-endemic area of Bangladesh," *PLoS Neglected Tropical Diseases*, vol. 4, no. 10, p. e832, 2010.

[11] K. M. Rahman, S. Islam, M. W. Rahman et al., "Increasing incidence of post-kala-azar dermal leishmaniasis in a population-based study in Bangladesh," *Clinical Infectious Diseases*, vol. 50, no. 1, pp. 73–76, 2010.

[12] R. N. Rai, M. Kumar, A. Srivastava et al., "Clinico-epidemiological profiles of post-kala-azar dermal leishmaniasis in Varanasi," *Journal of Communicable Diseases*, vol. 21, no. 3, pp. 214–217, 1989.

[13] C. P. Thakur, A. Kumar, G. Mitra et al., "Impact of amphotericin-B in the treatment of kala-azar on the incidence of PKDL in Bihar, India," *Indian Journal of Medical Research*, vol. 128, no. 1, pp. 38–44, 2008.

[14] G. Yee and A. M. Al Aboud, *Tinea Corporis*StatPearls Publishing, Treasure Island, FL, USA, 2020, https://pubmed.ncbi.nlm.nih.gov/31335080/.

[15] D. Taplin, "Dermatophytosis in Vietnam," *Cutis*, vol. 67, no. 5, pp. 19-20, 2001.

[16] M. L. Elgart, "Tinea incognito," *Dermatologic Clinics*, vol. 14, no. 1, pp. 51–55, 1996.

[17] V. Panasiti, R. G. Borroni, V. Devirgiliis et al., "Comparison of diagnostic methods in the diagnosis of dermatomycoses and onychomycoses," *Mycoses*, vol. 49, no. 1, pp. 26–29, 2006.

[18] M. F. Shalaby, A. N. El-Din, and M. A. El-Hamd, "Isolation, identification, and *in vitro* antifungal susceptibility testing of dermatophytes from clinical samples at Sohag University Hospital in Egypt," *Electronic Physician*, vol. 8, no. 6, pp. 2557–2567, 2016.

[19] A. N. Ates, K. Ozcan, and M. T. Ilkit, "Diagnostic value of morphological, physiological and biochemical tests in distinguishing *Trichophyton rubrum* from *Trichophyton mentagrophytes* complex," *Medical Mycology*, vol. 46, no. 8, pp. 811–822, 2008.

[20] A. Al Borzi, M. Rasouli, Z. Nademi, M. R. Kadivar, and B. Pourabbas, "Evaluation of rK39 strip test for the diagnosis of visceral leishmaniasis in infants," *Eastern Mediterranean Health Journal*, vol. 12, no. 3-4, pp. 294–299, 2006.

[21] N. Verma, D. Singh, K. Pandey et al., "Comparative evaluation of PCR and imprint smear microscopy analyses of skin biopsy specimens in diagnosis of macular, papular, and mixed papulo-nodular lesions of post-kala-azar dermal leishmaniasis," *Journal of Clinical Microbiology*, vol. 51, no. 12, pp. 4217–4219, 2013.

[22] A. M. Musa, E. A. Khalil, B. M. Younis et al., "Treatment-based strategy for the management of post-kala-azar dermal leishmaniasis patients in the Sudan," *Journal of Tropical Medicine*, vol. 2013, Article ID 708391, 5 pages, 2013.

[23] M. D. Sadick, F. P. Heinzel, V. M. Shigekane, W. L. Fisher, and R. M. Locksley, "Cellular and humoral immunity to leishmania major in genetically susceptible mice after in vivo depletion of L3T4+ T cells," *Journal of Immunology*, vol. 139, no. 4, pp. 1303–1309, 1987.

[24] K. Kemp, L. Hviid, A. Kharazmi, and M. Kemp, "Interferon-γ production by human T cells and natural killer cells in vitro in response to antigens from the two intracellular pathogens *Mycobacterium tuberculosis* and leishmania major," *Scandinavian Journal of Immunology*, vol. 46, no. 5, pp. 495–499, 1997.

[25] E. E. Zijlstra, "The immunology of post-kala-azar dermal leishmaniasis (PKDL)," *Parasites & Vectors*, vol. 9, no. 1, p. 464, 2016.

[26] M. G. Pitta, A. Romano, S. Cabantous et al., "IL-17 and IL-22 are associated with protection against human kala azar caused by *Leishmania donovani*," *Journal of Clinical Investigation*, vol. 119, no. 8, pp. 2379–2387, 2009.

[27] S. Gasim, A. M. Elhassan, A. Kharazmi, E. A. G. Khalil, A. Ismail, and T. G. Theander, "The development of post-kala-azar dermal leishmaniasis (PKDL) is associated with acquisition of leishmania reactivity by peripheral blood mononuclear cells (PBMC)," *Clinical & Experimental Immunology*, vol. 119, no. 3, pp. 523–529, 2000.

[28] S. R. Almeida, "Immunology of dermatophytosis," *Mycopathologia*, vol. 166, no. 5-6, pp. 277–283, 2008.

[29] V. Upadhyay, A. Kumar, A. K. Singh, and J. Pandey, "Epidemiological characterization of dermatophytes at a tertiary care hospital in Eastern Uttar Pradesh, India," *Current Medical Mycology*, vol. 5, no. 1, pp. 1–6, 2019.

[30] R. K. Topno, V. N. Rabi Das, M. Kumar, M. Madhukar, K. Pandey, and N. Verma, "Advanced case of PKDL due to delayed treatment: a rare case report," *PLoS Neglected Tropical Diseases*, vol. 14, no. 3, Article ID e0008052, 2020.

[31] S. Gawade, M. B. Nanaware, R. M. Gokhale, and P. S. Adhav, "Visceral leishmaniasis: a case report," *Australasian Medical Journal*, vol. 5, no. 2, pp. 130–134, 2012.

[32] D. Srivastava, M. C. R. Vyas, and C. K. Joshi, "Clinico-epidemiological study of cutaneous leishmaniasis in Bikaner (Rajasthan)," *Journal of Communicable Diseases*, vol. 19, no. 4, pp. 326–331, 1987.

18

A Rare Cutaneous Manifestation: Leukocytoclastic Vasculitis after Pfizer-BioNTech COVID-19 Vaccination

Yaritza Serrano Gomez ,[1] Brittney Grella,[2] and Hongbei Wang[3]

[1]*Department of Family Medicine, Northwell Health Glen Cove Hospital, Glen Cove, New York, USA*
[2]*Department of Medicine, Northwell Health Huntington Hospital, Huntington, New York, USA*
[3]*Department of Pathology, Northwell Health, New Hyde Park, New York, USA*

Correspondence should be addressed to Yaritza Serrano Gomez; yaritza.serrano@hotmail.com

Academic Editor: Hristo Dobrev

There is growing evidence that vaccines against SARS-CoV-2 can cause various skin reactions, many of which have autoimmune origins. These specific vaccine-induced autoimmune conditions with cutaneous manifestations include lupus erythematosus, bullous pemphigoid, vitiligo, alopecia areata, and leukocytoclastic vasculitis (LCV). In particular, LCV, which is also called hypersensitivity vasculitis, is an inflammation of small blood vessels. We present a case of an 81-year-old male evaluated in the emergency department for a bilateral purpuric non-blanching rash that appeared ten days after receiving the Pfizer-BioNTech booster vaccine against SARS-CoV-2. Results of a skin biopsy indicated LCV, and the rash completely resolved three weeks after clinical presentation.

1. Introduction

Vasculitis refers to inflammation of blood vessels leading to tissue destruction with or without organ damage. Vasculitis is classified as small, medium, or large vessel vasculitis and may be either idiopathic or associated with an underlying disease [1]. Leukocytoclastic vasculitis (LCV) is a small-vessel vasculitis characterized histopathologically by immune complex-mediated vasculitis of the dermal capillaries and venules [1, 2]. This condition can be idiopathic or associated with infections, neoplasms, autoimmune disorders, certain drugs, and the administration of vaccines, including those for influenza, hepatitis B virus (HBV), Bacille Calmette–Guérin (BCG), and human papillomavirus (HPV) [3]. LCV has been also identified as a rare extraintestinal skin manifestation of ulcerative colitis and more commonly occurs after the UC diagnosis in 59% of cases, and 68% of patients have active intestinal disease at the time of LCV diagnosis [4]. Clinical features of LCV include palpable purpura, small vessel inflammation, and extracutaneous involvement in approximately 30 percent of affected individuals [3]. In this report, we present a case of LCV after the patient received the Pfizer-BioNTech COVID-19 vaccine.

2. Case Presentation

An 81-year-old male with a past medical history of atrial fibrillation, hypertension, and hypothyroidism presented to the emergency department for evaluation of a bilateral lower extremity purpuric non-blanching rash that appeared two days prior. He had received the Pfizer-BioNTech booster vaccine against SARS-CoV-2 ten days before developing the rash. He reported having a similar rash after the second dose of the Pfizer-BioNTech COVID-19 vaccine six months before evaluation that was self-limited and resolved without further intervention. Physical examination was remarkable for purpuric 1 to 3 mm macules, some barely palpable and located in the shin and anterior and medial thighs of the lower extremities (Figures 1(a) and 1(b)). There was sparing of the abdomen, back, chest, upper extremities, and neck. Initial laboratory tests showed WBC 9.35×10^9/L, Hgb

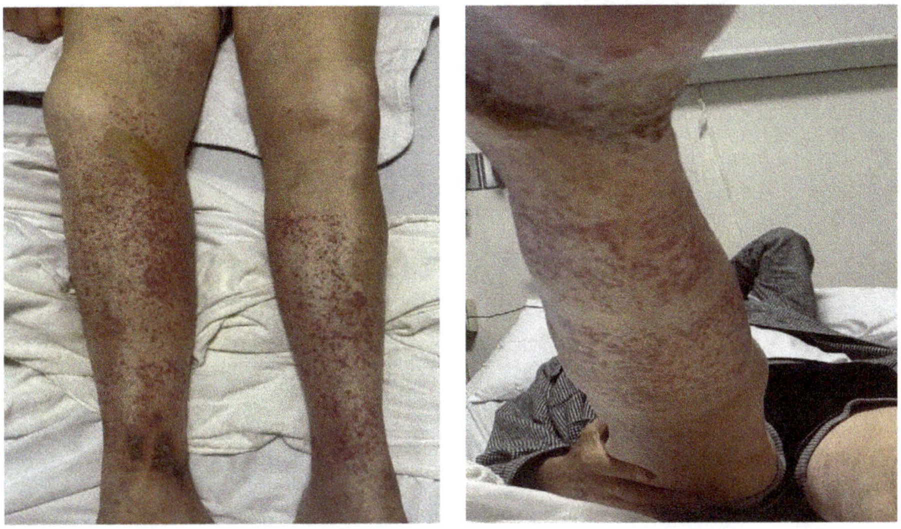

(a) (b)

Figure 1: (a, b) Purpuric 1–3 macules located in the lower extremities extending to the anterior and medial thighs.

13.3 g/dL, HCT 41.9%, Na 137 mEq/L, K 3.9 mmol/L, Cr 1.09 mg/dL, AST 18 U/L, ALT 16 U/L, CRP 9 mg/L, ESR 16 mm/hr, C3 120 mg/dL, and C4 20 mg/dL. Urinalysis was normal and without evidence of proteinuria or microhematuria. Additional laboratory tests were negative and included cANCA, pANCA, ANA, Hep C, and B serologies, syphilis screen, and Lyme antibodies. Ultrasound of the lower extremities was also performed and showed no evidence of venous thrombosis. Patient home medications included aspirin, finasteride, levothyroxine, and metoprolol tartrate. He denied the use of any new medications and any additional symptoms, including abdominal pain, vomiting, nausea, melena, hematochezia, hematuria, myalgia, arthralgia, fatigue, headache, fever, and chills.

The patient was admitted to the medicine floor for further investigation of the bilateral lower extremities' purpuric rash. During hospitalization, the dermatology and rheumatology specialists evaluated the patient and recommended performing a skin biopsy. A skin biopsy was performed and showed extravasation of erythrocytes, perivascular infiltrate of neutrophils, nuclear dust, and eosinophils, consistent with LCV and negative direct immunofluorescence (Figures 2(a) and 2(b)). The consensus decision was to treat conservatively without the use of systemic corticosteroids or any additional treatment and the patient was discharged home. In the outpatient follow-up, the patient reported complete resolution of the rash three weeks after the symptoms first appeared, and there was no need for any further testing or treatment.

3. Discussion

LCV is the histopathologic descriptor of a common form of small-vessel vasculitis involving arterioles, capillaries, and postcapillary venules [5]. The disease can be confined to the skin or affect many organs, including the kidneys, central nervous system, heart, gastrointestinal tract, and lungs [6]. The incidence of cutaneous LCV ranges from 15 to 38 cases per million annually in the United States and appears to affect both sexes and all ages equally, although some studies have noted a slightly higher incidence in males and older individuals [5]. LCV presents as erythematous macules with palpable purpura that involve primarily the lower extremities, but dependent areas, such as the back and buttocks, may also be affected [3, 5]. Patients may be completely asymptomatic or complain of burning, itching, or pain in the involved skin. Systemic symptoms can appear in approximately 30% of patients and may include low-grade fever, malaise, weight loss, myalgias, arthralgias, blood in the urine or stool, abdominal pain, vomiting, cough, numbness, and weakness [7]. The cutaneous manifestations of LCV usually appear approximately 1 to 3 weeks after the triggering event and usually resolve over 2 to 3 weeks [3, 5].

Although history and physical examination are sometimes sufficient to establish a working diagnosis, systematic laboratory tests are usually warranted to perform the differential diagnosis [5]. Tests should include analysis for infectious diseases (e.g., HBV, HCV, and human immunodeficiency virus), serum protein electrophoresis, immunoglobulins (IgG, IgA, and IgM), an antinuclear antibody panel, rheumatoid factor, serum C3, and C4 complement levels, ANCAs, and cryoglobulins [5, 6]. The cornerstone of LCV diagnosis is a skin biopsy with direct immunofluorescence, which should be performed whenever possible for confirmation [3]. After diagnosis, the recommended treatment depends on two major factors: the etiology and the extent of the disease. If LCV is limited to the skin, the management strategy should primarily focus on symptomatic relief since most acute episodes of cutaneous small-vessel vasculitis are self-limited and do not recur, even without treatment [3, 5]. When the cause of LCV is obvious, such as infection or drugs, eliminating or treating the trigger, whenever possible is crucial and often sufficient. In contrast, treatment should generally include systemic corticosteroids when symptoms are severe, intractable, or recurrent [5].

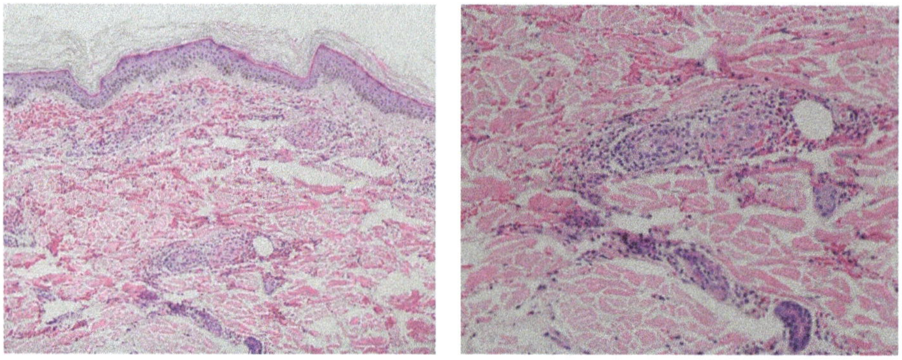

(a) (b)

Figure 2: (a, b) 100x low-power image (a) and 200x medium-power image (b) showing extravasation of erythrocytes, perivascular infiltrate of neutrophils, nuclear dusts, and eosinophils, and features of leukocytoclastic vasculitis.

Half of all cases of LCV are idiopathic but secondary causes such as infections and medications have been proposed as the most common triggers [7]. The medications commonly known to cause LCV are beta-lactams, erythromycin, clindamycin, quinolones, vancomycin, sulfonamide, furosemide, allopurinol, NSAIDs, amiodarone, beta-blockers, TNF-alpha inhibitors, SSRIs, metformin, and warfarin [2, 8]. In addition, several vaccines, including those against influenza, HBV, BCG, and HPV, have been implicated in the development of LCV [7, 9]. Including the case detailed here, there have been a few case reports of the development of LCV after administration of the Moderna and Pfizer-BioNTech COVID-19 vaccines [7]. The mechanism by which the SARS-CoV-2 vaccine induces this type of vasculitis is not completely clear, but could potentially be driven by off-target immune activation after vaccination [7, 9]. The SARS-CoV-2 vaccines are DNA/RNA-based vaccines that contain recombinant adenoviral vectors encoding the spike protein of SARS-CoV-2, stabilizers, and immune adjuvants [10]. It is possible that molecular mimicry might develop between the peptides that are expressed in the viral spike protein and host endothelial cells [10, 11]. It has been suggested that the SARS-CoV-2 spike protein can activate the alternative complement pathway, thereby leading to the inflammation of the cutaneous microvasculature.

Recent studies show evidence that the administration of the Moderna and Pfizer-BioNTech COVID-19 vaccines can lead to the development of cutaneous manifestations. These cutaneous manifestations ranged in a wide spectrum, including chilblain-like, urticarial eruptions, vesicular, morbilliform eruptions, livedoid, delayed large reactions, local injection site reactions, and vasculitis lesions [12, 13]. Delayed large local reactions are mostly found, followed by local injection site reactions, urticarial eruptions, and morbilliform eruptions [12, 13]. Additionally, fewer common reactions include pernio, cosmetic filler reactions, zoster, herpes simplex flares, and pityriasis rosea-like reactions [13]. Recent data shows that approximately 20% of patients receiving the Pfizer-BioNTech COVID- 19 vaccine reported skin reactions after the first dose only, 74% after the second dose only, and 6.0% after both doses, but there is insufficient evidence after the booster dose. The case presented here shows some new evidence of cutaneous manifestation after the booster vaccination. The patient in this case didn't have any systematic symptoms such as fever, abdominal pain, fever, arthralgia, or renal failure at the time of presentation, ruling out other forms of systemic vasculitis including IGA vasculitis, and suggesting more a cutaneous limited form of vasculitis like LCV. Although vasculitis development after SARS-CoV-2 vaccine administration could be worrisome, data suggest that cutaneous reactions to SARS-CoV-2 vaccination are generally minor and self-limited and should not discourage vaccination [13].

4. Conclusions

Vaccines against COVID-19 represent a pivotal and effective countermeasure to control the COVID-19 pandemic. This case reveals a potential association between the administration of a COVID-19 vaccine and the development of vasculitis. This could be secondary to complement activation or autoimmunity provoked by the vaccine's SARS-CoV-2 spike protein, leading to inflammation of the cutaneous microvasculature and resulting in vasculitis [3]. Although vasculitis may not be considered a contraindication of vaccination, further investigation is necessary to clarify the characteristics of vasculitis following COVID-19 vaccination.

Consent

The patient gave written informed consent for the publication of the case and accompanying images. The patient understood that his name and initial will not be published and due efforts will be made to conceal his identity.

Authors' Contributions

All named authors meet the International Committee of Medical Journal Editors (ICMJE) criteria for authorship for the manuscript, take responsibility for the integrity of the work, and have given final approval to the version to be published. Yaritza Serrano Gomez conceptualized the study, performed acquisition, interpreted the study, designed, and prepared the manuscript. Brittney Grella performed acquisition, edited and reviewed the article. Hongbei Wang performed histopathological imaging analysis and interpretation.

References

[1] J. C. Jennette, R. J. Falk, P. A. Bacon et al., "2012 revised international chapel hill consensus conference nomenclature of vasculitides," *Arthritis & Rheumatism*, vol. 65, no. 1, pp. 1–11, 2013.

[2] K. Nunez, "What you need to know about leukocytoclastic vasculitis," 2020, https://www.healthline.com/health/leukocytoclastic-vasculitis#:%7E:text=Leukocytoclastic%20vasculitis%20(LCV)%20refers%20to,break%20down%20and%20release%20debris.

[3] D. Baigrie, A. Goyal, and J. S. Crane, "Leukocytoclastic vasculitis," in *StatPearls*StatPearls Publishing, Treasure Island, FL, USA, 2022.

[4] I. Pantic, D. Jevtic, C. W. Nordstrom, C. Madrid, T. Milovanovic, and I. Dumic, "Clinical manifestations of leukocytoclastic vasculitis, treatment, and outcome in patients with ulcerative colitis: a systematic review of the literature," *Journal of Clinical Medicine*, vol. 11, no. 3, p. 739, 2022.

[5] P. Fraticelli, D. Benfaremo, and A. Gabrielli, "Diagnosis and management of leukocytoclastic vasculitis," *Internal and Emergency Medicine*, vol. 16, no. 4, pp. 831–841, 2021.

[6] A. B. Dicks and B. H. Gray, "Images in vascular medicine: leukocytoclastic vasculitis after COVID-19 vaccine booster," *Vascular Medicine*, vol. 27, no. 1, pp. 100-101, 2022.

[7] American Osteopathic College, "Leukocytoclastic vasculitis," 2022, https://www.aocd.org/page/LeukocytoclasticVas/Leukocytoclastic-Vasculitis.htm.

[8] S. Mahto, A. Sheoran, P. Verma, G. A. War, N. Agarwal, and A. Singh, "Leukocytoclastic vasculitis: an uncommon adverse effect of a common drug," *Journal of Family Medicine and Primary Care*, vol. 8, no. 6, pp. 2137–2139, 2019.

[9] S. R. Cohen, L. Prussick, J. S. Kahn, D. X. Gao, A. Radfar, and D. Rosmarin, "Leukocytoclastic vasculitis flare following the COVID-19 vaccine," *International Journal of Dermatology*, vol. 60, no. 8, pp. 1032-1033, 2021.

[10] E. Bostan, D. Gulseren, and O. Gokoz, "New-onset leukocytoclastic vasculitis after COVID-19 vaccine," *International Journal of Dermatology*, vol. 60, no. 10, pp. 1305-1306, 2021.

[11] W. J. Jin, S. W. Ahn, S. H. Jang, S. M. Hong, J. E. Seol, and H. Kim, "Leukocytoclastic vasculitis after coronavirus disease 2019 vaccination," *The Journal of Dermatology*, vol. 49, no. 1, pp. e34–e35, 2022.

[12] N. Khajavirad, M. Salehi, A. Haji Ghadery et al., "Serious events following COVID-19 vaccination with ChAdOx1 nCoV-19 vaccine (Vaxzevria): a short case series from Iran," *Clinical Case Reports*, vol. 10, no. 2, Article ID e05390, 2022.

[13] D. E. McMahon, E. Amerson, M. Rosenbach et al., "Cutaneous reactions reported after Moderna and Pfizer. COVID-19 vaccination: a registry-based study of 414 cases," *Journal of the American Academy of Dermatology*, vol. 85, no. 1, pp. 46–55, 2021.

19

L-Mesitran Foam: Evaluation of a New Wound Care Product

Segametsi Mary-Jane Mthanti,[1] **Gloria Pelle**,[2] **and Niels A. J. Cremers**[3,4]

[1]*Prime Cure Medical Centre, 1843 Tsubaki Street, Dube, Soweto 1801, Johannesburg, South Africa*
[2]*Safarmex, 85 Newton Road, Meadowdale, Germiston 1614, Johannesburg, South Africa*
[3]*Maastricht University Medical Centre, Department of Gynecology and Obstetrics, 6202AZ Maastricht, Netherlands*
[4]*Triticum Exploitatie BV, Sleperweg 44, 6222NK Maastricht, Netherlands*

Correspondence should be addressed to Niels A. J. Cremers; niels@mesitran.com

Academic Editor: Ravi Krishnan

Chronic wounds are a health problem that has devastating consequences for patients and their quality of life. Often, chronic wounds are stuck in the inflammatory phase or burdened with an infection. Therefore, it is important to find alternative all-round wound care products that have both wound healing and antimicrobial activities. New wound care products are developed constantly, implementing the latest knowledge and advances in wound care. Honey-based wound care formulations and foam dressings are increasingly used in the clinic. L-Mesitran Foam is a novel product in which a foam dressing is precoated with medical-grade honey. Here, we describe our first experiences with L-Mesitran Foam in the clinic. In this case report, a 57-year-old woman with diabetes mellitus type 2 and hypertension presented with a chronic diabetic venous leg ulcer on her leg. Treatments over six months with different treatments, including povidone-iodine, silver dressings, and compression therapy, were ineffective and subsequently switched to L-Mesitran Foam. The dressing choice was based on the wound type and complied with the instructions for use. Wound healing progressed nicely on different aspects and led to complete healing on day 23. No side effects or pain was experienced during treatment. The presented case supports the safety and efficacy of L-Mesitran Foam and serves as a proof of concept.

1. Introduction

Wounds that are stagnated for 4 weeks or are present for more than 8 weeks are considered to be chronic [1, 2]. Chronic wounds are a health problem that has devastating consequences for patients and their quality of life [3, 4]. With chronic wounds accounting for approximately 1–4% of the total healthcare expenditure, it has a major economic impact [3, 4]. Moreover, the expectations are that this will further rise because the number of patients likely increases due to longevity and increased incidences of comorbidities such as diabetes and morbidity [2, 4]. For example, the prevalence of diabetes mellitus has increased from 171 million in 2000 to 451 million in 2017 and is predicted to further increase to 693 million in 2045 [5, 6]. Although wounds in most cases eventually heal by themselves, if there are no underlying pathologies, wound healing can often be improved. Patients frequently use go-to products to disinfect wounds and use regular bandages to keep them clean. For example, the use of povidone-iodine is common practice for most patients to keep the wounds free of pathogens, and this product is often the first go-to product for wounds arising in and around people's homes. Povidone-iodine is an antiseptic and used to disinfect wounds; however, what most patients and nurses do not realize is that it does not promote healing [7]. Some people may still think that dry wounds heal faster, but the research of George Winter proved the concept that moist wounds heal faster than wet or dry wounds [8]. Unfortunately, wound care training in hospitals and universities is limited, and therefore, proper training and more publications about wound care regimens may improve doctors' and nurses' competencies [9, 10].

It is important to find alternative all-round wound care products that have both wound healing and antimicrobial activities. New wound care products are developed constantly, implementing the latest knowledge and understandings and advances in wound care. A new product that has very recently been launched is L-Mesitran Foam. L-Mesitran Foam is a foam dressing that on the one side is coated with L-Mesitran Soft gel. L-Mesitran Soft is a medical-grade honey (MGH)-based wound care formulation. Honey has been used for more than four millennia for wound care [11]. L-Mesitran Foam combines the potent antimicrobial and wound healing effects of MGH together with the strong absorbency capacity of the foam dressing. Both MGH and foam dressings are more and more used for wound care as can be seen by the steadily increased number of publications in PubMed over the last two decades. The search term "honey AND wounds" would yield a maximum of 14 papers per year before the year 2000, while there were 34 publications in 2005, 54 in 2010, and 103 in 2020. For the search term "foam AND dressing," a maximum of 12 papers about this topic were published before 2000, 19 in 2005, 37 in 2010, and 79 in 2020. We will present our experience on the use of L-Mesitran Foam and support it with a clinical case report.

1.1. About the L-Mesitran Foam Dressing: A Combination of Foam with L-Mesitran Soft Foam Layer. L-Mesitran Foam is a hydrophilic foam dressing with high absorption and retention characteristics [12, 13]. The sterile foam dressing can be applied as a primary or secondary dressing for wounds with moderate to high exudate and is covered on the one side with L-Mesitran Soft gel (Figure 1(a)). The polyurethane foam forms a cushioning layer that protects the wound from mechanical stress while allowing drainage to pass [12, 13]. Simultaneously, this physical barrier prevents pathogens from entering the wound, while it absorbs excess wound fluid and maintains a moist wound environment [13]. A schematic presentation of these mechanisms is shown in Figure 1(b).

1.2. Medical-Grade Honey (MGH)/L-Mesitran Soft Layer. L-Mesitran Foam is coated with L-Mesitran Soft gel and forms good protection to invading pathogens while killing any bacterial loads that are already present [11, 14]. L-Mesitran Soft is known for its antimicrobial and wound healing properties [13, 15, 16] and even exerts prophylactic activity [17, 18]. The antimicrobial effects are orchestrated by its osmotic activity, low pH, the release of hydrogen peroxide, and the presence of several antimicrobial molecules [13, 19, 20]. It has consistently been reported that the supplemented ingredients (such as vitamins C and E) in L-Mesitran Soft enhance the antimicrobial activity of MGH [15, 16, 21, 22]. L-Mesitran Soft has the strongest antimicrobial activity among different honey-based wound care products [13, 16]. The L-Mesitran Soft layer in L-Mesitran Foam creates a moist wound environment which stimulates healing as moist wounds heal faster than dry or wet wounds [8, 23]. Dry wounds result in scabs that disturb healing, while wet wounds lead to maceration and delayed healing [8].

The addition of L-Mesitran Soft to polyurethane foam results in bioactive dressing and establishes regenerative environment [12, 13]. The beneficial antimicrobial and healing properties of L-Mesitran Soft enhance the wound healing process [13, 16]. The introduction of MGH to the wound creates an osmotic effect which further stimulates the release of exudate that is subsequently absorbed and retained by the foam layer [12, 13]. Moreover, during dressing changes, the viscous nature of the MGH layer provides an interface between the wound bed and the foam part and subsequently prevents reopening of the freshly formed granulation tissue [23, 24].

1.3. Indications. According to the instructions for use of L-Mesitran Foam, the dressing can be used in the treatment of a wide variety of exuding wounds, such as (diabetic) ulcers, pressure ulcers, superficial and partial thickness burns, fungating wounds, donor sites, chronic wounds, and postoperative wounds.

2. Case Presentation

2.1. Patient History. A 57-year-old woman with diabetes mellitus type 2 and hypertension presented to the healthcare clinic with a superficial wound on the anterior aspect of the leg (Figure 2(a)). The diabetes is well-controlled, and the patient compliant with her treatments. The patient reported that the wound was caused by bumping into and being scratched by a steel surface. She has been treating it for six months with different treatments, including compression therapy, povidone-iodine, and silver dressings. Since the wound was becoming bigger and more painful throughout a 6-month period, the patient presented to our clinic providing specialized wound care services after hearing of it.

Originally, the wound was classified as a diabetic ulcer, as the patient is a known diabetic. In our clinic, the wound and patient's conditions were further analyzed, and since the wound was present for six months and there was venous insufficiency, we classified it as chronic diabetic venous leg ulcer. Signs of venous insufficiency included hemosiderin deposit, varicose veins presence, gravity-induced edema, and champagne bottle appearance and were confirmed using Doppler and an ankle-brachial pressure index score of 1.3. The wound was covered with a slimy sloughy looking tissue, suggestive to be a biofilm and being infected, as shown in Figure 2(b), day 0. The dimensions of the wound were about 5.5 cm in length and 3 cm in width.

2.2. Methods. The wound was treated with L-Mesitran Foam and compression therapy continued. The dressing choice was based on the wound type. The wound bed showed signs of granulation, low exudate level, presence of low-grade slough, and low odor, with suspicion of infection and the constant shiny appearance suggesting a biofilm. In addition, the wound did not respond to previous treatments and increased in size while not improving the wound edges. The L-Mesitran Foam was introduced as new dressing and was offered to us for testing. Based on its indications for use and our positive experience with the range of other L-Mesitran

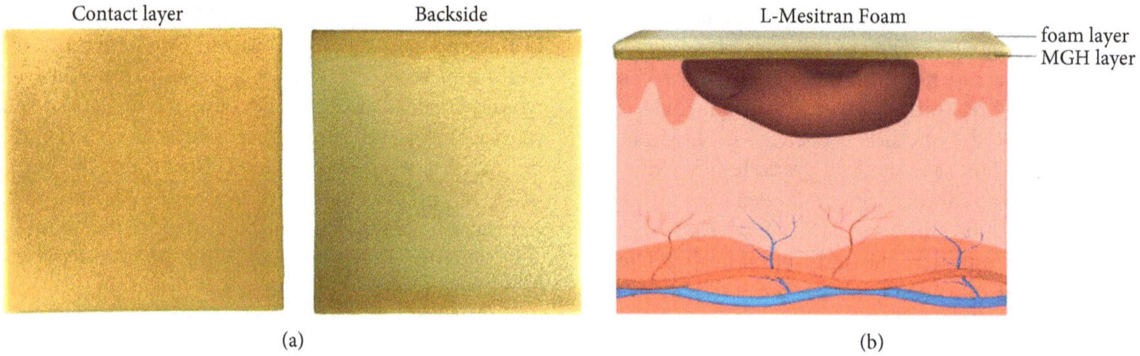

FIGURE 1: L-Mesitran Foam dressing. (a) Picture of the L-Mesitran Foam dressing showing the two layers: contact layer covered with L-Mesitran Soft and the backside being the foam dressing. The dimensions of the dressing are 10 cm in length, 10 cm in width, and 3 mm thick. (b) Schematic presentation of L-Mesitran Foam covering a wound. The MGH layer creates a moist wound environment and attracts the exudate towards the foam layer which subsequently absorbs it. The foam forms a physical barrier for invading pathogens and protects the wound from mechanical stress.

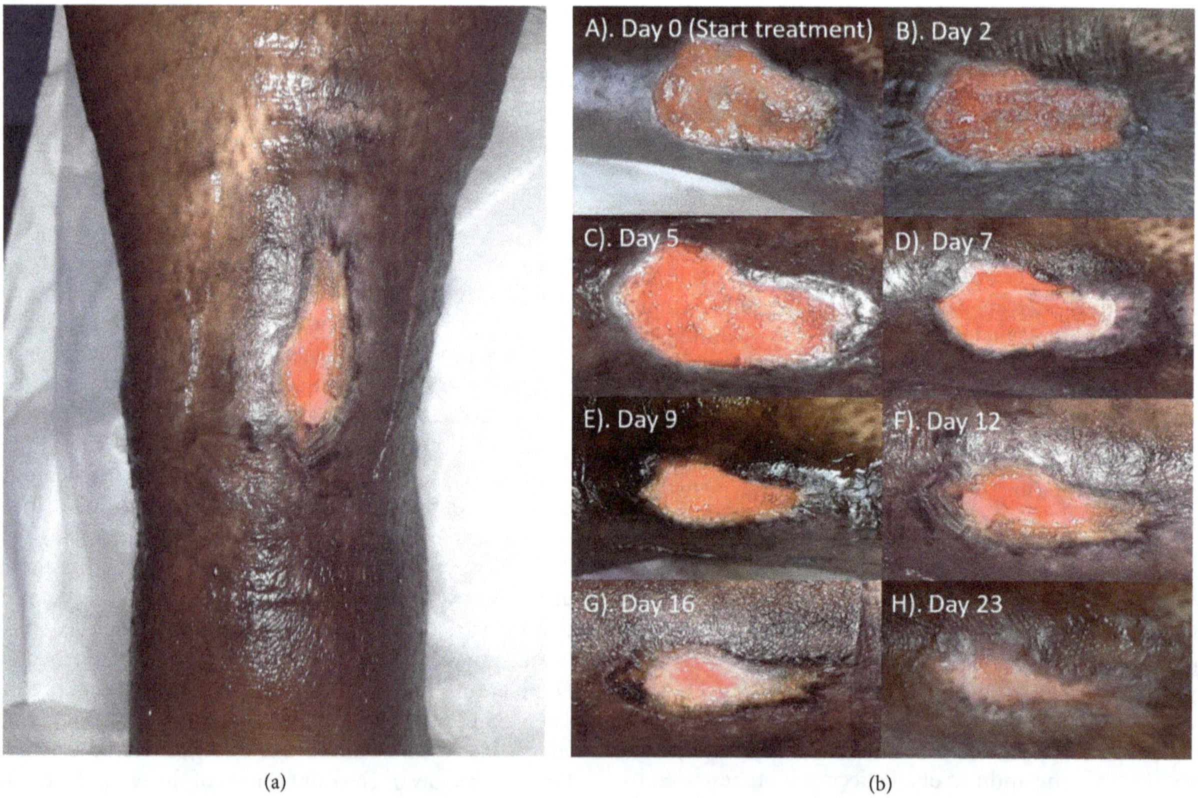

FIGURE 2: (a) Photo of the wound illustrating the location on the leg. (b) Evaluation of L-Mesitran Foam dressing for the treatment of a chronic diabetic venous leg ulcer. After each dressing change, a picture was taken to monitor the wound progression.

MGH-based wound care products, we selected the dressing to assess its efficacy in this wound.

The frequency of dressing changes was dependent on the volume of exudate produced. The dressings were initially changed every two to three days for the first two weeks, followed by longer periods up till one week at the end of the treatment. This was to first assess the dressing's ability to absorb and hold the exudate, to monitor the saturation of the dressing, and to enable checking of the wound progression. In the end, dressings were changed once a week because signs of infection disappeared and of the absence of exudate and clear wound healing progression.

The wound size was measured using ImageJ (National Institute of Health, USA, version 1.53k) by setting the scale at 5.5 cm (the original length of the wound) and subsequently performing a "freehand selection" of the wound to determine the area in square cm. Due to the angle of the pictures, there may be a small deviation from the actual area.

The relative closure was calculated by dividing the areas of the wounds by the wound area at the start.

3. Results

Since the wound did not heal for a 6-month period following different treatments, it was decided to treat the wound, which was presumably covered with biofilm and being infected, with L-Mesitran Foam (Figure 2(b), day 0). Because of the signs of venous insufficiency, the dressing was used in conjunction with compression with 40 mmHg. Since there were only local signs of infection, no systemic antibiotics were provided. Diabetic treatment continued as normal, and blood glucose levels were not affected by the treatment with L-Mesitran Foam. Already after one dressing (Figure 2(b), day 2), the sloughy tissue almost completely disappeared, and odor and pain levels strongly decreased. On day five, new granulation tissue was clearly formed, and the first signs of reepithelialization were visible at the edges. Moreover, the tissue looked more vital (Figure 2(b), day 5). After the third dressing (Figure 2(b), day 7), the wound was clean, and reepithelialization was further increased around the edges. The red color supports the tissue to be more vital and neovascularization was evident throughout the new tissue. After 9 days of MGH treatment (Figure 2(b), day 9), reepithelialization and formation of granulation tissue clearly progressed, which continued over the next days (Figure 2(b), days 12 and 16, respectively). The change of color from red into pink shows the wound is further healing and becoming more superficial. After just 23 days, the wound was almost completely closed (Figure 2(b), day 23). The relative wound closure was determined from the pictures and is shown in Figure 3. No side effects or pain were experienced due to the dressing change or use of the L-Mesitran Foam.

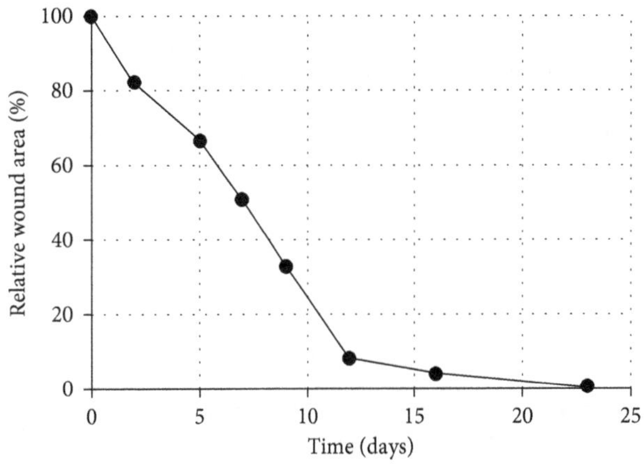

FIGURE 3: Relative wound closure in time, as quantified using ImageJ in relation to the wound area at the start of L-Mesitran Foam treatment.

4. Discussion

L-Mesitran Foam is a hydrophilic foam dressing which is coated on the one side with L-Mesitran Soft. L-Mesitran Soft has antimicrobial activity against a wide range of microorganisms and multiple mechanisms that are responsible for promoting wound healing. In combination with the foam dressing, L-Mesitran promotes the absorption of exudate by its osmotic activity. This osmotic activity attracts wound exudate and lymph fluid from deeper tissue, creating an outflow of fluid [25, 26]. The attracted wound fluid will subsequently be absorbed and retained by the dressing. The L-Mesitran Foam creates the optimal level of moisture and prevents maceration as may happen in wet wounds. L-Mesitran Foam delivers L-Mesitran Soft to the wound bed to foster its wound healing promoting activities. These activities include keeping the wound moist, promoting autolytic debridement, and stimulating granulation tissue formation and reepithelialization [11, 14, 23, 24]. The MGH forms an important nutrient source for the proliferating skin cells [14], but by its stimulatory effect on neovascularization, the transport of nutrients and oxygen from the body will also be improved [25, 26]. The L-Mesitran Foam is user and patient-friendly and can easily be cut to the size of the wound where the soft contact material can serve to protect wound edges and against external mechanical forces by forming a cushioning layer [13]. No pain or discomfort was experienced during the application or change of the dressings. The L-Mesitran Soft layer prevents newly formed granulation tissue to grow into the dressing and allows pain-free removal without reopening of the wound [13, 23, 24]. Even in preterm neonates, the L-Mesitran wound care products are used safely and effectively [11]. Although different L-Mesitran products (Soft, Ointment, Tulle, Hydro, and Net) were already successfully used in a previous study on patients with diabetic venous leg ulcers after previous therapies had failed, the L-Mesitran Foam was not used there [13]. The combination of L-Mesitran Soft with a foam dressing is of added value and can be used to manage a wide variety of exuding wounds. The fast healing of the presented stagnated wound indicates its potential. Despite the convincing results in only one patient and our experience teaching us the wide and efficacious applicability of MGH, the findings should be substantiated in larger patient groups, preferably in double-blinded randomized controlled trials.

5. Conclusion

The medical-grade honey of L-Mesitran has strong antimicrobial and wound healing activities. L-Mesitran Foam combines these excellent properties of L-Mesitran Soft with the technology of foam dressings. This fosters the opportunity to absorb and retain wound exudate and to protect the wound from external stressors. The presented case of a chronic diabetic venous leg ulcer serves as a proof of concept of L-Mesitran Foam.

References

[1] Y.-K. Wu, N.-C. Cheng, and C.-M. Cheng, "Biofilms in chronic wounds: pathogenesis and diagnosis," *Trends in Biotechnology*, vol. 37, no. 5, pp. 505–517, 2019.

[2] J. Lu, L. Turnbull, C. M. Burke et al., "Manuka-type honeys can eradicate biofilms produced byStaphylococcus aureus-strains with different biofilm-forming abilities," *PeerJ*, vol. 2, p. e326, 2014.

[3] M. Olsson, K. Järbrink, U. Divakar et al., "The humanistic and economic burden of chronic wounds: a systematic review," *Wound Repair and Regeneration*, vol. 27, no. 1, pp. 114–125, 2019.
[4] C. K. Sen, "Human wound and its burden: updated 2020 compendium of estimates," *Advances in Wound Care*, vol. 10, no. 5, pp. 281–292, 2021.
[5] N. H. Cho, J. E. Shaw, S. Karuranga et al., "IDF Diabetes Atlas: global estimates of diabetes prevalence for 2017 and projections for 2045," *Diabetes Research and Clinical Practice*, vol. 138, pp. 271–281, 2018.
[6] P. Saeedi, I. Petersohn, P. Salpea et al., "Global and regional diabetes prevalence estimates for 2019 and projections for 2030 and 2045: results from the international diabetes federation diabetes atlas, 9th edition," *Diabetes Research and Clinical Practice*, vol. 157, Article ID 107843, 2019.
[7] S. A. Kramer, "Effect of povidone-iodine on wound healing: a review," *Journal of Vascular Nursing*, vol. 17, no. 1, pp. 17–23, 1999.
[8] G. D. Winter, "Formation of the scab and the rate of epithelization of superficial wounds in the skin of the young domestic pig," *Nature*, vol. 193, no. 4812, pp. 293-294, 1962.
[9] P. Kamath, N. Agarwal, C. J. Salgado, and R. Kirsner, "Wound healing elective: an opportunity to improve medical education curriculum to better manage the increasing burden of chronic wounds," *Dermatology Online Journal*, vol. 25, no. 5, 2019.
[10] E. Kielo-Viljamaa, R. Suhonen, M. Ahtiala et al., "The development and testing of the C/WoundComp instrument for assessing chronic wound-care competence in student nurses and podiatrists," *International Wound Journal*, vol. 18, no. 1, pp. 62–78, 2021.
[11] E. Smaropoulos and N. A. J. Cremers, "Medical grade honey for the treatment of extravasation-induced injuries in preterm neonates – a case series," *Advances in Neonatal Care*, vol. 21., 2020 in press.
[12] https://mesitran.com/products/.
[13] H. K. R. Nair, N. Tatavilis, I. Pospíšilová, J. Kučerová, and N. A. J. Cremers, "Medical-grade honey kills antibiotic-resistant bacteria and prevents amputation in diabetics with infected ulcers: a prospective case series," *Antibiotics*, vol. 9, no. 9, 2020.
[14] E. Smaropoulos and N. A. J. Cremers, "The pro-healing effects of medical grade honey supported by a pediatric case series," *Complementary Therapies in Medicine*, vol. 45, pp. 14–18, 2019.
[15] T. de Groot, T. Janssen, D. Faro, N. A. J. Cremers, A. Chowdhary, and J. F. Meis, "Antifungal activity of a medical-grade honey formulation against Candida auris," *Journal of Fungi (Basel)*, vol. 7, no. 1, 2021.
[16] C. C. F. Pleeging, T. Coenye, D. Mossialos et al., "Synergistic antimicrobial activity of supplemented medical-grade honey against *Pseudomonas aeruginosa* biofilm formation and eradication," *Antibiotics*, vol. 9, no. 12, p. 866, 2020.
[17] K. Gustafsson, A. J. Tatz, R. A. Slavin et al., "Intra-incisional medical grade honey decreases the prevalence of incisional infection in horses undergoing colic surgery: a prospective randomised controlled study," *Equine Veterinary Journal*, vol. 53, 2020.
[18] H. H. Mandel, G. A. Sutton, E. Abu, and G. Kelmer, "Intralesional application of medical grade honey improves healing of surgically treated lacerations in horses," *Equine Veterinary Journal*, vol. 52, no. 1, pp. 41–45, 2020.
[19] J. Majtan, "Honey: an immunomodulator in wound healing," *Wound Repair and Regeneration*, vol. 22, no. 2, pp. 187–192, 2014.
[20] M. D. Mandal and S. Mandal, "Honey: its medicinal property and antibacterial activity," *Asian Pacific Journal of Tropical Biomedicine*, vol. 1, no. 2, pp. 154–160, 2011.
[21] R. Hermanns, N. A. J Cremers, J. P Leeming, and E. T van der Werf, "Sweet relief: determining the antimicrobial activity of medical grade honey against vaginal isolates of Candida albicans," *Journal of fungi (Basel, Switzerland)*, vol. 5, no. 3, 2019.
[22] A. M. P. Oliveira, J. S. P. Devesa, and P. B. Hill, "In vitro efficacy of a honey-based gel against canine clinical isolates of Staphylococcus pseudintermedius and Malassezia pachydermatis," *Veterinary Dermatology*, vol. 29, no. 3, pp. 180–e65, 2018.
[23] E. Smaropoulos and N. A. Cremers, "Medical grade honey for the treatment of paediatric abdominal wounds: a case series," *Journal of Wound Care*, vol. 29, no. 2, pp. 94–99, 2020.
[24] E. Smaropoulos and N. A. J. Cremers, "Treating severe wounds in pediatrics with medical grade honey: a case series," *Clinical Case Reports*, vol. 8, no. 3, pp. 469–476, 2020.
[25] F. Gottrup, "Oxygen in wound healing and infection," *World Journal of Surgery*, vol. 28, no. 3, pp. 312–315, 2004.
[26] K. Rossiter, A. J. Cooper, D. Voegeli, and B. A. Lwaleed, "Honey promotes angiogeneic activity in the rat aortic ring assay," *Journal of Wound Care*, vol. 19, no. 10, pp. 442–446, 2010.

20

Giant Muscle Invasive Dermatofibroma Clinically Mimicking a Malignant Tumor

Hideyuki Kinoshita[1] **Takeshi Ishii,**[1] **Hiroto Kamoda,**[1] **Toshinori Tsukanishi,**[1] **Sumihisa Orita**[2] **Kazuhide Inage**[2] **Seiji Ohtori**[2] **and Tsukasa Yonemoto**[1]

[1]*Department of Orthopedic Surgery, Chiba Cancer Center, 666-2 Nitonacho, Chuo-ku, Chiba 260-8717, Japan*
[2]*Department of Orthopaedic Surgery, Graduate School of Medicine, Chiba University, 1-8-1 Inohana, Chuo-ku, Chiba 260-8670, Japan*

Correspondence should be addressed to Hideyuki Kinoshita; kinoshi1783@yahoo.co.jp

Academic Editor: Alireza Firooz

Dermatofibromas are common benign fibrohistiocytic lesions, usually appearing as slow growing firm dermal nodules with a predilection for the extremities (mostly the lower legs). They are found mostly in middle-aged women and are usually smaller than 2 cm in diameter. Giant dermatofibromas exceeding 5 cm in diameter are rare. In recent years, reports have suggested a relationship between the primary size of dermatofibromas and rates of local recurrence and metastases after surgery. This relationship is however debated. The present report describes the case of a giant muscle invasive tumor in a 51-year-old female patient who presented with a large ulcerated mass in the right upper arm. The tumor appeared clinically malignant, measuring approximately 12 cm × 6 cm in size, with ulceration and invasion of surrounding muscle. Wide resection of the tumor was performed with myocutaneous flap-plasty. Histopathological examination showed evidence of a dermatofibroma. No recurrence, metastases, or other complications were noted at 5 years after surgery. The present case demonstrates that although dermatofibromas are essentially benign, they may present with atypical features including large size, ulceration, and muscle invasion, clinically mimicking malignant tumors.

1. Introduction

Dermatofibromas, also known as benign fibrous histiocytomas, are common harmless cutaneous nodules arising from reactive fibroblastic proliferation of unknown etiology. They are most frequently found in the extremities and are more common in women [1]. They usually present as red-brown or yellow-brown papules on the limbs, particularly in the thighs and lower legs, measuring less than 2 cm in diameter [2]. The tumor is typically located in the skin, involving the subcutaneous fat, dermis, and epidermis, without invasion to surrounding muscles. However, atypical clinical findings have been reported in recent years, including giant tumor size, associated ulceration, and the occurrence of metastases [3, 4]. These atypical tumors may be clinically difficult to distinguish from malignant tumors, leading to a possibility of misdiagnoses. Appropriate histological evaluation is an important tool to prevent misdiagnoses, allowing distinction between benign dermatofibromas and malignant tumors such as dermatofibrosarcoma protuberans (DFSP) [5].

Here we present a case of giant muscle invasive dermatofibroma, clinically suspicious of a malignant tumor. Successful wide resection was performed, and the patient remains healthy without recurrence for 5 years.

2. Case Presentation

A 51-year-old female patient presented to our orthopedic outpatient department with a rapidly enlarging ulcerated right upper arm swelling which was growing gradually over the past six months. She recalled that it had been a pea-sized lesion and had remained the same size over the past 30 years. No history of preceding episodes of trauma or local irritation was found. The initially asymptomatic lesion had recently become painful and pruritic with slight bleeding. On examination, a large nodulo-ulcerative plaque was noted

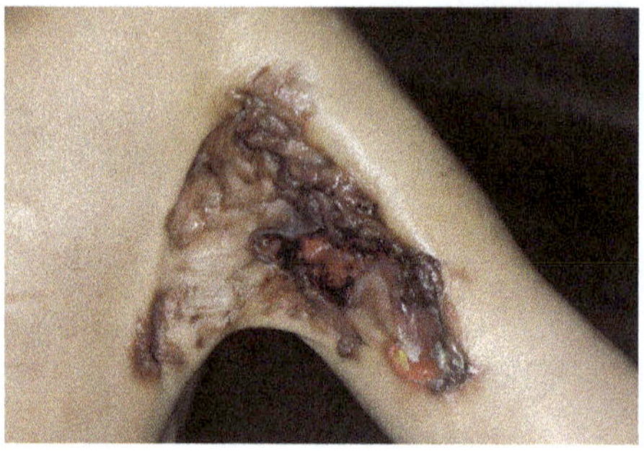

FIGURE 1: The large nodulo-ulcerative plaque with bleeding seen on frontal view; located at the back of the right upper arm, measuring 12 cm × 6 cm.

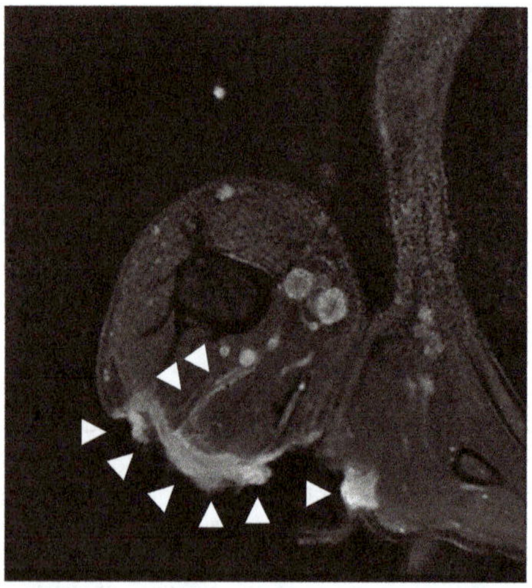

FIGURE 2: Axial view of the dermatofibroma (arrowhead) on magnetic resonance imaging; invasion to the deltoid and triceps brachii muscles is seen.

on the right upper arm, measuring approximately 12 cm × 6 cm in size (Figure 1). Magnetic resonance imaging (MRI) revealed a mass measuring 12 cm × 6 cm × 1.5 cm, invading the deltoid and triceps brachii muscles (Figure 2). Examination of the needle biopsy specimen demonstrated the proliferation of spindle cells in a storiform arrangement in the dermis. Results of tests for CD34 and factor VIII were negative, suggesting the possibility of a benign tumor. However, the clinical findings, which included muscle invasion, large tumor size, and rapid enlargement, suggested the possibility of malignancy, prompting the need for wide resection and myocutaneous flap-plasty. Intraoperatively, the tumor was found to have invaded the deltoid and triceps brachii muscles, as well as the cutaneous and subcutaneous tissue. Wide resection was achieved with a 3 cm margin. A latissimus dorsi musculocutaneous flap was needed to close the skin defect. The postoperative period was uneventful. Histopathological examination following hematoxylin and eosin stain revealed spindle cell proliferation with a vague storiform growth pattern and basal cell hyperplasia in the overlying epidermal cells (Figure 3(a)). The tumor tested negative for CD 34 on immunohistochemical staining but tested positive for SMA, CD 68, and factor XIIIa (Figures 3(b)–3(d)). Mitoses were inconspicuous in the lesion, and the Ki 67 labeling index was also low, at 1 to 2%. These findings were consistent with a diagnosis of dermatofibroma. In 5 years of follow-up, the patient did not experience any recurrence, metastases, or other complications.

3. Discussion

Dermatofibromas are common, usually benign, soft-tissue tumors often found on the extremities, particularly the lower limbs. They typically present as asymptomatic, firm, slow-growing, red-brown, or yellow-brown dome-shaped nodules, measuring between a few millimeters to 1 to 2 cm in diameter [2]. In the current case, the tumor measured 12 cm × 6 cm, which was large compared to a typical dermatofibroma. On attaining large sizes, these lesions are clinically called giant dermatofibromas. In their series of eight cases reported in 1994, Requena et al. reported the features that have been widely accepted to define "giant" dermatofibromas. These include (a) size of 5 cm or larger, (b) pedunculated lesions, (c) benign biological behavior despite their size, and (d) the same histopathological characteristics as conventional dermatofibromas [6]. Although the large dermatofibroma in the present case enlarged rapidly clinically mimicking malignancy, it did not meet all the mentioned defining criteria. Therefore, according to the mentioned criteria, the lesion in the present case could not be defined as a typical "giant dermatofibroma." Dermatofibromas are known to be benign lesions. It was believed that although they could recur locally, they lacked the capacity to metastasize [7]. However, in recent years, in addition to local recurrence, some dermatofibromas have been reported to have metastasized during postoperative follow-up. In their case series, Leona et al. reported series that metastases occurred several months to years after diagnosis, and the lungs, lymph nodes, soft tissues, and liver were the principal sites of metastasis. They also reported that the primary tumor size was related to the incidence of local recurrence and metastases after surgery [4]. Dermatofibromas are usually located in the skin, involving the subcutaneous fat, dermis, and epidermis. Although muscle invasive dermatofibromas have been reported in post-excision cases, muscle invasion prior to surgery is rare [8], and this finding is usually indicative of malignancy. In the present case, the tumor was very large, had overlying ulceration, invaded muscle, and was hemorrhagic, clinically suggestive of malignancy. Despite a needle biopsy diagnosis suggestive of a benign tumor, wide resection was performed with a musculocutaneous flap, based on a clinical suspicion of malignancy. Five years after surgery, the patient is well and has a healthy-looking scar with no signs of recurrence and metastasis, despite the giant preoperative tumor size and muscle invasion.

The differential diagnoses of dermatofibromas include other benign lesions such as nodular fasciitis, neurofibromas, and leiomyomas, as well as malignant tumors such as DFSP [5]. On immunostaining, dermatofibromas typically test negative for the CD 34 antibody (positive in 85% of DFSP)

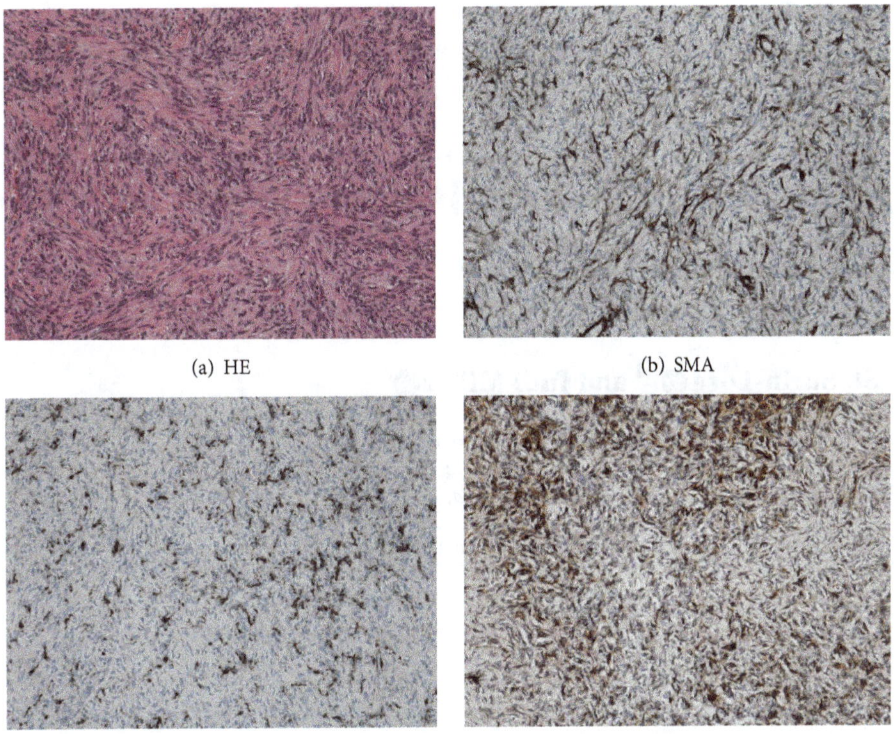

(a) HE (b) SMA

(c) CD68 (d) Factor XIIIa

FIGURE 3: (a) Proliferation of spindle cells with vague storiform growth pattern and basal cell hyperplasia of overlying epidermal cells noted on hematoxylin and eosin staining. (b–d) Immunohistochemical stain showing positivity for (b) SMA, (c) CD 68, and (d) factor XIIIa.

and positive for SMA, CD 68, and factor XIIIa [9]. In the case described, the immunohistochemical reactions were suggestive of a dermatofibroma, and mitoses were not conspicuous; Ki 67 labeling index was also low, suggestive of a benign tumor such as dermatofibroma. Therefore, a combination of these immunohistochemical reactions is necessary for an accurate diagnosis.

In conclusion, the present report describes the case of a giant muscle invasive dermatofibroma, which was clinically suspected to be malignant owing to its appearance. Giant dermatofibromas that invade the muscle may recur or metastasize after surgery. In these cases, adequate surgery, thorough histopathological examination, and careful follow-up are essential for better outcomes.

Consent

Written informed consent was obtained from the patient for publication of this case report and the accompanying images.

References

[1] L. C. Parish, S. Yazdanian, W. C. Lambert, and P. C. Lambert, "Dermatofibroma: a curious tumor," *Skinmed Journal*, vol. 10, no. 5, pp. 268–270, 2012.

[2] A. N. Mota, V. D. Tortelly, D. L. Obadia, and R. S. Silva, "Atrophic dermatofibroma," *Anais Brasileiros de Dermatologia*, vol. 88, no. 5, pp. 793–795, 2013.

[3] T. Karlidag, E. Keles, I. Orhan, M. E. Kaplama, and B. Cobanoglu, "Giant ulcerative dermatofibroma," *Case Reports in Otolaryngology*, vol. 2013, Article ID 254787, 2013.

[4] L. A. Doyle and C. D. Fletcher, "Metastasizing "benign" cutaneous fibrous histiocytoma: a clinicopathologic analysis of 16 cases," *The American Journal of Surgical Pathology*, vol. 37, no. 4, pp. 484–495, 2013.

[5] A. Szumera-Cieckiewicz and K. Ptaszynski, "Benign fibrous histiocytoma of the skin metastasizing to the inguinal lymph node," *Polish Journal of Pathology*, vol. 62, no. 3, pp. 183–186, 2011.

[6] L. Requena, M. C. Fariña, C. Fuente et al., "Giant dermatofibroma. A little-known clinical variant of dermatofibroma," *Journal of the American Academy of Dermatology*, vol. 30, no. 5, pp. 714–718, 1994.

[7] L. Guillou, S. Gebhard, M. Salmeron, and J. M. Coindre, "Metastasizing fibrous histiocytoma of the skin: a clinicopathologic and immunohistochemical analysis of three cases," *Modern Pathology*, vol. 13, no. 6, pp. 654–660, 2000.

[8] T. Mentzel, H. Kutzner, A. Rütten, and H. Hügel, "Benign fibrous histiocytoma (dermatofibroma) of the face: clinicopathologic and immunohistochemical study of 34 cases associated with an aggressive clinical course," *American Journal of Dermatopathology*, vol. 23, no. 5, pp. 419–426, 2001.

[9] K. J. Lang, S. Lidder, M. Hofer, C. Graham, and A. Taylor, "Rapidly evolving giant dermatofibroma," *Case Reports in Medicine*, vol. 2010, Article ID 620910, 2010.

21

Topical Treatment of Truncal Acne with Tretinoin Lotion 0.05% and Azelaic Acid Foam

Sharleen St. Surin-Lord [1,2] **and Judi Miller** [3]

[1]*Howard University College of Medicine, 520 W St NW, Washington, DC 20059, USA*
[2]*Visage Clinical Research LLC, 1400 Mercantile Lane, Suite 110, Largo, MD 20774, USA*
[3]*Strategic Pharmaceutical Advisors, 1750 Tysons Boulevard, Suite 1500 McLean, VA, USA*

Correspondence should be addressed to Sharleen St. Surin-Lord; derm@visagederm.com

Academic Editor: Ravi Krishnan

Truncal acne is present in approximately half of all patients with facial acne but is also occasionally seen in isolation. Important considerations when selecting treatment options for adult female acne, whether on the face, back, chest, or shoulders, include patient compliance, treatment response time, tolerability of the treatment, and psychosocial impact of the disease. Oral antibiotics are widely prescribed for truncal acne due to the challenges of applying topical therapy to such an extensive body surface area. In cases of severe inflammatory and nodular acne vulgaris, this may be a reasonable consideration; however, oral antibiotics should only be used for short durations. Overprescription contributes to microbial resistance and may cause disruption of the gastrointestinal microbiome. In many cases of mild, moderate, or even severe truncal acne, combinations of topical therapies may be valid alternatives. The introduction of foam formulations with enhanced percutaneous absorption and tretinoin lotion formulations that incorporate moisturizing/hydrating agents challenges the previously held idea that effective and tolerable treatment of truncal acne requires oral treatment. This case series describes four female African-American patients with truncal acne successfully treated with a combination of tretinoin lotion 0.05% and azelaic acid 15% foam.

1. Introduction

Acne vulgaris (AV) is characterized by lesions resulting from inflammation of pilosebaceous units [1]. Areas with the highest density of these units include the face, chest, and back. Cutibacterium acnes (C. acnes) is the major occupant of the pilosebaceous unit, accounting for up to 90% of the microbiota [2], and its overproliferation was previously thought to contribute to inflammatory acne. However, a rapidly expanding body of research indicates both the presence of a gut-brain-skin axis and that indigenous microbes of the skin and gut may be vital to the immunological, hormonal, and metabolic equilibrium of the host [3]. Thus, an efficacious and tolerable topical alternative to oral antibiotics in the treatment of AV warrants some investigation.

Truncal acne refers to AV affecting the chest and/or back and is present in approximately 50% of patients with facial acne [4]. In patients with acne, approximately 3% suffer only from truncal acne [5]. Pathophysiologically, truncal acne is no different from acne on the face, although the effects of pressure, occlusion, friction, and heat produced by clothing, shoulder pads, and other sporting equipment may contribute to exacerbation of acne on the chest, back, and shoulders [6]. Truncal acne can have a significant impact on sexual and bodily self-consciousness of appearance in both men and women [7].

Although truncal acne is expected to respond to therapy in a similar manner as acne on the face, the challenges of topical application, particularly to the back, are obvious, making patient compliance a challenge. As such, dermatologists have frequently resorted to prescribing oral antibiotics for these large and hard-to-reach body areas in contravention of the American Academy of Dermatology guidelines [8] and potentially increasing the growing problem of antibiotic resistance. It is currently estimated that more than 50% of C. acnes strains are resistant to topical macrolide antibiotics [9]; therefore, physicians have a duty to evaluate and prescribe appropriate alternative treatments.

2. Case Series

Patient 1 is a 30-year-old female who presented with a three-year history of severe back acne, frequent breakouts, and concerns regarding the dark spots they leave behind. She had seen a dermatologist in the past and had been treated with oral erythromycin, which improved but did not stop her breakouts. Switching to oral doxycycline did not help at all, nor did the use of adjuvant daily adapalene lotion 0.1%.

At baseline, the patient had no facial acne or hyperpigmentation, and the skin was smooth, soft, and radiant. AV was predominant on her chest and her back. Hyperpigmented macules were noted on her chest and back, along with hyperpigmented papules and pustules on her back (Figure 1(a)).

Since this patient had previously failed therapy with two oral antibiotics and adapalene, a retinoid of higher potency was required. Tretinoin lotion 0.05% (Altreno®, Ortho Dermatologics) was prescribed for its tretinoin concentration (0.05%), particle size (85% less than 10 microns), and homogenous distribution as well as its unique formulation with added hyaluronic acid and collagen, which we hoped would decrease dryness and irritation.

She was also prescribed azelaic acid foam 15% for twice daily use on her back in an effort to treat hyperpigmentation. Azelaic acid foam is indicated for rosacea and is known to have a lightening effect on the skin. It is an alternative for patients who wish to avoid hydroquinone.

The patient was followed up at 4 weeks. At this time, she verbalized satisfaction with the treatment. She stated that the dark spots looked much lighter and that she had not had an eruption since the initial visit. On physical exam, the postinflammatory hyperpigmentation was noticeably lightened. There was one pustule, one skin-colored papule, and one hyperpigmented papule. The patient denied any itching or burning sensations where the tretinoin 0.05% lotion had been applied, and there was no evidence of retinoid dermatitis or xerosis in the treatment areas. (Figure 1(b)).

At 12-week follow-up, there was no evidence of acne and sustained improvement of postinflammatory hyperpigmentation (Figure 1(c).

Patient 2 is a 33-year-old female with a history of acne for several years prior to her initial visit, as well as seborrheic dermatitis and mild atopic dermatitis. She had been on numerous over-the-counter (OTC) mediations and prescription medications for acne in the past. Initially, clindamycin phosphate and benzoyl peroxide gel 1.2%/2.5% (Acanya®, Coria Laboratories) was prescribed for her facial acne along with doxycycline 150 mg oral daily and azelaic acid foam 15% twice daily for her truncal acne. At 3-month follow-up, she complained that although the initial regimen helped, she was still experiencing eruptions on both her face and back. She was then treated with a benzefoam 9.8% topical foaming short contact cleanser for her face and chest, azelaic acid 15% foam for her chest, clindamycin phosphate and benzoyl peroxide gel 1.2%/3.75% (Onexton®, Ortho Dermatologics) for her face daily, and adapalene and benzoyl peroxide 0.3%/2.5% (Epiduo®, Galderma) topical gel nightly. She was prescribed hydroquinone 4% lotion twice daily for the hyperpigmentation on her chest and back. Three months later, she stated that the oral antibiotics were no help at all, and they were discontinued. Adapalene 0.1% lotion was prescribed for application to the chest and back once daily.

This regimen successfully controlled the facial and truncal acne for over 6 months, until the truncal acne recurred. At this time, she was commenced on minocycline 115 mg orally daily, but as this did not control the truncal acne well enough, the patient utilized a recommended 10% glycolic acid cleanser to her chest and back three times per week and a 2% glycolic and 2% salicylic acid solution to spray on her trunk along with the adapalene 0.1% lotion.

The hyperpigmentation on the patient's chest, shoulders, and back remained quite remarkable, and the patient became frustrated with the dyspigmentation. The oral antibiotic was discontinued, and a series of 20% salicylic acid chemical peels were performed monthly for a total of 5. These were effective in lightening the hyperpigmented macules and controlling the truncal acne at first; however, upon follow-up, truncal acne and dark spots prevailed over facial acne. Therapy with tretinoin lotion 0.05% was initiated twice daily, along with azelaic acid 15% foam. The patient was asked to return in 4 and then 8 weeks. Truncal acne was well controlled, as was postinflammatory hyperpigmentation. The patient denied any itching or burning sensations where the tretinoin lotion was applied, and there was no evidence of retinoid dermatitis or xerosis in the treatment areas.

Patient 3 is a 24-year-old female who presented with a history of moderate facial acne since age 13. She stated that since starting oral contraceptives two months before, her skin had become sensitive to touch and that acne bumps had become bigger. A change in diet helped mildly but breakouts remained consistent. Two weeks prior, she had a severe flare with lumps all over her neck, jawline, and chest. Her cellphone camera photos were reviewed which revealed numerous inflamed papules on the face and nodules on the neck. On physical examination, there were erythematous papules on the nuchal scalp and thick flakes with some erythema. There were inflamed papules, some atrophic skin, and pustules on the cheeks, with significant pustules and inflamed papules on her chin. There was some scarring, acne cysts, and erythematous macules on the neck, with many hyperpigmented macules. The patient's chest had erythematous papules and macules, while her back and shoulders had many erythematous papules and hyperpigmented macules (Figures 2(a)–2(c)).

The patient declined oral isotretinoin at this time. Due to the inflammatory nature of this patient's presentation, she was initially prescribed tazarotene 0.1% (Fabior®, Mayne Pharma) foam nightly with clindamycin phosphate and benzoyl peroxide gel 1.2%/3.75% in the morning for her facial acne. She was instructed to use Neutrogena Hydro

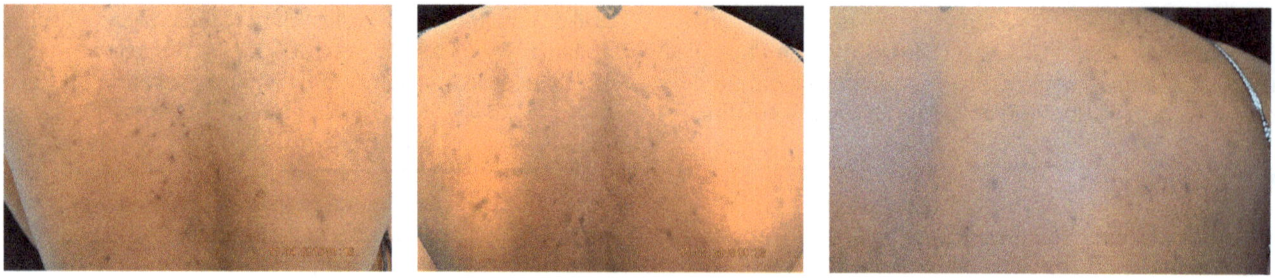

(a) (b) (c)

FIGURE 1: Patient 1: (a) pretreatment; (b) after 4 weeks treatment with tretinoin and azelaic acid; and (c) after 12 weeks treatment with tretinoin lotion and azelaic acid.

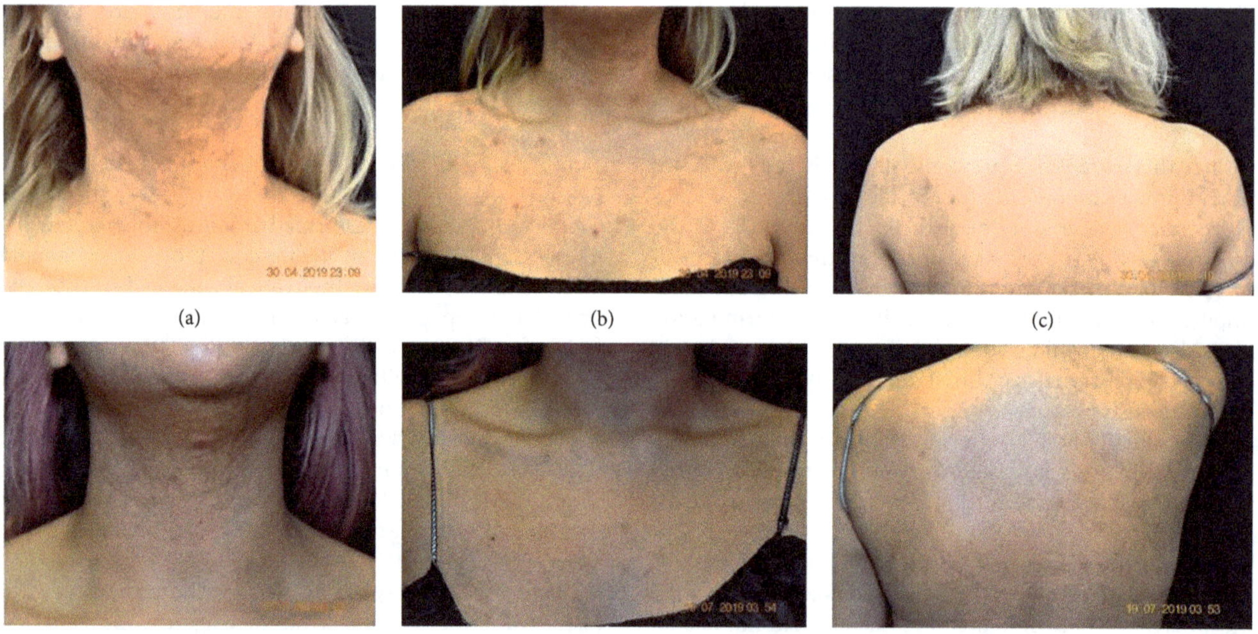

(a) (b) (c)

(d) (e) (f)

FIGURE 2: Patient 3: (a) pretreatment (chin and neck); (b) pretreatment (chest); (c) pretreatment (back); (d) after 12 weeks treatment with tretinoin lotion and azelaic acid (chin and neck); (e) after 12 weeks treatment with tretinoin lotion and azelaic acid (chest); and (f) after 12 weeks treatment with tretinoin lotion and azelaic acid (back).

Boost to treat any dry skin or flaking. For the truncal acne, she was instructed to apply tretinoin 0.05% lotion nightly to the chest, neck, shoulders, and back and azelaic acid 15% foam twice daily to the chest, shoulders, and back. She did not wish to treat the seborrheic dermatitis. She was also prescribed sarecycline 100 mg by mouth daily. The patient presented 7 days later complaining of a generalized pruritic eruption. On physical examination, there were still inflamed papules and cysts on the patient's facial skin, and her chest, back, arms, and legs had developed a morbilliform eruption. The sarecycline was discontinued, and the patient was placed on a short course of oral corticosteroids as well as fluocinonide 0.05% topical cream for twice daily use and instructed to never take oral tetracyclines again. 3 weeks later, the patient stated that her skin was clear from drug eruption. The Neutrogena Hydro Boost that was recommended to use in case of dryness caused a burning sensation on her face after using azelaic acid foam at night, so she changed foam frequency to every other night but continued using the foam twice daily and tretinoin lotion 0.05% every night on her chest and back. Upon physical exam, the following were noted: scales on the scalp and some cysts, inflamed papules, and hyperpigmented macules on the face but less than before. On the chest, shoulders, and back, there were fewer acne papules than at the previous visit. The patient stated that she was satisfied with her current regimen; however, glycolic acid 10% wipes were recommended for morning application to better control facial acne. This patient was seen one month later, at which time her face, chest, and neck were clear. (Figure 2(d))

Patient 4 is a 32-year-old female who has been treated for moderate facial acne for the past three years with a regimen that included tazarotene 0.1% gel, dapsone 7.5% gel, and clindamycin phosphate and benzoyl peroxide gel 1.2%/3.75%.

Despite this aggressive topical regimen, this patient never completely cleared. In 2017, she sought treatment for her truncal acne as she began to notice eruptions on her chest and back after she began to work out. Physical examination revealed erythematous papules and inflamed papules on her cheeks, forehead, and chin, as well as skin-colored and hyperpigmented papules on her chest, back, and shoulders. She was advised to shower immediately after workouts, and the following were added to her treatment regimen: benzefoam 9.8% topical to the chest and back and azelaic acid foam 15% daily to the face. She continued to flare over the next three months with erythematous papules and inflamed papules on her cheek, forehead, and chin and notably with skin-colored and hyperpigmented papules on her chest, back, and shoulders. She declined any oral medications, so it was advised that she uses Cetaphil cleansing cloths immediately after working out to cleanse her skin and then shower with the benzefoam short contact cleanser soon after. Subsequently, she agreed to try minocycline 115 mg orally daily and adapalene 0.1% lotion on her back once daily. At 2-month follow-up, the flares were under control and the patient only had hyperpigmentation on her back, shoulders, and chest. Minocycline was changed to doxycycline, but 4 months later, truncal acne began to flare again. The patient was offered, but declined, isotretinoin therapy. Over the next 12 months, the patient continued to flare on her face and trunk and also developed atopic dermatitis. She eventually admitted to not being adherent to oral regimens and stated she preferred topical regimens, so tretinoin lotion 0.05% once daily at bedtime and azelaic acid 15% foam twice daily were initiated for her truncal acne. At one-, two-, and 3-month follow-ups, she expressed satisfaction with not having to use oral medications and stated she had broken out less between visits.

3. Discussion

Although AV is principally a disorder of adolescence, research suggests that the prevalence of adult acne is increasing, especially in females [10]. In this population, persistent acne, i.e., acne that continues from adolescence into adulthood is seen in about 80% of cases. Important considerations when selecting a treatment for adult female acne, whether on the face or trunk, are the slower response to treatment, increased likelihood of skin irritation, and greater psychosocial impact of the disease [11]. Oral antibiotics, although widely prescribed for the back and truncal acne, should be used only when absolutely necessary and for short durations. Not only does overprescription contribute to microbial resistance, antibiotics can disrupt gut flora and the gut-skin axis and the resulting intestinal dysbiosis, and worsening of acne [12].

Topical retinoids are highly effective and are recommended as first line therapy in mild-to-moderate acne; however, they can be associated with significant skin dryness, erythema, and even development of dermatitis [13]. As such, successful treatment must always balance efficacy against tolerability, and less irritating formulations may provide the best results. In the author's experience, many patients have not tolerated higher-dose retinoids on the chest and back, making adapalene 0.1% lotion a good option. However, when this is not effective, one must consider other, more potent, and tolerable treatment options. The most recent of these is a topical lotion formulation of tretinoin 0.05% together with sodium hyaluronate, soluble collagen, glycerin, and small amounts of mineral oil. These moisturizing/hydrating agents have been shown to enhance efficacy, alleviate dryness and improve skin comfort, and accelerate the healing process [14].

While previous studies have shown that azelaic acid therapy can enhance efficacy and improve patient satisfaction when used in combination with other topical medications such as benzoyl peroxide 4% gel, clindamycin 1% gel, tretinoin 0.025% cream, and erythromycin 3%/benzoyl peroxide 5% gel [15], this is the first report documenting the use of a combination of once daily application of topical tretinoin 0.05% lotion and twice daily azelaic acid 15% foam in truncal acne. In addition to the treatments noted, all patients were instructed to use a sunscreen with SPF 50 on the chest and back if those areas were ever exposed and daily on the face, except patient 1 who only had truncal acne.

It should be noted that none of these patients were taking hormone based therapies, i.e., combined oral contraceptives and/or spironolactone as part of their adult acne treatment regimen, although Patient 3 was taking a combined norgestimate and ethinyl estradiol pill as an oral contraceptive. We acknowledge that while hormonal therapies are usually highly effective for patients with severe seborrhea, flare-ups before menstruation, endocrine abnormalities, and persistent inflammation recalcitrant to treatment, they are not without side effects and spironolactone is not approved for use in acne in the US.

In the four female adult patients reported here, this combination of tretinoin 0.05% lotion and azelaic acid 15% foam resulted in sustained improvement of their long-standing, previously treatment refractory truncal acne during the follow-up observation period. Nevertheless, we acknowledge that these results may be limited by the relatively short follow-up, especially as adult female acne tends to be more chronic and relapse more frequently than adolescent acne, and that prolonged maintenance treatment will likely be essential. Additionally, these results need to be confirmed in a larger patient population.

Consent

The subjects in this case series all gave written informed consent to publish their case details, including photographic images.

Acknowledgments

The work was supported by Ortho Dermatologics. Article processing charges will be covered by Ortho Dermatologicals.

References

[1] M. Toyoda and M. Morohashi, "Pathogenesis of acne," *Medical Electron Microscopy*, vol. 34, no. 1, pp. 29–40, 2001.

[2] E. A. Grice, H. H. Kong, S. Conlan et al., "Topographical and temporal diversity of the human skin microbiome," *Science*, vol. 324, no. 5931, pp. 1190–1192, 2009.

[3] Y. B. Lee, E. J. Byun, and A. H. S. Kim, "Potential role of the microbiome in acne: a comprehensive review," *Journal of Clinical Medicine*, vol. 8, no. 7, p. 987, 2019.

[4] J. K. Tan, J. Tang, K. Fung et al., "Prevalence and severity of facial and truncal acne in a referral cohort," *Journal of Drugs in Dermatology*, vol. 7, no. 7, pp. 551–556, 2008.

[5] J. Q. Del Rosso, J. B. Bikowski, E. Baum, J. Smith, and S. Hawkes, "A closer look at truncal acne vulgaris: prevalence, severity, and clinical significance," *Journal of Drugs in Dermatology*, vol. 6, no. 6, pp. 597–600, 2017.

[6] R. S. Basler, "Acne mechanica in athletes," *Cutis*, vol. 50, no. 50, pp. 125–128, 1992.

[7] J. Hassan, S. Grogan, D. Clark-Carter, H. Richards, and V. M. Yates, "The individual health burden of acne: appearance-related distress in male and female adolescents and adults with back, chest and facial acne," *Journal of Health Psychology*, vol. 14, no. 8, pp. 1105–1118, 2009.

[8] B. L. Adler, H. Kornmehl, and A. W. Armstrong, "Antibiotic resistance in acne treatment," *JAMA Dermatology*, vol. 153, no. 8, pp. 810-811, 2017.

[9] T. R. Walsh, J. Efthimiou, and B. Dréno, "Systematic review of antibiotic resistance in acne: an increasing topical and oral threat," *The Lancet Infectious Diseases*, vol. 16, no. 3, pp. e23–e33, 2016.

[10] G. K. Kim and B. B. Michaels, "Post-adolescent acne in women: more common and more clinical considerations," *Journal of Drugs in Dermatology*, vol. 11, no. 11, pp. 708–713, 2012.

[11] B. Dréno, A. Layton, C. C. Zouboulis et al., "Adult female acne: a new paradigm," *Journal of the European Academy of Dermatology and Venereology*, vol. 27, no. 9, pp. 1063–1070, 2013.

[12] M. A. Dagnelie, E. Montassier, A. Khammari, C. Mounier, S. Corvec, and B. Dréno, "Inflammatory skin is associated with changes in the skin microbiota composition on the back of severe acne patients," *Experimental Dermatology*, vol. 28, no. 8, pp. 961–967, 2019.

[13] L. Culp, S. Moradi Tuchayi, H. Alinia, and S. R. Feldman, "Tolerability of topical retinoids:are there clinically meaningful differences among topical retinoids?" *Journal of Cutaneous Medicine and Surgery*, vol. 19, no. 6, pp. 530–538, 2015.

[14] L. H. Kircik, Z. D. Draelos, and D. S. Berson, "Polymeric emulsion technology applied to tretinoin," *Journal of Drugs in Dermatology*, vol. 18, no. 4, pp. S148–S154, 2019.

[15] G. Webster, "Combination azelaic acid therapy for acne vulgaris," *Journal of the American Academy of Dermatology*, vol. 43, no. 2, pp. S47–S50, 2000.

22

Verruca Vulgaris and Seborrheic Keratosis Exacerbated by Immunosuppression

Shohei Iida, Kyoko Sugioka, Makoto Kondo, Yoshiaki Matsushima, Kento Mizutani, Koji Habe, and Keiichi Yamanaka

Department of Dermatology, Mie University, Graduate School of Medicine, 2-174 Edobashi, Tsu, Mie 514-8507, Japan

Correspondence should be addressed to Keiichi Yamanaka; yamake@clin.medic.mie-u.ac.jp

Academic Editor: Jacek Cezary Szepietowski

Verruca vulgaris is an infectious disease caused by the human papillomavirus and characterized by hyperkeratotic papules or plaques with a clear boundary. Seborrheic keratosis is a commonly encountered lesion on the face, trunk, or extremities and is described as seborrheic verruca because of its clinical similarity to warts; furthermore, it is occasionally associated with immune suppression, especially in cases of Leser-trélat syndrome. Although these diseases are frequently found in healthy individuals, they typically show a good response to cryotherapy. However, cases in immunosuppressed patients are intractable to therapy. Overall immune status is evaluated via complete blood count (CBC); however, white blood count does not show the exact immune ability, and NK cell activity is often decreased in cases of malignancy. Here, we present two cases of exacerbated verruca vulgaris and seborrheic verruca observed in patients with malignancy. Although the patients seemed to be in good condition and had a normal CBC, immunosuppression was suspected based on the degree of skin rashes. NK cell activity was decreased in both patients, and both cases had malignancy. The measurement of NK cell activity may be a useful approach to evaluate immune status.

1. Introduction

Verruca vulgaris is a benign proliferation of the stratified squamous epithelium resulting in a papillary or verrucous exophytic mass. Depending on the inoculation titer, an incubation period of 3 weeks to 8 months is required before lesions become apparent [1]. Lesions are easily seen on the hands, arms, and legs; however, they can also appear on the surface of the skin in any region of the body or, more rarely, on mucous membranes [2]. Seborrheic verruca is an asymptomatic benign epidermal keratinocytic tumor commonly seen in elderly patients. It may also act as an acquired cutaneous lesion predisposing individuals to the development of other dermatoses. Seborrheic verruca is also observed in patients with benign neoplasms, pregnancy, or human immunodeficiency virus infections.

Several treatments are available for eradicating verruca lesions including surgery, cryotherapy, electrocauterization, laser, or topical agents; however, the treatment strategy varies depending on disease location and severity, as well as the patient's immune status [3]. These are silent and slow growing lesions in healthy individuals, but can result in serious and rapid growth in immunosuppressed patients. Here we present two cases of verruca vulgaris and seborrheic verruca observed in patients with malignancy.

2. Case Presentation

2.1. Case 1. A 61-year-old Japanese man visited our department for a verrucous formation on his lip that was growing rapidly and invading his palate (Figure 1). He also showed verrucous vegetation characterized by pigmentation, and a blackish brown mass with pruritus gradually developed on his axilla, posterior neck, and face. He had a history of hypertension, hyperuricemia, hyperlipidemia, gastrectomy and cholecystectomy for gastric cancer and was actively receiving chemotherapy for the treatment of multiple metastases. We diagnosed malignant acanthosis nigricans and verruca vulgaris. We intended to perform a skin

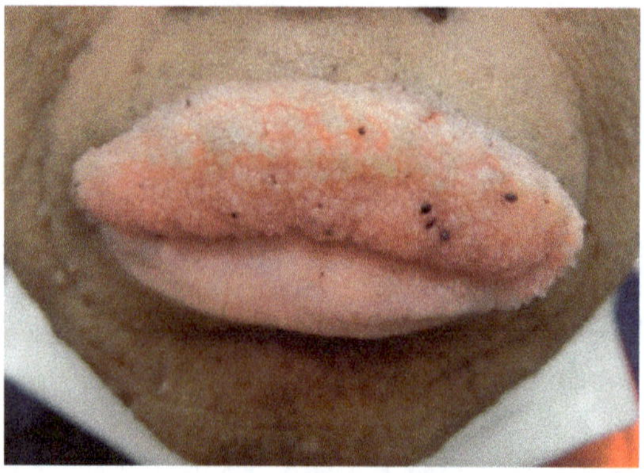

Figure 1: A rapidly growing papillomatous verruca originating on the lip and invading the palate.

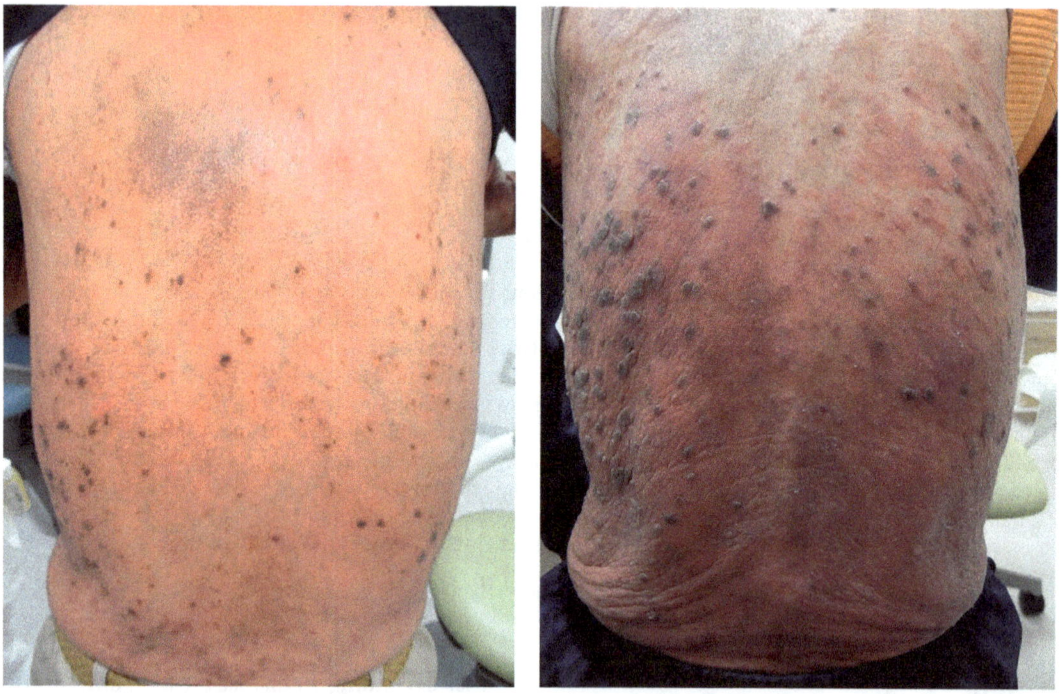

(a) (b)

Figure 2: (a) Multiple flat black spots on the patient's back three months prior to admission. (b) Multiple seborrheic verruca on the patient's back on admission.

biopsy of a patient with verrucous vulgaris to exclude verrucous carcinoma, squamous papilloma, condyloma acuminatum, and multifocal epithelial hyperplasia, but we could not obtain consent from the patient. The verruca was treated with cryotherapy without any response. Due to the serious phenotypes of his skin manifestations, we were anxious about the patient's immune status; however, his immune condition had been evaluated as "normal" by his physician on the basis of laboratory data including a complete blood count (CBC). Although his neutrophil function in phagocytosis and sterilization fell within the normal range, his natural killer (NK) cell activity was 0.3% (normal range: 8.9–29.5%). We issued a warning about his immunosuppressed status, but the patient died due to pneumonia and multiple organ failure.

2.2. Case 2. A 77-year-old man with a 37-year history of pustular psoriasis being treated with brodalumab, a human monoclonal antibody that binds to interleukin (IL) 17 receptor A (IL17R) with high affinity, was hospitalized for erythroderma and high fever. Chest computed tomography revealed pneumonia, a lung tumor, and mediastinal lymphadenopathy. Biopsy of the mediastinal lymph node with immunohistochemical study revealed lung adenocarcinoma. Furthermore, a head MRI revealed a brain metastasis. His performance status was 4, and he was not a candidate for chemotherapy.

Multiple black-colored seborrhoic verruca appeared on his back, which rapidly increased in number and size within 3 months (Figures 2(a) and 2(b)). We speculated that these seborrhoic verruca were related to his lung cancer, a phenomenon known as the Leser-trélat sign. Although his CBC, including absolute neutrophil and lymphocyte counts, was within the normal range, his natural killer (NK) cell activity was 2.3% (normal range: 8.9–29.5%). We speculated the patient was in an immunosuppressed state. The patient's medical condition rapidly declined and he died within 2 months.

3. Discussion

NK cells are critical components of the innate immune system and do not express the T-cell receptor; they function in nonspecific cytotoxicity to virus-infected cells and cancer cells. NK cell receptors consist of activating and inhibitory receptors that determine susceptibility to virus infection. Inhibitory receptors recognize MHC-class I and, upon binding, will prevent cytotoxicity. Since virus-infected cells and cancer cells show down-regulated MHC-class I, NK cells attack target cells. One study found the percentages of NK cells were significantly decreased in patients with gastric cancer, and the percentages of tumor-infiltrating NK cells were positively correlated with survival and disease progression [4]. Brodalumab is an anti-IL-17RA antibody and hampers IL-17 signaling by blocking its receptor. IL-17 not only plays an oncogenic role in tumorigenesis by regulating tumor angiogenesis and enhancing tumor immune evasion but also exerts anti-tumor functions by enhancing NK cells and cytotoxic T lymphocyte (CTL) activation [5]. In the second case, brodalumab may have contributed to the measured reduction in NK cell activity.

Immune status is evaluated by checking CBC including white blood cells, but we often encounter viral infections such as cytomegalovirus in patients receiving anti-cancer drugs even with normal CBC. In these two cases, the CBC was within the normal range, but NK cell activity was low. By measuring NK cell activity, we noticed the fatal risk of lung infection in the first case, and we suspected seborrheic verruca related to lung cancer in the second case. Although CBC is normal, NK cell activity may be low in patients with abrogative skin rash, suggesting the importance of measuring NK cell activity.

Disclosure

Shohei Iida and Kyoko Sugioka are equal first authors.

Authors' Contributions

SI, KS, YM, KM, KH, and KY took care of the patients. SI, KS, and KY wrote the manuscript. Shohei Iida and Kyoko Sugioka contributed equally to this work.

References

[1] J. Doorbar, N. Egawa, H. Griffin, C. Kranjec, and I. Murakami, "Human papillomavirus molecular biology and disease association," *Reviews in Medical Virology*, vol. 25, no. 1, pp. 2–23, 2016.

[2] M. M. Lipke, "An armamentarium of wart treatments," *Clinical Medicine & Research*, vol. 4, no. 4, pp. 273–293, 2006.

[3] D. Bzhalava, P. Guan, S. Franceschi, J. Dillner, and G. Clifford, "A systematic review of the prevalence of mucosal and cutaneous human papillomavirus types," *Virology*, vol. 445, no. 1-2, pp. 224–231, 2013.

[4] L.-s. Peng, J.-y. Zhang, Y.-s. Teng et al., "Tumor-associated monocytes/macrophages impair NK-cell function via TGFβ1 in human gastric cancer," *Cancer Immunology Research*, vol. 5, no. 3, pp. 248–256, 2017.

[5] X. Qian, H. Chen, X. Wu, L. Hu, Q. Huang, and Y. Jin, "Interleukin-17 acts as double-edged sword in anti-tumor immunity and tumorigenesis," *Cytokine*, vol. 89, pp. 34–44, 2017.

23

Surgery of Kerion, a Nightmare for Nondermatologists

Vikash Paudel

Department of Dermatology, National Medical College, Birgunj, Parsa, Nepal

Correspondence should be addressed to Vikash Paudel; vikashpoudel@iom.edu.np

Academic Editor: Sergio A. Cuevas Covarrubias

Kerion is an inflammatory type of tinea capitis characterized by swelling and alopecia of the scalp, which could be mistaken as bacterial infection. It occurs most frequently in children. We report a 10-year-old child whose kerion was misdiagnosed as bacterial abscess and unnecessarily incised. Later, her condition was rediagnosed as kerion based on clinical appearance and potassium hydroxide wet mount. The lesions resolved completely with systemic antifungal treatment, griseofulvin, leaving residual scarring alopecia. The delay in the proper diagnosis and inappropriate treatment of this patient resulted in permanent scarring alopecia. Thus, clinicians must have a high index of suspicion for tinea capitis when dealing with inflammatory scalp lesions.

1. Introduction

Kerion is an inflammatory fungal infection of the hair follicle of the scalp, characterized by boggy swelling, purulent discharge, alopecia, and lymphadenopathy. It is more common among children. Different pathogens have been implicated to cause kerion, and the predominant are dermatophytes of genus Trichophyton and Microsporum [1]. Because of its clinical presentation, it might be mistaken for pyoderma, especially an abscess [2, 3].

We report a case of kerion of a child which was misdiagnosed and mismanaged as pyoderma with incision and drainage under local anesthesia, resulting in delayed specific treatment, unnecessary economic burden, risk of anesthesia and surgery, and severe morbidity of scarring alopecia. Thus, we recommend that patients especially children who present with boggy swelling on the scalp should be seen by dermatologists for its appropriate management.

2. Case Presentation

It is a story of a 10-year-old female child who presented with mild, tender, itchy, and boggy swelling of the scalp for one-month duration. The lesions started as a small tender nodule over the vertex which gradually increased in size to cover a larger area of vertex. It was associated with areas of hair loss and easily pluckable hairs and infrequent purulent discharge. For this, she visited a nearby surgeon who mistook it as a bacterial abscess and underwent incision and draining under local anesthesia. During surgical procedures, the scalp tissue was very friable to leave a chunk of depression, which could not be sutured and was referred to us for further management.

Examination revealed a localized area of hair loss at the vertex of scalp (6×5 cm) with dispersed multiple boggy nodules and polygonal incised ulcer (3 cm $\times$ 1.5 cm) with friable edges at the middle of alopecia. Areas of purulent discharge and patchy hair loss were also noted at the periphery of lesions (Figure 1(a)). The left anterior cervical lymph nodes were palpable and tender. Wood's lamp examination revealed yellow-green fluorescence over the affected area. Potassium hydroxide (KOH) wet mount was performed in hair samples and scalp scrapings, which showed multiple branching hyphae from skin lesion and ectothrix in hair follicles (Figures 2(a) and 2(b)). A provisional diagnosis of kerion with secondary ulcer was made, and the patient was prescribed oral griseofulvin 250 mg daily and ketoconazole shampoo for 6 weeks along with oral flucloxacillin, analgesics, and Condy's crystal solution of 1 : 10000 of potassium permanganate for 1 week. She was advised to follow up frequently until the lesion subsides.

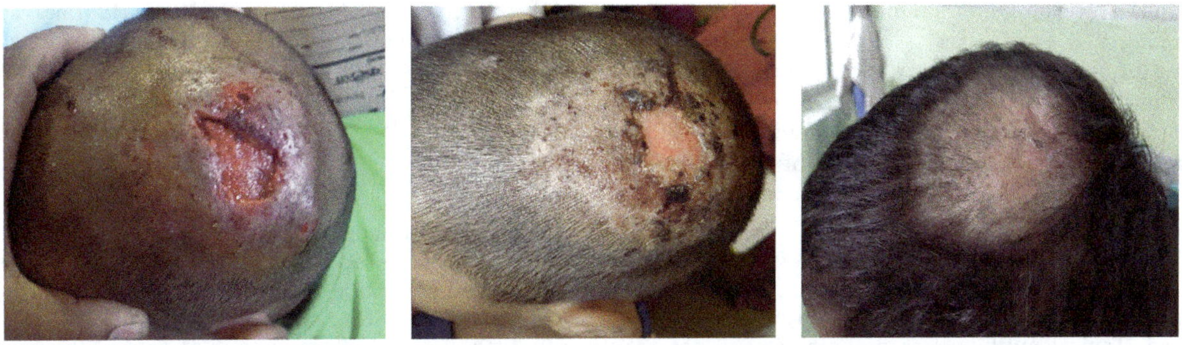

(a) (b) (c)

FIGURE 1: (a) Initial lesion of tinea capitis after surgical incision. (b) Two weeks after starting oral griseofulvin. (c) Eight weeks after starting oral griseofulvin.

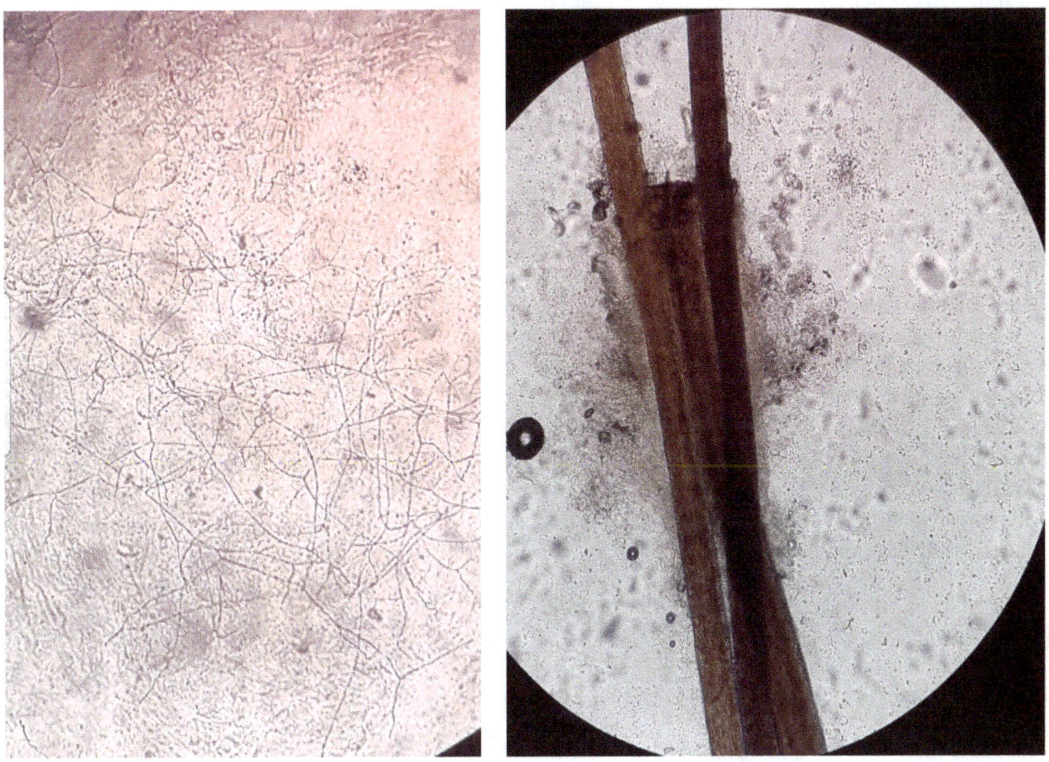

(a) (b)

FIGURE 2: (a)Branching hyphae under KOH wet mount (10x). (b) Ectothrix shown in hair follicle in KOH wet mount (40x).

Eight weeks later, the lesions healed leaving residual scarring alopecia in the incised region (Figures 1(b) and 1(c)).

3. Discussion

Tinea capitis is a common and easily transmitted childhood fungal scalp infection. Kerion is a type of inflammatory tinea capitis associated with tender boggy swelling, purulent discharge, alopecia, and regional lymphadenopathy [1]. It is common among children but can be seen from newborn to elderly [4]. Its improper management could lead to permanent scarring alopecia. The most common pathogen responsible for kerion in humans is *Microsporum* and *Trichophyton*, which are zoophilic dermatophytes. Potassium hydroxide (KOH) wet mount, Wood lamp examination, and dermoscopy aid in diagnosis, whereas the fungal culture helps to identify species which might not be always positive [5]. Because of bogginess of the kerion, discharge, and regional lymphadenopathy, it could be confused with bacterial pyoderma, especially by nondermatologist where the clinical exposure of fungal infection (tinea capitis) is limited. In our patient, the diagnosis of kerion was missed by the surgeon, and thus incision and drainage were unnecessarily performed.

Our diagnosis was based on typical clinical features and KOH mount. Fungal culture and species identification were not possible because of unavailability of advanced laboratories facilities. The standard treatment of tinea capitis is systemic antifungal therapy for two to six weeks with oral terbinafine, griseofulvin, or itraconazole, whereas with griseofulvin, mycological cure and efficacy rates are generally high, so it is commonly preferred [6]. The duration of therapy could be extended until clinical clearance is achieved. Topical antifungal as monotherapy is not recommended as these agents are unable to penetrate the hair follicle adequately. Adjunctive topical therapies such as selenium sulphide or clotrimazole or ketoconazole shampoo or creams reduce disease transmission and shorten treatment duration [7]. Antihistamines might be helpful for pruritus and in reducing dissemination of spores due to scratching. Antibiotic treatment is not recommended unless there is a chance of secondary bacterial infection or lesion is traumatized. There is no role of surgical incision and debridement in the case of kerion [8, 9]. There is a controversial role of oral steroids in management of kerion, and thus they are usually not recommended as part of routine care for kerion [10]. As there is no strong recommendation in the use of oral steroid and the patient had history of surgical manipulation of the lesions, oral steroid was not considered in our case.

As illustrated in this case, kerion could easily be misdiagnosed as a bacterial infection due to its clinical presentation. Only the systemic antifungal therapy is the foundation of treatment, and surgical incision is unnecessary and is associated with hazards. In the absence of laboratory facilities, a trial of oral antifungal agents is justified while monitoring the treatment response. Clinicians should have a high index of suspicion for tinea capitis when dealing with inflammatory scalp lesions.

References

[1] R. J. Hay, "Tinea capitis: current status," *Mycopathologia*, vol. 182, no. 1-2, pp. 87–93, 2017.

[2] E. S. Martin and B. E. Elewski, "Tinea capitis in adult women masquerading as bacterial pyoderma," *Journal of the American Academy of Dermatology*, vol. 49, no. 2, pp. 177–S179, 2003.

[3] L. L. Stein, E. G. Adams, and K. Z. Holcomb, "Inflammatory tinea capitis mimicking dissecting cellulitis in a postpubertal male: a case report and review of the literature," *Mycoses*, vol. 56, no. 5, pp. 596–600, 2013.

[4] C. Fremerey and P. Nenoff, "Tinea capitis in a newborn," *New England Journal of Medicine*, vol. 378, no. 21, p. 2022, 2018.

[5] A. K. C. Leung, K. L. Hon, K. F. Leong, B. Barankin, and J. M. Lam, "Tinea capitis: an updated review," *Recent Patents on Inflammation & Allergy Drug Discovery*, vol. 14, no. 1, pp. 58–68, 2020.

[6] M. L. Bennett, A. B. Fleischer, J. W. Loveless, and S. R. Feldman, "Oral griseofulvin remains the treatment of choice for tinea capitis in children," *Pediatric Dermatology*, vol. 17, no. 4, pp. 304–309, 2000.

[7] A. K. Gupta, R. R. Mays, S. G. Versteeg et al., "Tinea capitis in children: a systematic review of management," *Journal of the European Academy of Dermatology and Venereology*, vol. 32, no. 12, pp. 2264–2274, 2018.

[8] E. Thoma-Greber, S. Zenker, M. Röcken, H. Wolff, and H. C. Korting, "Surgical treatment of tinea capitis in childhood. Fallbericht. Chirurgische behandlung der tinea capitis im kindesalter," *Mycoses*, vol. 46, no. 8, pp. 333–354, 2003.

[9] L. v. Laer Tschudin, E. Laffitte, F. Baudraz-Rosselet, G. Dushi, J. Hohlfeld, and A. S. de Buys Roessingh, "Tinea capitis: no incision nor excision," *Journal of Pediatric Surgery*, vol. 42, no. 8, pp. E33–E36, 2007.

[10] S. Ali, T. A. D. Graham, and S. E. D. Forgie, "The assessment and management of tinea capitis in children," *Pediatric Emergency Care*, vol. 23, no. 9, pp. 662–668, 2007.

24

Long-Term Medical Follow-Up (for More than 15 Years) of a Patient with Stage IA Mycosis Fungoides Originally Presenting in Childhood: Remission for >15 Years with Localised Beam Therapy

Eric Bessell[1], **Martin Dalton**[2] **and John David Parry**[2]

[1]*Department of Clinical Oncology, Nottingham City Hospital, Nottingham, UK*
[2]*The Surgery, Ravenshead, Nottinghamshire, UK*

Correspondence should be addressed to Eric Bessell; ebessell@hotmail.co.uk

Academic Editor: Bhushan Kumar

A man now aged 80 years has received specialist care for stage 1A mycosis fungoides for 58 years. The disease developed in childhood. Long-term follow-up (>30 years) of patients with mycosis fungoides is infrequently described in the world literature. The disease in this patient was limited to 5 areas, but these were large (up to 25 cm in diameter). The rest of the skin was normal clinically. All 5 areas were treated separately with electron beam therapy (3–4 MeV) to a dose of 30 Gy in 15 fractions over 3 weeks between 2000 and 2005. Complete regression was obtained in all 5 areas, and the patient has been in complete remission for 15 years after living with the disease previously for over 40 years.

1. Introduction

Mycosis fungoides (MF) is the most frequent type of primary cutaneous T-cell lymphoma but is uncommon with an annual incidence of 4 cases per million [1]. The average age at diagnosis is 59 years [2], and it rarely occurs in children [3]. There is therefore little opportunity to follow patients for very long periods. Long-term follow-up has been reported by the Italian Study Group for Cutaneous Lymphoma [2]. Twenty-seven Italian centres were involved in reporting follow-up information on patients treated between 1975 and 2010 with MF, and the median follow-up was 14.5 years (range: 1–35 years). The 10-year survival rate for early-stage disease (1A) was 93%, and the disease progression at 30 years was 13%. Patients in this study with stage 1A/1B disease had an annual rate of progression to stage IIB disease of 1–2% which was maintained for 15 years from diagnosis. Long-term follow-up of MF and Sezary syndrome has also been reported from Stanford University School of Medicine in the USA [4]. They reported on 525 patients treated between 1958 and 1999. The 30-year overall survival for 155 patients with stage 1A MF was 54%, and the disease-specific survival for these patients was 98%. The annual rate of progression to more advanced disease was similar to the Italian study (1–2% for 15 years).

2. Case Report

A man now aged 80 years presented with a rash in childhood (at the age of 3 years, in 1944, according to his mother). All correspondence and clinical notes relating to MF since 1962 have been reviewed by the authors. The rash remained unchanged according to the patient, and no specific diagnosis was made until 1962 when he was 21 years old. A diagnosis of parapsoriasis [5] was then made by a dermatologist, but the skin condition was not described in detail; it was called a long-standing skin eruption. He was treated with triamcinolone in Eucerin (1 in 10) ointment. The rash remained unchanged until 1971 when the patient was described as developing raised infiltrated lesions particularly involving his upper left thigh. A biopsy was then taken which showed early MF, and he was treated with betamethasone ointment. Again, there was no significant change in the patches/plaques, and when systemic PUVA was introduced in Nottingham in 1982, he received a short course of PUVA which resulted in intense irritation of the involved skin. He continued with betamethasone until this reaction resolved. In 1991, a further biopsy confirmed early MF, and he was treated with clobetasone cream intermittently for the next 9 years. During that time, the plaques on his left wrist and left inguinal region became more prominent.

In 2000, he was referred by a dermatologist to an oncologist for consideration of localised electron beam therapy because of progression of MF in the skin of the left wrist and left inguinal region. On examination, there were multiple plaques in the skin of the left inguinal region 15 × 15 cm in overall dimension (Figure 1) and a plaque 8.6 × 6.0 cm on the anterior left wrist (Figure 2). In addition, there was a large (25 × 15 cm) area on the lateral aspect of his right thigh which had not changed in recent years, a 3 cm area on the lateral aspect of his left thigh, and a patch 13 × 8 cm in the posterior left thigh extending down to the popliteal fossa. There were, therefore, a total of five areas of skin involvement.

There were no visible areas elsewhere in the skin, and no lymph nodes were palpable. A skin biopsy in the left inguinal region showed a hyperkeratotic, parakeratotic, acanthotic epidermis with the superficial dermis bearing a dense lymphoid infiltrate of predominantly T-cells (CD 34+, CD4+, and CD8−). The MIB1 labelling index was low, but a clonal T-cell receptor gene arrangement was demonstrated consistent with MF. The stage was IA with less than 10% of the skin involved (TNM staging: T1b) [6].

A treatment strategy was discussed with the patient, and the plan was to treat the most active areas (left wrist and left inguinal region) first to establish whether a complete response could be obtained rather than treating all five areas at the same time. Total skin electron beam therapy was considered, but the MF had been limited to defined areas for many years.

Therefore, in November 2000, electron beam therapy (4 MeV) was given to the skin of the anterior left wrist (30 Gy in 15 fractions over 23 days), and in January 2001, the same treatment was given to the skin of the left inguinal region. Complete regression of both these areas of MF was achieved. A biopsy of the area on the lateral aspect of the right thigh in March 2001 confirmed patch stage MF, and progression of this disease in the skin of the right thigh was observed during 2001. The large area increased in size with new adjacent lesions developing with soreness as a prominent symptom. The whole area in the lateral right thigh was treated with electron beam therapy in the same way as the previous areas in the left inguinal region and left wrist. Again, complete regression was achieved in the skin of the lateral right thigh. The remaining areas of patch disease in the lateral and the posterior left thigh were observed over the next 4 years, and no significant change was seen. The area in the skin of the lateral left thigh had been present since the 1960s. A decision was then made with the patient in 2005 to treat both these areas (the lateral and the left posterior thigh) so that all visible diseases would have been treated (there had been no

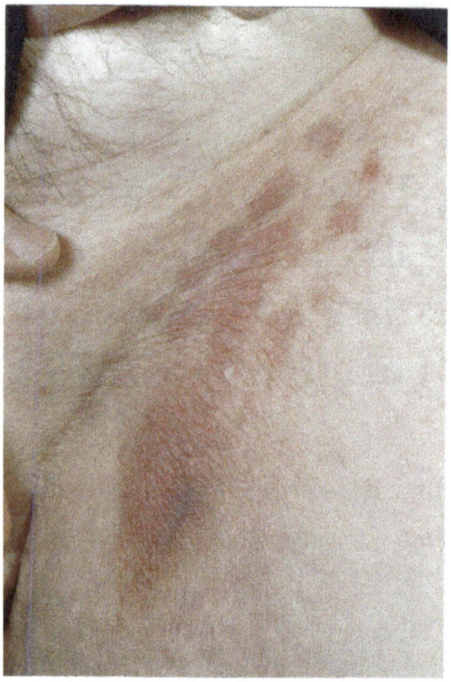

Figure 1: Multiple plaques of mycosis fungoides in the skin of the left inguinal region.

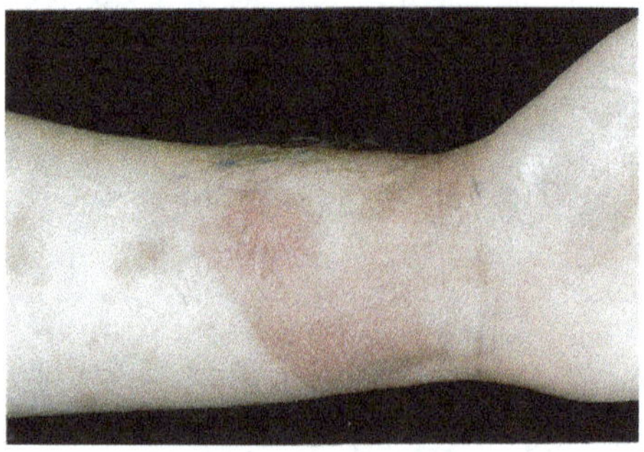

Figure 2: Plaque of mycosis fungoides on the anterior left wrist.

recurrence of the three previously treated areas of MF). Electron beam therapy (2.7 MeV) was given in October 2005 to both areas (30 Gy in 15 fractions over 21 days), and again, complete remission was obtained in the skin of the lateral and the left posterior thigh.

In 2020, he remained in complete remission from MF with no recurrence of any of the five treated areas and no new lesions developing. After living with MF for over 40 years, he has now been in remission for 15 years.

3. Discussion

A case report demonstrating over 50 years of follow-up and treatment for MF has not been published in the world literature before presumably because MF is rare in childhood. There is considerable stress associated with living with cutaneous lymphoma for decades and much relief when complete remission is achieved [7]. This case shows that long-term remission can be achieved with IA disease as has been shown in the Italian and American long-term studies.

The key decision is when to start definitive treatment with electron beam treatment.

The British Association of Dermatologists and UK Cutaneous Lymphoma Group guidelines for the management of primary cutaneous lymphomas were published in 2018 [8]. No guidance is given addressing the age at which treatment with electron beam therapy should be started. In the guidance, it stated that MF is a multifocal disease, and whilst local control with radiotherapy is readily achievable, this is usually a palliative approach. In addition, it was stated that rarely, MF can present as a solitary patch or plaque, and local radiotherapy can be used with curative intent (20–30 Gy in 2 Gy fractions). This dose (30 Gy in 2 Gy fractions) was used for the patient described in this case report with curative intent but to 5 areas rather than one. The European Organisation for Research and Treatment recommendation (2017) is 20–24 Gy in this situation [9]. The patient in this case report has been in remission from MF for more than 15 years.

There should be a detailed discussion with patients with stage IA MF, whose disease involves more than one site, but has not changed over many years, about the possibility of potentially curative treatment with localised electron beam therapy. This discussion could have been started when the patient was in their 40s or 50s rather than at age 60 years as in this case if the curative potential of radiotherapy was better understood.

4. Conclusion

Localised electron beam therapy can be used with curative intent in stage IA MF with more than one lesion if the multiple patches and plaques have been unchanged for several years.

Consent

The patient gave his informed consent for this publication (including the images) and is one of the authors of this case report.

Authors' Contributions

All authors were involved in the collection of medical records over the long time period involved, revised the article, and gave final approval to the submitted manuscript.

References

[1] P. T. Bradford, S. S. Devesa, W. F. Anderson, and J. R. Toro, "Cutaneous lymphoma incidence patterns in the United States: a population-based study of 3884 cases," *Blood*, vol. 113, no. 21, pp. 5064–5073, 2009.

[2] P. Quaglino, N. Pimpinelli, E. Berti et al., "Time course, clinical pathways, and long-term hazards risk trends of disease progression in patients with classic mycosis fungoides," *Cancer*, vol. 118, no. 23, pp. 5830–5839, 2012.

[3] P. M. Laws, N. H. Shear, and E. Pope, "Childhood mycosis fungoides: experience of 28 patients and response to phototherapy," *Pediatric Dermatology*, vol. 31, no. 4, pp. 459–464, 2014.

[4] Y. H. Kim, H. L. Liu, S. Mraz-Gernhard, A. Varghese, and R. T. Hoppe, "Long-term outcome of 525 patients with mycosis fungoides and Sezary syndrome: clinical prognostic factors and risk for disease progression," *Archives of Dermatology*, vol. 139, no. 7, pp. 857–866, 2003.

[5] S. Menni, R. Piccinno, L. Crosti, and E. Berti, "Parapsoriasis in two children: a clinical, immunophenotypic, and immunogenotypic study," *Pediatric Dermatology*, vol. 11, no. 2, pp. 151–155, 1994.

[6] J. Scarisbrick, "Staging of mycosis fungoides and Sezary syndrome: time for an update?" *EMJ Hematology*, vol. 6, no. 1, pp. 92–100, 2018.

[7] F. Sampogna, M. Frontani, G. Baliva et al., "Quality of life and psychological distress in patients with cutaneous lymphoma," *British Journal of Dermatology*, vol. 160, no. 4, pp. 815–822, 2009.

[8] D. Gilson, S. J. Whittaker, F. J. Child et al., "British association of dermatologists and UK cutaneous lymphoma group guidelines for the management of primary cutaneous lymphomas 2018," *British Journal of Dermatology*, vol. 180, no. 3, pp. 496–526, 2019.

[9] F. Trautinger, J. Eder, C. Assaf et al., "European organisation for research and treatment of cancer consensus recommendations for the treatment of mycosis fungoides/Sézary syndrome-update 2017," *European Journal of Cancer*, vol. 77, pp. 57–74, 2017.

25

Trichotemnomania in an Adolescent Girl: A Case Report of an Asian Child and Literature Review

V. Thadchanamoorthy,[1] Markandu Thirukumar,[1] Kavinda Dayasiri,[2] N. Thamilvannan,[3] and Judy Jeyakumar[4]

[1]*Faculty of Health Care Sciences, Eastern University, Sri Lanka*
[2]*Base Hospital, Mahaoya, Sri Lanka*
[3]*Teaching Hospital, Batticaloa, Sri Lanka*
[4]*Department of Psychiatry, Base Hospital, Valaichenai, Sri Lanka*

Correspondence should be addressed to Kavinda Dayasiri; kavindadayasiri@gmail.com

Academic Editor: Alireza Firooz

Trichotemnomania (TT) refers to cutting or shaving of one's own hair as a compulsive act. This condition is reported rarely and may be indicative of an underlying obsessive-compulsive disorder. TT may be misdiagnosed with trichotillomania or other disorders such as alopecia areata, tinea capitis, and postinflammatory scars. The diagnosis of trichotemnomania is confirmed by dermoscopic assessment, histopathological changes of hair, and correlation of these findings with clinical history. A fourteen-year-old adolescent girl presented with focal hair loss over forehead for duration of two-weeks and periodic abnormal breathing and poor sleep for 2-month duration. Besides, she had also lost some of pubic hair and hair on the forearm over preceding 24 hours. This patient was assessed by a team including a paediatrician, gynecologist, dermatologist, and psychiatrist to gather focused medical history and to perform physical examination, laboratory investigations, and dermoscopic assessment. It was revealed that she used to shave or cut regularly following stressful situations across various aspects of her life and hyperventilate as a means of relieving her stress. Eventually, she was diagnosed to have trichotemnomania and was started oral sertraline 50 mg/day for one month. Clinical features and her behaviour improved with regular cognitive behavioural therapy, and hairs were demonstrated to grow up normally with change in behaviour. Currently, she does well at school and is off medications and being followed up at the child guidance clinic. Trichotemnomania is a very rare disorder which is characterised by cutting or shaving of one's own hairs as a compulsive habit. The condition needs careful and detailed assessment by a team of specialists to identify coexisting psychiatric disorders and offer treatment.

1. Background

Trichotemnomania (TT) is an extremely rare and under-assessed condition [1]. It is defined as shaving or cutting of one's own hair anywhere in the body using scissors or a razor, and it has been considered as obsessive-compulsive behaviour [2]. Although trichotillomania has been well-described since 1987 under the Diagnostic and Statistical Manual of Mental Disorders [1], trichotemnomania is rarely reported and likely misdiagnosed. The name trichotemnomania stems from Greek words: thrix (hair), temnein (cut), and mania (madness) [3]. In contrast to trichotemnomania, children with trichotillomania pull their own hairs. Both conditions are self-induced and not convinced to change their routine behaviour [4]. Children with this condition are ashamed due to their behaviour and have psychological pain in them [4]. Unless clinicians have a greater degree of suspicion and perform dermoscopic examination, there is a high probability that the diagnosis remain unexposed and may be misdiagnosed as trichotillomania. The dermatoscopic examination demonstrates healthy-looking hair shafts and is helpful to differentiate trichotemnomania from other similar conditions mimicking the morphological appearance yet with a different pathological diagnosis [4–6]. Only a very limited number of cases with trichotemnomania have been reported in medical literature including three adolescent children [2–7]. The authors present an adolescent girl who had the habit of cutting and shaving her own hair as a means of relieving stress, and the diagnosis of trichotemnomania was confirmed based on clinical history, dermoscopy examination of hair, and histopathological examination by a multidisciplinary group of specialist health professionals. The reported child also was diagnosed to have obsessive-compulsive disorder and currently being followed up in the child guidance clinic under the same multidisciplinary team.

2. Case Presentation

A 14-year-old previously healthy child was referred to the paediatrician by the gynecologist as she had unexplained hair loss on the left side of forehead for two-week duration. She did not have hair loss at any other sites of her body initially. In addition, parents also reported that she had poor sleep at night and also had witnessed abnormal fast breathing from time to time for two months. Her school performance was above average. Family history revealed that her parents were elderly and overprotective but had no similar illness or any other psychiatric illnesses in the family. The patient reported that parents had never allowed this child to have friends or share her problems with friends. Except during school hours, she had no association with her friends. As there was the pandemic of COVID-19, she did not attend school and was missing her school friends.

Physical examination revealed that she is active, pink, and well-grown. There was oval-shaped patch of hair loss on the left forehead (Figure 1). No other hair loss was noted. All other systems examination was normal. The dermatologist suspected the possibility that hair had likely been shaved rather than pulled (trichotillomania) or lost spontaneously. The dermoscopy examination revealed uniform loss of hair with all the hair follicular openings filled with black hair shafts (Figure 2). Furthermore, there was no erythema, tenderness, ulcers, or scaring, and it was confirmed that hair loss was caused by shaving with a blade upon careful history taking. The hair-pull test was negative. Her parents were advised about the nature of her problem, but parents were not convinced at all initially. She was referred to the psychiatrist for further assessment. While waiting for psychological assessment in one-week time, her mother again reported that there was hair loss in the pubic region and hand on the next day (Figure 3). These patches of hair loss were also confirmed to be secondary to shaving rather than pulling of her hairs. The child denied the act of shaving. However, parents were convinced this time and were advised to observe the child as to whether she had any shaving razors or been using her father's shaving razor. Subsequently, the mother could find a razor in her bed room.

The psychiatrist further assessed her and found that she had clinical features of obsessive-compulsive disorder and anxiety behaviour. The final diagnosis was made as trichotemnomania secondary to obsessive-compulsive disorder following multidisciplinary assessment. She was started on sertraline at a dose of 50 mg/day and behaviour modification counselling.

After 3 months of treatment, the medication could be tailed off. Currently, she has been under follow-up at the child guidance clinic and off all medications. As school had been restarted following control of COVID-19 outbreak in the country, she now has an opportunity to make new friends. Her hyperventilation and sleep disorder have also resolved.

3. Discussion

The reported patient had obsessive-compulsive disorder, which is defined as having recurrent, persistent, irresistible thoughts, ideas, impulses, or sensations (obsessions) that make one to feel doing an act repeatedly (compulsive behaviour) to relieve anxiety [8]. Trichotemnomania is induced by anxiety with purpose of avoiding stress. Trichotemnomania is defined as hair loss precipitated by disturbing thoughts and excessive emotional turmoil as patient tries to stop the action and feeling of satisfaction when they do the action [9]. Similar act has been noticed in trichotillomania [10]. These patients may feel ashamed due to their act and appearance, and also they may have feelings of doing this act as a mistake [11]. Patients with trichotemnomania usually have a fair degree of insight [12].

The reported child denied the act which made her parents to consult various specialist health professionals, and clinicians suspected various causes for her hair loss including endocrinological aetiologies. Unexplained symptoms have the potential to make clinicians to perform unnecessary investigations including invasive procedures such as biopsy to exclude other possible differential diagnosis [4–6]. All the possible differentials including systemic lupus erythematous and endocrine abnormalities were ruled out in this child.

As reported in literature [7], this child did not worry about her hair loss and suggested interventions unlike her parents who were worried about their only daughter's future including marriage and physical appearance. She kept on cutting pubic hair and forearm hair even after her first consultation with paediatrician. She reported to her mother that she had hair loss in other sites the following day but denied that she shaved hair. Her act of rejection of the fact that she shaved might be due to feelings of guilty and discomfiture. Similar observations have been made in other reports [6]. Fortunately, she was not commenced on any medications although some clinicians suggested treatment with hematinics at the initial stage of her presentation.

The literature reveals that patches of hair loss in trichotemnomania are often seen in scalp, although it is possible that other sites can be involved including pubis, eye lashes, eyebrows, and axilla [6, 13]. When hair is cut or shaved, dermatoscopy shows presence of the follicle opening with filled hair shaft and an otherwise healthy-looking scalp with no signs of inflammations such as erythema, tenderness ulcers, and scaring. Hair-pull test is negative for

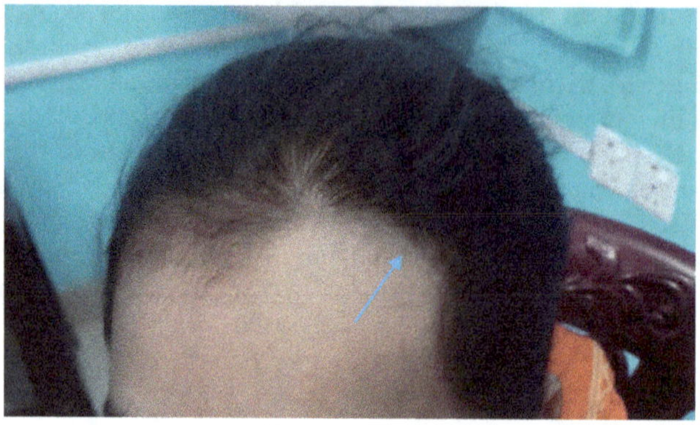

FIGURE 1: Hair loss over the forehead.

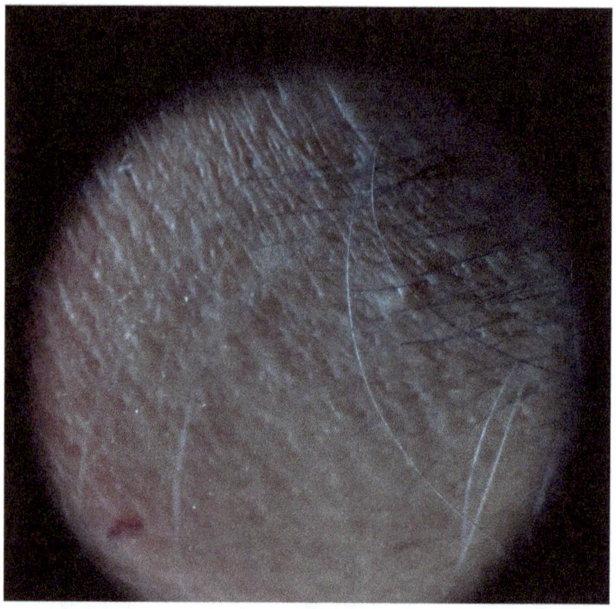

FIGURE 2: Dermoscopic appearance of forehead.

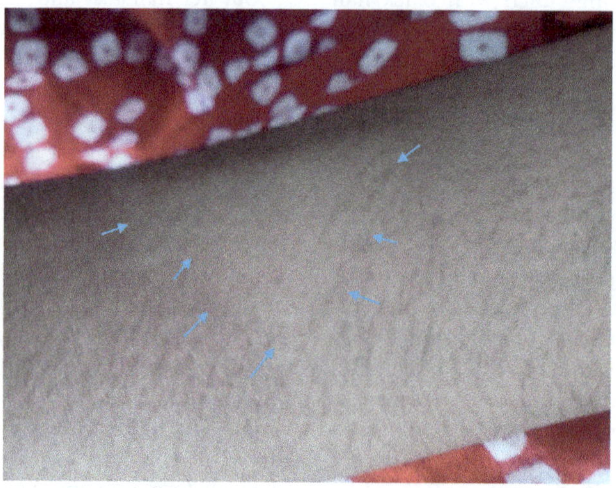

FIGURE 3: Dermoscopic appearance of forearm.

trichotemnomania [3, 4]. Hairs preserve normal pigmentation and texture on the cleanly cut surfaces [14]. The reported child had lesions in forehead, followed by pubic area and forearm, and the dermatoscopic findings are compatible with trichotemnomania.

The differential diagnosis of trichotemnomania includes trichotillomania, trichoteiromania, trichodagonomania, and alopecia areata which all share similar phenotypic appearance, although histopathological findings are different. The only way to differentiate was either dermatoscopic assessment or histopathological assessment [2].

Trichotillomania is common in scalp and occurs also in other sites [6, 13]. The physical appearance comprises irregular and bald patches containing varying lengths of hairs, and histology reveals an increased number of catagen hair follicles with pigment cast, follicular plugging, and trichomalasia [4, 15]. Trichoteiromania is described as hair loss secondary to psychiatric disorders. The affected patient tries to break their hairs by rubbing or scratching of hairs [16]. Their hairs appear as bald spots with different hair lengths as if they were cut by scissors, and white tips associated with distal splitting is a histological feature. The appearance is described as brush-like spitting at the end of the hair shaft on the light microscopy [16, 17]. Tricodagonamania is also another psychiatric disorder, which leads to compulsive habit of biting their own hair and hair loss is not located in the head, and therefore, no loss of hair is present in scalp [18]. Alopecia areata is another differential diagnosis and occurs secondary to autoimmune disease. It can affect any part of the body with patchy boldness over a period of time. Hair-pull test would be positive in alopecia areata. Trichoscopy examination shows yellow dots (hyperkeratotic plugs), small exclamation-mark hairs, and black dots (destroyed hairs in the follicle opening) [19]. Hairs upon regrowth appear to be blonde or white hairs with no pigmentation [14]. Tinea capitis present with single or multiple patchy hair loss secondary to cutaneous fungal infection. It usually accompanies inflammation, scaring, pustules, and itching often leaving black dots. Wood-lamp examination and microscopy can identify the organism [20, 21]. The postinflammatory and posttraumatic scars can also mimic the trichotemnomania following patchy infection or trauma.

The management of obsessive-convulsive disorder prevents the act of compulsive cutting of hairs. The main treatment modality is cognitive-behavioural therapy combined with pharmacological treatment to control obsessive-compulsive behaviour [22]. The reported child was started on both drug treatment and cognitive behavioral therapy. She responded to treatment successfully over 3 months.

Trichotemnomania is a rare, yet underdiagnosed and underreported, condition according to available literature. The clinicians should explore all children presenting with unexplained focal loss of hair in-depth by focused history, and physical examination before an extensive list of investigations would be carried out to arrive at a diagnosis of an underlying organic disorder. The management of trichotemnomania in children is multidisciplinary and involves paediatrician, dermatologist, psychiatrist, and psychologist.

Abbreviations

COVID-19: Coronavirus disease-2019
FSH: Follicular stimulating hormone
LH: Luteinizing hormone
ANA: Antinuclear nuclear antibody.

Consent

Written informed consent was obtained from the patient's legal guardian for publication of this case report.

Authors' Contributions

VT, MT, NT, and JJ performed clinical management of the patient. VT, MT, and KD performed literature survey and wrote and edited the manuscript. All authors read and approved the final version of the manuscript.

Acknowledgments

The authors would like to thank Dr. Dharshini Dilakumar, Consultant Endocrinologist, Teaching Hospital, Batticaloa, for organizing to arrange hormonal assessment for this child.

References

[1] S. R. Chamberlain, B. L. Odlaug, V. Boulougouris, N. A. Fineberg, and J. E. Grant, "Trichotillomania: neurobiology and treatment," *Neuroscience & Biobehavioral Reviews*, vol. 33, no. 6, pp. 831–842, 2009.

[2] S. Gallouj, S. Rabhi, H. Baybay et al., "Trichotemnomanie associée à une trichotillomanie: intérêt diagnostique de la dermoscopie," *Annales de Dermatologie et de Vénéréologie*, vol. 138, no. 2, pp. 140-141, 2011.

[3] O. Braun-Falco and V. P. Trichotemnomania, "A special skin manifestation of a cerebral-organic psycho-syndrome," *Hautarzt*, vol. 19, pp. 551–553, 1968.

[4] J. Orgaz-Molina, H. Husein-ElAhmed, M. Soriano-HernÃ ¡ndez, and S. Arias-Santiago, "Trichotemnomania: hair loss mediated by a compulsive habit not admitted by patients," *Acta Dermato Venereologica*, vol. 92, no. 2, pp. 183-184, 2012.

[5] H. Meiers, "Trichotemnomania," *Hautarzt*, vol. 22, pp. 335–337, 1971.

[6] R. Happle, "Trichotemnomania: obsessive-compulsive habit of cutting or shaving the hair," *Journal of the American Academy of Dermatology*, vol. 52, no. 1, pp. 157–159, 2005.

[7] Ş. Eray and b Bilge Ateş, "Three adolescent cases of a very rare disorder: *Trichotemnomania*," *Psychiatry and Clinical Psychopharmacology*, vol. 29, no. 2, pp. 212–215, 2019.

[8] "Obsessive-compulsive disorder," in *American Psychiatric Association: Diagnostic and Statistical Manual of Mental Disorders*p. 457, American Psychiatric Association, Washington, DC, 2000.

[9] G. A. Christenson and S. J. Crow, "The characterization and treatment of trichotillomania," *The Journal of Clinical Psychiatry*, vol. 57, pp. 42–49, 1996.
[10] J. A. Cotteril, "Trichotillomania: a manipulative alopecia?" *International Journal of Dermatology*, vol. 32, pp. 182-183, 1993.
[11] G. J. Diefenbach, D. F. Tolin, S. Hannan, J. Crocetto, and P. Worhunsky, "Trichotillomania: impact on psychosocial functioning and quality of life," *Behaviour Research and Therapy*, vol. 43, no. 7, pp. 869–884, 2005.
[12] T. H. Zhu, M. Nakamura, B. Farahnik et al., "Obsessive-compulsive skin disorders: a novel classification based on degree of insight," *Journal of Dermatological Treatment*, vol. 28, no. 4, pp. 342–346, 2017.
[13] A. Chiriac, P. Brzezinski, T. Pinteala, A. E. Chiriac, and L. Foia, "Common psychocutaneous disorders in children," *Neuropsychiatric Disease and Treatment*, vol. 11, pp. 333–337, 2015.
[14] D. J. Cline, "Changes in hair color," *Dermatologic Clinics*, vol. 6, no. 2, pp. 295–303, 1988.
[15] S. A. Muller and R. K. Winkelmann, "Trichotillomania," *Archives of Dermatology*, vol. 105, no. 4, pp. 535–539, 1972.
[16] P. Freyschmidt-Paul, R. Hoffmannn, and R. Happle, "Trichoteiromania," *European Journal of Dermatology*, vol. 11, pp. 369–371, 2001.
[17] S. Reich and R. M. Trüeb, "Trichoteiromanie," *JDDG: Journal der Deutschen Dermatologischen Gesellschaft*, vol. 1, no. 1, pp. 22–28, 2003.
[18] M. Jafferany, J. Feng, and R. L. Hornung, "Trichodaganomania: the compulsive habit of biting one's own hair," *Journal of the American Academy of Dermatology*, vol. 60, no. 4, pp. 689–691, 2009.
[19] L. Rudnicka, M. Olszewska, A. Rakowska, E Kowalska-Oledzka, and M Slowinska, "Trichoscopy: a new method for diagnosing hair loss," *Journal of Drugs in Dermatology: JDD*, vol. 7, no. 7, pp. 651–654, 2008.
[20] I. M. Freedberg and T. B. Fitzpatrick, *Fitzpatrick's Dermatology in General Medicine*, p. 645, McGraw-Hill, Medical Pub. Division, New York, NY, USA, 2003.
[21] S. Ali, T. A. D. Graham, and S. E. D. Forgie, "The assessment and management of tinea capitis in children," *Pediatric Emergency Care*, vol. 23, no. 9, pp. 662–665, 2007.
[22] J. S. Phillip and E. Hollander, "Management of obsessive-compulsive disorder F1000Prime," *Rep*, vol. 6, p. 68, 2014.

26

Dercum's Disease: A Case Report of a Patient having Both Type 1 and Type 2 Dercum's Disease

Cameron Moattari,[1] Richard A. Giovane,[2] and Stephanie DiGiovanni Kinsely[3]

[1]*State University of New York Downstate Medical Center, Brooklyn, NY 11203, USA*
[2]*Regional Medical Center of Central Alabama, Family Medicine, 29L V Stabler Drive, Greenville, AL 36037, USA*
[3]*University of Alabama, Department of Family Medicine, 801 Campus Drive, Tuscaloosa, AL 35487, USA*

Correspondence should be addressed to Richard A. Giovane; richardgiovane357@gmail.com

Academic Editor: Sergio A. Cuevas Covarrubias

Dercum's disease, or adiposis dolorosa, is a rare disorder which consists of multiple, painful lipomas within the subcutaneous tissue and has a distribution mainly in the abdomen and extremities. Dercum's disease can be defined as in combination with chronic painful adipose tissue. Although the etiology of Dercum's disease is not clear, it is thought to be a combination of a neurological and endocrine disorder. Treatment for this disease is centered at managing pain. Although there is no standard of care for managing pain, there are different pain management regimes that are promising.

1. Introduction

Dercum's disease is a rare disorder characterized by chronic pain due to multiple lipomas in the adipose tissue [1]. Epidemiology for the condition is not defined, but the literature suggests a higher prevalence in obese females, aged 35–50 [1].The disease is often accompanied by a number of associated symptoms such as weakness, fatigue, depression, and dementia [2]. The painful adipose tissue can be diffuse and generalized or concentrated in palpable lipomas [3]. The most commonly affected locations are the extremities, the trunk, the pelvic area, and the buttocks [4].The diagnosis of Dercum's disease is a diagnosis of exclusion and is made clinically, although imaging can be helpful. Effective treatment for patients with Dercum's disease is currently lacking as there is no effective long term treatment. The approach to management of Dercum's disease involves pain control through oral medications or direct injections or surgical removal. Surgical interventions, however, such as liposuction and lipectomy have varying outcomes [5, 6], and direct lidocaine injections into the lipomas have been shown to provide only short-term pain relief [7]. Many case reports of treatment with various medications such as corticosteroids and experimental therapies exist in the literature, but large-scale studies are lacking.

2. Case Presentation

We present a case of a 48-year-old female who presented to the clinic for established care. The patient had just been discharged from hospice care due to chronic pain secondary to Dercum's disease. Upon chart review, the patient had a medical history of type 2 diabetes, Hashimoto's disease, migraines, and obesity. Regarding her diagnosis of Dercum's disease, a chart review revealed that the patient began having episodic bouts of generalized pain starting at the age of 40. The pain rate was 7–10/10 during her episodes and could last minutes to days, with the longest episode of generalized pain lasting for 32 days. She also began experiencing migraines along with the pain, accompanied by auras as well as blurry vision and photophobia. Her episodes of pain became more frequent, and she began noticing tender lumps around her abdomen. During one episode, she went to the emergency room due to severe pain. Although her medical records could not be obtained, according to her husband, her lab tests were unremarkable; however, a CT scan of her abdomen revealed many small masses in her subcutaneous tissue. Attempts to obtain the CT scan images were not successful as her husband could not recall the specific emergency room she went to. Subsequent biopsies of the masses revealed histopathologic characteristics of lipomas. The patient's clinical picture was in favor of the diagnosis of Dercum's disease. The patient was discharged and was told to follow-up with her primary care doctor, as well as she was given an appointment with an endocrinologist. The patient saw the endocrinologist for further evaluation, and the patient was diagnosed as having both type I and type II Dercum's disease as she initially had widespread pain in her adipose tissue and then developed painful lipomas. She was referred to physical therapy and was managed in an outpatient setting for years for her pain control which included oxycodone 10 mg BID, ibuprofen 800 mg TID, and alprazolam 0.5 mg TID PRN for anxiety. Upon presentation at the clinic, the patient was accompanied by her husband for established care. The patient reported severe constant diffuse pain, poor appetite, and difficulty sleeping because of the pain. A physical exam revealed multiple mobile, tender masses on her neck, arms, chest, and abdomen. The patient was referred to pain management and hospice care for further evaluation and management. Eventually, the patient was lost to follow-up, and means of communication went unanswered

3. Discussion

Dercum's disease, or adiposis dolorosa, is a rare disorder consisting of multiple, painful lipomas subcutaneously distributed mainly on the trunk and extremities [1]. Historically, the associated symptoms in Dercum's disease include easy bruisability, sleep disturbances, impared memory, depression, difficulty concentrating, anxiety, diabetes, fatigue, weakness, and joint aches, yet these symptoms are not always present [2]. The minimum definition of Dercum's disease proposed by Hansson et al. is generalized as overweight or obesity in combination with chronic (>3 months) painful adipose tissue [2]. Dercum's disease has been suggested to be classified into 4 distinct variants: type I—the generalized diffuse form presenting with widespread painful adipose tissue with no apparent lipomas; type II—the generalized nodular form presenting with widespread, painful adipose tissue with increased pain surrounding lipomas; type III—the localized nodular form presenting with pain strictly surrounding lipomas; and type IV—the juxta-articular form, presenting as painful adipose tissue near large joints, usually the medial knee [2]. Most cases of Dercum's disease occur sporadically although several reports suggest an autosomal dominant inheritance pattern with a possible genetic heterogeneity favoring women [2]. In the case presented, our patient was diagnosed with having both type I and type II per the endocrinologist in which she saw. It was supported by the fact that she initially had widespread painful tissue which then developed painful lipomas.

Diagnosis of Dercum's disease is based mainly on physical examination after other diagnoses have been ruled out. Such differential diagnoses to consider are fibromyalgia, lipoedema, panniculitis, endocrine disorders, primary psychiatric disorders, multiple symmetric lipomatosis, familial multiple lipomatosis, and adipose tissue tumours. Imaging may aid in diagnosis. MRI may demonstrate multiple small, oblong, fatty lesions in the subcutaneous tissue with a nodular increased fluid signal that appears "blush-like." Ultrasound may show hyperechoic nodules [4]. There are no clear laboratory markers for the condition. ESR or CPR may be elevated, while autoimmune disease markers are usually negative [2]. One study found that adipose IL-6 and IL-13 levels were significantly elevated in women with Dercum's disease compared to matched controls, while Fractalkine and MIP-1b levels were significantly lower. IL-6, IL-13, Fractalkine, and MIP-1b are glycoproteins and chemokines that are proinflammatory. The clinical significance of these findings is unclear [8]. Regional bioimpedance measures can help in distinguishing lipoedema from Dercum's disease [9].

The etiology of Dercum's disease is not clear. Several theories have been proposed, yet none demonstrates clear evidence. Endocrine and nervous system dysfunction have been suspected but never proven to be implicated. Stretching and pressure on nerves from growing lipomas has been suggested but never shown histopathologically [2]. Lipid metabolism has also been suggested as fatty acid composition determined by gas chromatography/mass spectrometry showed a statistically significantly lower vaccenic acid/stearic acid desaturation index of subcutaneous adipose tissue between participants with Dercum's disease compared with control participants [7]. Inflammation has also been suggested but not been shown to vary significantly on histopathology between fat biopsies of painful and non-painful areas in patients with Dercum's disease, or compared with obese control patients [10].

Treatment for Dercum's disease revolves around managing pain. Currently, there is no standard of therapy but several options described in numerous case reports exist for reducing symptoms. Lifestyle interventions such as diet and exercise have not been shown to reduce painful fatty tissue. Surgical interventions such as liposuction or lipectomy subjectively improve pain measurements, although this effect diminishes over time. One case report showed reduced pain and increased mobility in 4 patients with the juxta-articular form after dermolipectomy of the medial knee [8]. The utility of surgery in relation to the inherent risks has been called into question, and further research is required [8–10]. Lidocaine injection directly into lipomas has been shown to provide pain relief for up to 4 months [11]. Moreover, intravenous lidocaine showed improvement of pain for up to 9 months [12]. Many medications have been shown to improve pain. NSAIDs were traditionally thought to be ineffective, but a study by Herbst et al. showed reduced pain in 89% of patients with Dercum's disease ($n = 89$) [2, 13, 14]. Corticosteroids given orally or through injection have not been shown to provide any benefit, and one case study showed a link between corticosteroid use and the development of Dercum's disease [15]. In addition, case reports exist supporting the potential use of pregabalin [16], D-amphetamine [16], metformin [17], interferon alfa-2b [18], infliximab, and methotrexate [19] in managing pain. Several novel and noninvasive procedures have also been described as beneficial. Treatment with transcutaneous frequency rhythmic electrical modulation system over 6 months improved pain assessment and reduced subcutaneous adipose tissue in one man with Dercum's disease [20]. A group of 10 patients with Dercum's disease reported improvement in pain after 5 days of rapidly cycling hypobaric pressure [21]. Four weeks of subcutaneous adipose tissue therapy, a form of deep tissue massage, demonstrated a significant decrease in weight but no change in pain scores in several women with Dercum's disease [22]. Randomized, controlled trials are needed to confirm the data described in these studies.

4. Conclusion

Dercum's disease is a rare condition that is characterized by painful lipomas and other nonspecific symptoms. Patients with this condition are difficult to diagnose due to its rarity and differing presentations. Managing patients with this condition can prove to be difficult as there is no standard of care for symptom control.

Abbreviations

CT: Computed tomography
IL-6/13: Interleukin-6/13
MIP-1b: Macrophage inflammatory protein-1b
MRI: Magnetic resonance imaging.

References

[1] K. L. Herbst and S. Asare-Bediako, "Adiposis dolorosa is more than painful fat," *The Endocrinologist*, vol. 17, no. 6, pp. 326–334, 2007.

[2] E. Hansson, H. Svensson, and H. Brorson, "Review of dercum's disease and proposal of diagnostic criteria, diagnostic methods, classification and management," *Orphanet Journal of Rare Diseases*, vol. 7, no. 1, p. 23, 2012.

[3] E. Hansson, J. Manjer, H. Svensson, and H. Brorson, "Quality-of-life in patients with dercum's disease-before and after liposuction," *Journal of Plastic Surgery and Hand Surgery*, vol. 46, no. 3-4, pp. 252–256, 2012.

[4] D. Masic, E. Liang, C. Long, E. J. Sterk, B. Barbas, and M. A. Rech, "Intravenous lidocaine for acute pain: a systematic review," *Pharmacotherapy: The Journal of Human Pharmacology and Drug Therapy*, vol. 38, no. 12, pp. 1250–1259, 2018.

[5] B. J. Tins, C. Matthews, M. Haddaway et al., "Adiposis dolorosa (dercum's disease): MRI and ultrasound appearances," *Clinical Radiology*, vol. 68, no. 10, pp. 1047–1053, 2013.

[6] K. L. Herbst, A. D. Coviello, A. Chang, and D. L. Boyle, "Lipomatosis-associated inflammation and excess collagen may contribute to lower relative resting energy expenditure in women with adiposis dolorosa," *International Journal of Obesity*, vol. 33, no. 9, pp. 1031–1038, 2009.

[7] R. Crescenzi, P. M. C. Donahue, S. Weakley, M. Garza, M. J. Donahue, and K. L. Herbst, "Lipedema and dercum's disease: a new application of bioimpedance," *Lymphatic Research and Biology*, vol. 17, no. 6, pp. 671–679, August 2019.

[8] J. K. Yee, S. A. Phillips, K. Allamehzadeh, and K. L. Herbst, "Subcutaneous adipose tissue fatty acid desaturation in adults with and without rare adipose disorders," *Lipids in Health and Disease*, vol. 11, no. 1, p. 19, 2012.

[9] E. Hansson, H. Svensson, U. Stenram, and H. Brorson, "Histology of adipose tissue inflammation in dercum's disease, obesity and normal weight controls: a case control study," *Journal of Inflammation*, vol. 8, no. 1, p. 24, 2011.

[10] U. Wollina, B. Heinig, D. Langner, and A. Nowak, "Juxta-articular adiposis dolorosa (dercum's disease type IV): report of four cases and treatment by dermolipectomy," *Wiener Medizinische Wochenschrift*, vol. 165, no. 17-18, pp. 374–377, 2015.

[11] E. Hansson, H. Svensson, and H. Brorson, "Liposuction may reduce pain in dercum's disease (adiposis dolorosa)," *Pain Medicine*, vol. 12, no. 6, pp. 942–952, 2011.

[12] R. L. Atkinson, "Intravenous lidocaine for the treatment of intractable pain of adiposis dolorosa," *International Journal of Obesity*, vol. 6, no. 4, Article ID 7129748, 351–357 pages, 1982.

[13] U. Wollina, A. Goldman, and B. Heinig, "Microcannular tumescent liposuction in advanced lipedema and dercum's disease," *Giornale italiano di dermatologia e venereologia: organo ufficiale, Societa italiana di dermatologia e sifilografia*, vol. 145, no. 2, pp. 151–159, 2010.

[14] U. Lange, P. Oelzner, and C. Uhlemann, "Dercum's disease (lipomatosis dolorosa): successful therapy with pregabalin and manual lymphatic drainage and a current overview," *Rheumatology International*, vol. 29, no. 1, pp. 17–22, 2008.

[15] S. S. Greenbaum and J. Varga, "Corticosteroid-induced juxta-articular adiposis dolorosa," *ArchDermatol*, vol. 127, no. 2, Article ID 231233, 1991.

[16] S. Ghazala, J. Bilal, E. Ross, I. B. Riaz, B. Kalb, and K. L. Herbst, "Low-dose d-amphetamine induced regression of liver fat deposits in dercum disease," *The American Journal of Medicine*, vol. 131, no. 6, pp. 705–708, 2018.

[17] K. Łabuzek, S. Liber, D. Suchy, and B. Okopień, "A successful case of pain management using metformin in a patient with adiposis dolorosa," *International Journal of Clinical Pharmacology and Therapeutics*, vol. 51, no. 6, pp. 517–524, 2013.

[18] Z. Gonciarz, W. Mazur, J. Hartleb et al., "Interferon alfa-2b induced long-term relief of pain in two patients with adiposis dolorosa and chronic hepatitis C," *Journal of Hepatology*, vol. 27, no. 6, p. 1141, 1997.

[19] A. Singal, J. J. Janiga, N. M. Bossenbroek, and H. W. Lim, "Dercum's disease (adiposis dolorosa): a report of improvement with infliximab and methotrexate," *Journal of the European Academy of Dermatology and Venereology*, vol. 21, no. 5, p. 717, 2007.

[20] S. Martinenghi, A. Caretto, C. Losio, M. Scavini, and E. Bosi, "Successful treatment of dercum's disease by transcutaneous electrical stimulation: a case report," *Medicine (Baltimore)*, vol. 94, no. 24, p. e950, 2015.

[21] K. Herbst and T. Rutledge, "Pilot study: rapidly cycling hypobaric pressure improves pain after 5 days in adiposis dolorosa," *Journal of Pain Research*, vol. 3, pp. 147–153, 2010.

[22] M. Ibarra, A. Eekema, C. Ussery, D. Neuhardt, K. Garby, and K. L. Herbst, "Subcutaneous adipose tissue therapy reduces fat by dual X-ray absorptiometry scan and improves tissue structure by ultrasound in women with lipoedema and dercum disease," *Clinical Obesity*, vol. 8, no. 6, pp. 398–406, 2018.

27

A Rare Case of Porocarcinoma and Trichoblastoma Arising in a Nevus Sebaceus of Jadassohn

Drew C. Mitchell,[1] Gina J. Kuehn,[2] Glynis A. Scott,[2,3] Timothy D. Doerr,[4] and Francisco Tausk[2]

[1]*University of Rochester School of Medicine & Dentistry, 601 Elmwood Avenue Box 400, Rochester, NY 14642, USA*
[2]*Department of Dermatology, University of Rochester Medical Center, 40 Celebration Drive, Rochester, NY 14642, USA*
[3]*Department of Pathology, University of Rochester Medical Center, 601 Elmwood Avenue Box 626, Rochester, NY 14642, USA*
[4]*Department of Otolaryngology, University of Rochester Medical Center, 601 Elmwood Avenue Box 629, Rochester, NY 14642, USA*

Correspondence should be addressed to Drew C. Mitchell; dmitche2@bidmc.harvard.edu

Academic Editor: Sergio A. Cuevas Covarrubias

Nevus sebaceus of Jadassohn, or "organoid nevus," is a common, benign hamartoma of the skin consisting of epithelial and adnexal components. Its natural history and association with neoplastic growths is well documented. The majority of concomitant neoplasms are benign—trichoblastoma and syringocystadenoma papilliferum are most frequently discovered—but malignant tumors have been described. We present the case of a 58-year-old male with a congenital nevus sebaceus of Jadassohn on his left parietal scalp that had been enlarging, changing color, and bleeding over the prior year. Clinical exam and histology disclosed the presence of a trichoblastoma and porocarcinoma arising within the nevus sebaceus. Porocarcinoma is a rare, intermediately aggressive, malignant eccrine gland tumor that is frequently metastasized at presentation. Otolaryngology performed wide local resection with sentinel lymph node biopsy. This case highlights the diversity of tumors associated with nevus sebaceus of Jadassohn, potential for malignant expansion, and necessity for close monitoring and maintaining a low threshold for biopsy in evolving lesions.

1. Introduction

Nevus sebaceus of Jadassohn (NSJ), also known as "organoid nevus," is a common, benign hamartoma composed of abnormally developed hair follicles, papillomatous epidermal hyperplasia, and ectopic apocrine glands that presents at birth or in early childhood [1–4]. Typically, NSJ presents as a single, sharply demarcated yellow-orange plaque on the scalp, often with accompanying alopecia [3, 4]. It is identified in approximately 0.3% of neonates [4] and has an incidence of 0.05–1.0% in dermatology patients [2, 4].

The natural history of NSJ and its association with neoplastic growths is richly documented such that 'Tumoral' is the accepted final developmental stage [4]. Although the overwhelming majority of neoplasms that arise in NSJ are benign, malignancies have been consistently discovered, and the risk of neoplasia—benign or malignant—increases with age [1–3]; however, to the best of the authors' knowledge, this is the first multitumoral case involving a porocarcinoma. We report a rare case of porocarcinoma and trichoblastoma arising in an NSJ.

2. Case Report

A 58-year-old male presented for an evolving mass on his left scalp. The mass was noted at birth and had been enlarging, changing color, and bleeding over the past 12 months. On exam, a 3.0 cm × 3.0 cm yellow-to-tan verrucous, papulated plaque with central, large pink, and violaceous-to-blue nodules was present on the left posterior parietal scalp with overlying alopecia (Figure 1).

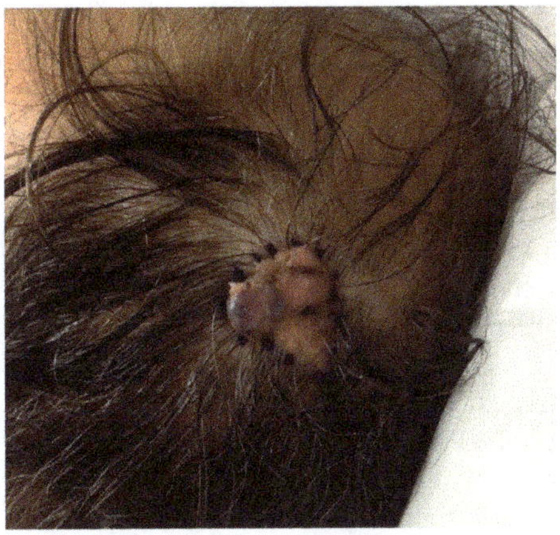

FIGURE 1: Clinical appearance of left parietal lesion at presentation to dermatology clinic.

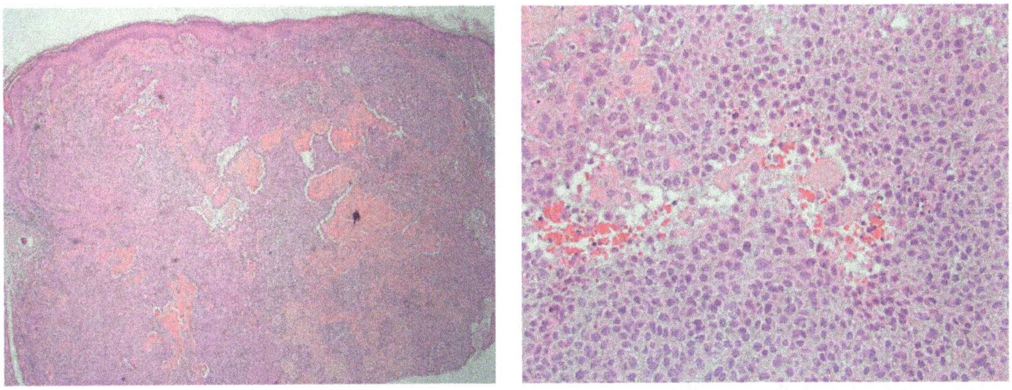

(a) (b)

FIGURE 2: (a) Scanning micrograph of the porocarcinoma shows an expansile tumor arising from the epidermis with extension deep into the reticular dermis (hematoxylin and eosin, 4x). (b) Higher power shows focal necrosis of the tumor which displays cytologic atypia, including mitotic figures (hematoxylin and eosin, 20x).

A shave biopsy of the entire lesion was performed. Pathology disclosed changes consistent with an organoid nevus with two distinct neoplasms within. A basaloid tumor arising from the epidermis with a focal ribbon and pigmented pattern consistent with trichoblastoma and an adjacent downgrowth of atypical squamous epithelium with dysplasia and easily identified mitotic figures with a glassy stroma and eccrine differentiation consistent with porocarcinoma (Figures 2(a) and 2(b)). Immunohistochemical stains against cytokeratin 7 highlighted portions of the tumor.

The patient was referred to otolaryngology for wide local resection with sentinel lymph node biopsy. There was no parotid gland enlargement or palpable anterior or posterior cervical lymphadenopathy. Wide local excision (6 cm × 6 cm with 1.5 cm to 2 cm margins) was performed with sentinel lymph node biopsy from the left tail of the parotid identified through nuclear medicine. Reconstruction was with opposing transposition flaps.

Surgical pathology revealed no residual porocarcinoma in the scalp specimen and negative sentinel lymph nodes; therefore, no further treatment, including chemotherapy, was indicated. Three years later, the patient remained disease free.

3. Discussion

Nevus sebaceus of Jadassohn is a common, congenital lesion that overwhelmingly presents on the head with a special affinity for the scalp and persists throughout life [1–3, 5]. Generally, it evolves from a smooth bald patch in infancy to a raised cerebriform lesion in adulthood [4]. While not fully elucidated, the etiology of NSJ is thought to result from stem cell genomic mosaicism that expands the distribution of the lines of Blaschko [3].

NSJ's association with secondary neoplasms is well established. It is estimated that 10–21% of NSJs develop a tumor [1, 2, 5]; however, since there are no prospective follow-up studies of NSJ, it is likely that this number is biased and overinflated. Moreover, greater than 90% of these tumors are benign [1–5].

Historically, it was thought that basal cell carcinomas (BCC) were the most common neoplasm complicating NSJ, but studies from the early 1990s and forward have confirmed that what was previously believed to be BCC were, in fact, misdiagnosed trichoblastomas [1, 5]. It is now accepted that trichoblastoma and syringocystadenoma papilliferum are the two most common neoplasms in NSJ, each occurring in approximately 5% of NSJ [1, 2, 4, 5]. BCC is the most common malignant neoplasm associated with NSJ [2, 5]. NSJs are often surgically removed for cosmesis but due to low rates of tumor development, especially malignant, prophylactic removal is no longer recommended [3, 4].

Porocarcinoma is the most common malignant eccrine gland tumor and accounts for an estimated 0.005–0.01% of all cutaneous tumors [6, 7]. Its etiology is poorly understood, but it can arise primarily or secondarily; preexisting eccrine poroma, exposure to chemical agents, chronic light exposure, and immunosuppression are all thought to be potential contributing factors for its genesis [7, 8].

Porocarcinomas present as a solitary nodule or mass involving the lower extremities—head/neck and upper extremity lesions are seen about equally [6–9]. The scalp is an uncommon site of presentation with less than 20 reported cases in the literature [9]. There is a strong predilection toward older age groups (7th-8th decade of life) and inconsistent reports regarding gender preference [7–9].

Porocarcinomas are an intermediately aggressive tumor with metastatic disease at presentation in up to 31% of cases, most frequently involving regional lymph nodes (60%) and the lungs (13%) [6–8]. When metastases are discovered, mortality is high: 80% in distant disease and 65–67% when lymph nodes are involved [6, 7]. Wide local resection is the mainstay of treatment with adjuvant chemoradiotherapy added for metastatic disease or local recurrence [6–9]. Despite therapy, there is a 20% recurrence rate [7, 9].

The only case describing a porocarcinoma developing in an NSJ was reported in 1985 by Tarkhan and Domingo where the lesion also arose on the scalp but had postauricular extension and metastasis [10]. Previous reports of porocarcinomas document that those located on the head/neck had the lowest incidence of lymph node metastasis at the time of diagnosis, as compared with other anatomical locations [7]. It is unclear if porocarcinomas arising within NSJ obey the same tendencies as those developing elsewhere. Additionally, NSJs on the scalp are more regularly complicated by neoplastic growths than NSJs in other locations [5].

In our case, the patient demonstrated a porocarcinoma that arose adjacent to a trichoblastoma. There are several reports of multiple neoplasms developing in a single NSJ [1, 2], and trichoblastoma is the tumor most likely to cooccur with another neoplasm [2]. Although the relationship of trichoblastoma to multiple neoplastic growths may simply be a function of its relatively high incidence in NSJ, this would not explain why it is seen more commonly than in syringocystadenoma papilliferum. To the best of our knowledge, this is the first reported case of the simultaneous appearance of a porocarcinoma and another tumor arising in an NSJ.

This case highlights the potential for malignant expansion in NSJ, the diversity of tumors that arise within it, and the clinical necessity of closely monitoring the evolution of these lesions and maintaining a low threshold for biopsy.

Disclosure

All authors, except Drew Mitchell, were employed by the University of Rochester Medical Center. Drew Mitchell was a medical student at the University of Rochester School of Medicine and Dentistry.

References

[1] G. Jaqueti, L. Requena, and E. Sánchez Yus, "Trichoblastoma is the most common neoplasm developed in nevus sebaceus of Jadassohn: a clinicopathologic study of a series of 155 cases," *The American Journal of Dermatopathology*, vol. 22, no. 2, pp. 108–118, 2000.

[2] M. H. Idriss and D. M. Elston, "Secondary neoplasms associated with nevus sebaceus of Jadassohn: a study of 707 cases," *Journal of the American Academy of Dermatology*, vol. 70, no. 2, pp. 332–337, 2014.

[3] D. B. Eisen and D. J. Michael, "Sebaceous lesions and their associated syndromes: part I," *Journal of the American Academy of Dermatology*, vol. 61, no. 4, pp. 549–560, 2009.

[4] M. A. Muñoz-Pérez, M. J. García-Hernandez, J. J. Ríos, and F. Camacho, "Sebaceus naevi: a clinicopathologic study," *Journal of the European Academy of Dermatology and Venereology*, vol. 16, no. 4, pp. 319–324, 2002.

[5] B. Cribier, Y. Scrivener, and E. Grosshans, "Tumors arising in nevus sebaceus: a study of 596 cases," *Journal of the American Academy of Dermatology*, vol. 42, no. 2, pp. 263–268, 2000.

[6] A. M. Salih, F. H. Kakamad, R. A. Essa et al., "Porocarcinoma: a systematic review of literature with a single case report," *Journal of Surgery Case Reports*, vol. 30, pp. 13–16, 2017.

[7] A. Nazemi, S. Higgins, R. Swift, G. In, K. Miller, and A. Wysong, "Eccrine porocarcinoma," *Dermatologic Surgery*, vol. 44, no. 10, pp. 1247–1261, 2018.

[8] A. M. Salih, F. H. Kakamad, H. O. Baba et al., "Porocarcinoma; presentation and management, a meta-analysis of 453 cases," *Annals of Medicine and Surgery*, vol. 20, pp. 74–79, 2017.

[9] W. Melgandi, R. Benson, A. Hakin, and S. Bhasker, "Porocarcinoma scalp with high risk features treated with surgery and adjuvant radiotherapy: a case report and review of literature," *Journal of the Egyptian National Cancer Institute*, vol. 28, no. 3, pp. 195–198, 2016.

[10] I. I. Tarkhan and J. Domingo, "Metastasizing eccrine porocarcinoma developing in a sebaceous nevus of Jadassohn. Report of a case," *Archives of Dermatology*, vol. 121, no. 3, pp. 413–415, 1985.

Use of Reflectance Confocal Microscopy for Hidrocystomas: An Emerging, Cost-Effective and Powerful Tool

Amanda Walker[1] **Vikram Nath Sahni**[2] **Dev Ram Sahni**[3] **and Julia Curtis**[3]

[1]*University of Utah, School of Medicine, Salt Lake City, UT 84132, USA*
[2]*Drexel University, College of Medicine, Philadelphia, PA 19129, USA*
[3]*University of Utah School of Medicine, Department of Dermatology, Salt Lake City, UT 84132, USA*

Correspondence should be addressed to Dev Ram Sahni; sahnidr@vcu.edu

Academic Editor: Hristo Dobrev

Reflectance confocal microscopy (RCM) is an emerging and noninvasive imaging tool in dermatological practice. Benefits of this modality include differentiation between benign and malignant skin lesions, prevention of unnecessary biopsies, and cost effectiveness. However, RCM findings for benign lesions are rarely reported in the literature. We describe a case of reflectance confocal microscopy findings of a hidrocystoma and review potential applications of this imaging technique in everyday clinical practice.

1. Introduction

In vivo reflectance confocal microscopy (RCM) is a powerful and noninvasive imaging tool. RCM can be utilized in conjunction with dermoscopy to differentiate between malignant and benign cutaneous lesions. However, because most benign lesions are rarely imaged, the differentiation between malignant and benign skin lesions such as hidrocystomas when using RCM can be difficult.

Hidrocystomas are benign cystic tumors composed of eccrine or apocrine sweat glands [1, 2]. Eccrine hidrocystomas are located in the periorbital and malar regions and have a female predilection. Apocrine hidrocystomas present on the head, neck, and eyelid margin and occur equally in both genders [1, 2]. Hidrocystomas typically present as dome-shaped papules. Eccrine hidrocystomas are flesh-colored to light blue and smaller in size (1–6 mm), whereas apocrine hidrocystomas are dark blue to black and larger in size (3–15 mm) [1, 2]. Although these lesions are benign clinically, they are often mistaken for basal cell carcinoma, syringomas, milia, and blue nevi [1, 2]. Additionally, hidrocystomas can sometimes share similar dermoscopic features with basal cell carcinoma such as a blue-gray hue, making diagnosis without biopsy difficult [3, 4].

Through utilization of RCM, providers can detect smaller malignant neoplasms and avoid unnecessary painful and scarring biopsies, as well as prevent further morbidity from missed neoplastic diagnoses [5]. We describe a case of RCM findings of a hidrocystoma and explain the utility and application of this tool in clinical practice.

2. History of the Present Illness

A patient presented to the clinic for a skin check. On exam, there was a 3–4 mm grey shiny papule on the left medial lower eyelid. Dermoscopic exam revealed few vessels and a grey hue. RCM revealed a homogenous tubular cyst-like structure (Figure 1). Cutaneous biopsy revealed a cystic structure lined by a double layer of epithelial cells with decapitation secretion, confirming the diagnosis of hidrocystoma (Figure 2).

3. Discussion

Reflectance confocal microscopy can be a cost-effective, sensitive, and specific tool and is gaining popularity in ophthalmological and dermatological practice. RCM is more sensitive than slit-lamp examination for identification of

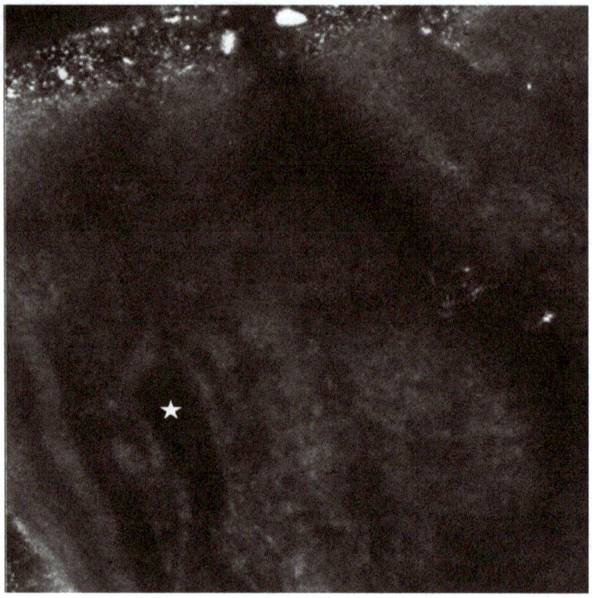

FIGURE 1: Homogenous tubular cyst-like structure (indicated by the star). The CaliberID 3000 handheld device was utilized. The depth of this image was taken at 60 μm.

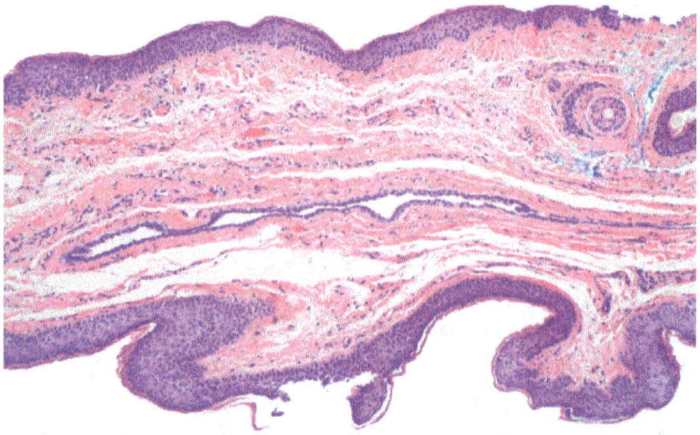

FIGURE 2: A cystic space lined by two layers of epithelial cells. Decapitation secretion can also be seen in the cyst-like space (100x H and E).

basal cell carcinoma involving the eyelid margin and conjunctiva [6]. Furthermore, reflectance confocal microscopy was in concordance with histopathologic findings in 48 of 49 BCCs, demonstrating a sensitivity of 98% for the diagnosis of basal cell carcinoma [6]. While RCM findings for BCC are well known in the literature, those for hidrocystomas are severely lacking. RCM features of hidrocystomas include homogenous cystic structures adjacent to normal-appearing adnexal structures lacking tumor islands or silhouettes [2]. The most common clinical differential diagnosis for hidrocystomas includes basal cell carcinoma, syringomas, blue nevi, and milia. While clinical similarity can make the diagnosis challenging, RCM can aid in differentiation between hidrocystomas and these entities. Characteristic RCM findings for BCC include elongated cells with polarized nuclei intermixed with inflammatory cells, dark silhouettes, bright tumor islands, and abundant vasculature and pleomorphism of the overlying epidermis [7, 8]. RCM findings for syringomas include round to oval highly refractive and relatively monomorphous masses with dark line structures correlating to the ductal lumina [9]. Milia demonstrate refractive global keratin in the superficial dermis [9]. Blue nevi exhibit hyperreflective cells with plump cellular bodies and long dendrites intermingled with elongated collagen fibers [10].

The clinical benefits of utilizing RCM include prevention of unnecessary biopsies, decreased pain, improved cosmetic outcomes, and enhanced surveillance for recurrent malignancy [5]. Systematic use of RCM in a hospital setting reduced over 70% of the excisions of benign nevi vs. melanoma [5]. Assuming a stable number of diagnoses of melanoma over one year, this equates to a total of 3,053 unnecessary excisions that could be avoided. RCM also reduced the number needed to excise (NNE) from 19.41 with dermoscopy alone to 6.25 in combination with RCM [5]. Projected cost savings of 260,000 euros were attributed to prevention of unnecessary biopsies [5]. RCM and clinical exam can diagnose melanoma together in a single visit and result in excision concurrently, which improves patient outcomes from those lost to follow-up [11].

RCM imaging of the skin was granted codes for reimbursement by the US Centers for Medicare and Medicaid Service in 2016 and may be utilized as a cost-effective tool in dermatology [12]. However, additional imaging and training in the identification of benign and malignant lesions needs to occur. We provide further evidence for the utility of RCM in clinical practice and report a case of RCM findings of a hidrocystoma.

References

[1] K. Sarabi and A. Khachemoune, "Hidrocystomas—a brief review," *MedGenMed : Medscape General Medicine*, vol. 8, no. 3, p. 57, 2006.

[2] K. Willard, K. E. Warschaw, and D. L. Swanson, "Use of reflectance confocal microscopy to differentiate hidrocystoma from basal cell carcinoma," *Dermatologic Surgery*, vol. 37, no. 3, pp. 392–394, 2011.

[3] P. Zaballos, P. Serrano, G. Flores et al., "Dermoscopy of tumours arising in naevus sebaceous: a morphological study of 58 cases," *Journal of the European Academy of Dermatology and Venereology*, vol. 29, no. 11, pp. 2231–2237, 2015.

[4] P. Zaballos, J. Bañuls, C. Medina, E. Salsench, P. Serrano, and N. Guionnet, "Dermoscopy of apocrine hidrocystomas: a morphological study," *Journal of the European Academy of Dermatology and Venereology*, vol. 28, no. 3, pp. 378–381, 2014.

[5] G. Pellacani, A. Witkowski, A. M. Cesinaro et al., "Cost-benefit of reflectance confocal microscopy in the diagnostic performance of melanoma," *Journal of the European Academy of Dermatology and Venereology*, vol. 30, no. 3, pp. 413–419, 2016.

[6] E. Cinotti, A. Singer, B. Labeille et al., "Handheld in vivo reflectance confocal microscopy for the diagnosis of eyelid margin and conjunctival tumors," *JAMA Ophthalmology*, vol. 135, no. 8, pp. 845–851, 2017.

[7] S. Gonzalez and Z. Tannous, "Real-time, in vivo confocal reflectance microscopy of basal cell carcinoma," *Journal of the American Academy of Dermatology*, vol. 47, no. 6, pp. 869–874, 2002.

[8] A. L. Agero, K. J. Busam, C. Benvenuto-Andrade et al., "Reflectance confocal microscopy of pigmented basal cell carcinoma," *Journal of the American Academy of Dermatology*, vol. 54, no. 4, pp. 638–643, 2006.

[9] M. Gao, Y. Lin, L. Wang et al., "The differential diagnosis of syringoma and milia based on the imaging of reflectance confocal microscopy," *Skin Research and Technology*, vol. 26, no. 6, pp. 951–953, 2020.

[10] E. Cinotti, C. Couzan, J. L. Perrot et al., "Reflectance confocal microscopy for the diagnosis of vulvar naevi: six cases," *Journal of the European Academy of Dermatology and Venereology*, vol. 30, no. 1, pp. 30–35, 2016.

[11] G. Pellacani, P. Pepe, A. Casari, and C. Longo, "Reflectance confocal microscopy as a second-level examination in skin oncology improves diagnostic accuracy and saves unnecessary excisions: a longitudinal prospective study," *British Journal of Dermatology*, vol. 171, no. 5, pp. 1044–1051, 2014.

[12] M. Rajadhyaksha, A. Marghoob, A. Rossi, A. C. Halpern, and K. S. Nehal, "Reflectance confocal microscopy of skin in vivo: from bench to bedside," *Lasers in Surgery and Medicine*, vol. 49, no. 1, pp. 7–19, 2017.

29

A Case Report of a Patient with Turner Syndrome, Multiple Comorbidities and Pustular Psoriasis: Correlation or Coincidence?

Andjela Egger, Andrea Maderal, Hadar Lev-Tov, and Olivera Stojadinovic

Dr Phillip Frost Department of Dermatology and Cutaneous Surgery, University of Miami Miller School of Medicine, 1600 NW 10th Ave #1140, Miami, FL 33136, USA

Correspondence should be addressed to Andjela Egger; axn404@med.miami.edu

Academic Editor: Tak-Wah Wong

Turner syndrome (TS) is one of the most common chromosomal abnormalities. Patients with TS are at an increased risk for the development of metabolic syndrome, hypertension (HTN), diabetes mellitus type II (DM2), hyperlipidemia (HLD), obesity, and cardiovascular disease. The association between psoriasis and the aforementioned conditions including metabolic syndrome, HTN, HLD, obesity, and cardiovascular disease has also been established. Although the mechanism for heightened risk in TS patients is yet to be elucidated, patients suffering from TS and cardiometabolic diseases are likely to be at an even higher risk for developing psoriasis than patients suffering from TS alone. We present a case of a 53-year-old Hispanic woman with a mosaic TS and multiple comorbidities who presented with pustular psoriasis. For this patient, management can be challenging considering her numerous medical comorbidities and the presence of both TS and psoriasis.

1. Introduction

Psoriasis is a chronic inflammatory disease commonly seen in dermatologic practice, and its pathogenesis is attributed to Th-1 and Th-17 cell dysregulation among others [1]. Besides the commonly seen rheumatologic issue of psoriatic arthritis, psoriasis has been shown to have an association with metabolic syndrome and its diagnostic components: obesity, insulin resistance, lipid abnormalities, high blood pressure, and related cardiovascular risk factors [2].

Particularly, this association has been found consistently in epidemiologic studies showing that patients with more severe psoriasis have an increased prevalence of metabolic syndrome than patients with mild psoriasis [1]. Turner syndrome (TS) is a genetic condition representing a constellation of characteristic physical features in combination with completely or partially missing X chromosome in a female. TS's associations with autoimmune diseases, including autoimmune skin disorders such as psoriasis [3], lichen planus [4], and alopecia areata [5], have previously been reported in the literature. Further, like psoriasis, TS has also been associated with multiple cardiovascular risks and comorbidities, including metabolic syndrome and DM2 especially in adults [6]. In the current report, we present an adult patient with TS and multiple comorbidities which include metabolic syndrome and DM2 who developed pustular psoriasis. We postulate that patients suffering from TS and cardiometabolic disease may be at a heightened risk for developing psoriasis. Moreover, patients suffering from TS who develop psoriasis may be at an increased risk for developing cardiovascular disease and complications. We believe that clinicians taking care of such patients should be aware of this heightened risk and proactively screen for conditions such as metabolic syndrome and DM2 as early and as efficiently as possible.

2. Case Presentation

A 53-year-old Hispanic woman with a mosaic Turner syndrome, presented with a one-week history of a sudden, mildly pruritic widespread rash. Prior to presenting at the University of Miami Department of Dermatology, the patient was seen in the emergency department and was discharged with a triamcinolone ointment which partially alleviated her symptoms. The patient denied a history of skin rashes, upper respiratory infection, constitutional symptoms, or arthralgias. She had numerous medical comorbidities, including hypertension (HTN), coronary artery disease (CAD) status-post stents, history of a cerebral vascular accident, hyperlipidemia (HLD), poorly controlled diabetes mellitus type II, and chronic kidney disease (CKD), which she took several medications for, including atenolol, rosuvastatin, clopidogrel, insulin, aspirin, losartan, ondansetron, and metformin. Yet, she denied any changes to her medication regimen for the past several years. Her past medical history was negative for multiple sclerosis, neurodegenerative disease, hepatitis, tuberculosis, or congestive heart failure.

The physical examination revealed a generalized eruption of well-demarcated pink papules and plaques, with fine scale and central clearing (Figures 1(a) and 1(b)), involving approximately 10% of the body surface area and mostly lower extremities, back, left axilla, and chest. No lymphadenopathy, nail or mucosal involvement was noted. There was no joint erythema or swelling. Notable laboratory findings included negative antistreptolysin O and anti-DNAse B antibodies and a normal level of serum calcium.

Skin biopsy was obtained and demonstrated scale/crust with a collection of neutrophils between parakeratotic layers, a mild psoriasiform hyperplasia with a reduced granular layer, and mild sparse chronic inflammatory infiltrate in dermis, which is consistent with pustular psoriasis.

The patient appeared to partially respond to topical therapy given at the emergency department, and her more affected areas were treated with clobetasol 0.05% ointment twice a day and her less bothersome areas were treated with triamcinolone 0.1% ointment twice a day. Moreover, treatment also included a narrow band UVB phototherapy which was administered twice a week, while additional work-up including hepatitis panel, quantiferon, CBC, and CMP was obtained in anticipation of potential biologic therapy. Screening labs for possible biologic therapies were negative; however, the patient demonstrated significant improvement and resolution of skin lesions and symptoms after seven narrow-band UVB phototherapy sessions, thus hindering the need for more aggressive treatment.

3. Discussion

Turner syndrome is associated with an increased prevalence of autoimmune conditions and increased risk of cardiometabolic diseases [7, 8]. Psoriasis is an immune-mediated disease supported by findings of deregulated response of T-cells, dendritic cells, and proinflammatory cytokines, which improves with immune modulation [9]. TS patients are at an increased risk for developing metabolic syndrome including HTN, DM2, HLD, obesity, and cardiovascular disease [8]. Moreover, TS patients are at an increased risk of developing psoriasis [2, 10, 11]. On the other hand, psoriasis may lead to insulin resistance through various inflammatory cytokines, including the TNF-alpha, which contributes to cell dysfunction and atherogenesis, leading to myocardial infarction and stroke [1]. In cases of TS, however, the mechanism of development of metabolic syndrome and accompanied conditions is yet to be fully understood [11]. Recently, Calcaterra et al. found the prevalence of metabolic syndrome in TS patients to be 4.7% (12.5% in obese and 4.3% in nonobese patients), and metabolic syndrome was associated with visceral adiposity ($P = 0.008$). They also reported that the 45,X karyotype is associated with an atherogenic profile [12, 13]. A couple of more recent studies also highlighted the higher prevalence of metabolic comorbidities in the 45,X karyotype [14] as well as the increased risk of metabolic syndrome in TS patients who were older and had weight gain [15]. Particularly, compared to 45,X, mosaicism seems to mitigate the cardiovascular risk factors in TS [16]. TS patients are at a significantly higher risk for developing DM2 than the rest of the population [17]; studies in Denmark have shown that the risk increased 3-4 times [6]. Moreover, there have been some postulations on how this may occur. It appears that the intrinsic genetic defect in TS may play the most important role in the pathogenesis although factors such as autoimmunity and unhealthy lifestyle choices may contribute to a lesser extent. Additionally, metabolic syndrome has been shown to have a significant and positive association with psoriasis development [2]. Considering this, it is possible that patients who suffer from TS and cardiometabolic disease have a higher propensity to develop psoriasis. Moreover, it is also possible that patients who suffer from TS and psoriasis are at an even greater risk of developing or worsening already present cardiometabolic comorbidities, which calls for greater awareness to risk assess and manage cardiovascular disease and metabolic syndrome in this patient population. Ito et al. reported a case of a patient with TS who was suffering from pustular psoriasis and subsequently developed dilated cardiomyopathy hypothesizing that chronic inflammation may be a predisposing factor for dilated cardiomyopathy in this patient population [18]. Davenport proposed management approaches to TS patients [19]; considering our patient suffered from TS and psoriasis, these approaches may have to be enhanced. Similarly, these proposed steps in management should be considered as early as possible as girls with TS are at a greater risk for cardiovascular disease and decreased beta-cell dysfunction than age- and standardized BMI-matched girls [20, 21]. Furthermore, psoriasis management in patients with TS and comorbidities associated with cardiovascular disease may be challenging given the possibility of altered drug metabolism in the liver and via renal clearance [22, 23]. These alterations may exclude therapies such as methotrexate, acitretin, or cyclosporine, especially if the patient has transaminitis, or consequences of CKD.

Our patient, had a history of CKD and a remote history of transaminitis, excluding possible treatment with several aforementioned oral agents. Fortunately, the patient responded well to topical and light therapy. However, a potential treatment with a biological agent was considered initially.

This report describes a case of pustular psoriasis developing in a female with a mosaic TS and multiple comorbidities. This case brings greater awareness to the risks

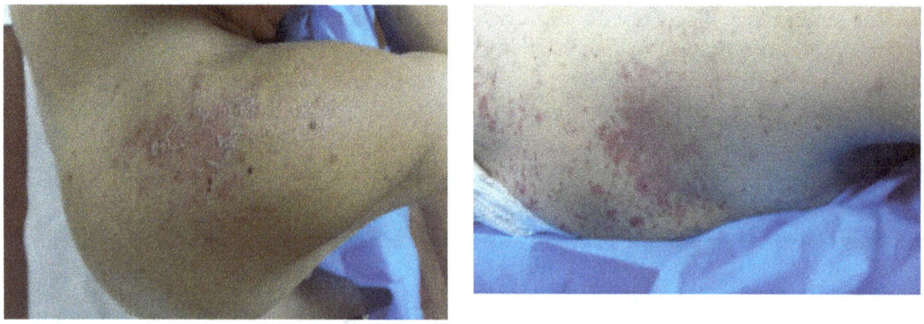

(a) (b)

Figure 1: Well-demarcated pink papules and plaques, with fine scale present on the patient's back (a) and chest (b).

of developing cardiovascular disease and metabolic syndrome in patients suffering from TS and their propensity for psoriasis development. It also highlights the association between TS, psoriasis, and cardiometabolic disease; we propose that patients suffering from TS who develop psoriasis may be at a greater risk for developing or worsening cardiovascular disease and its consequences. Despite having mosaic TS that appears to mitigate the cardiovascular risks compared to the monosomy genotype, our patient suffered from many cardiovascular and metabolic comorbidities and subsequently developed psoriasis. The patient responded well to topical and phototherapy treatment; however, role for biologics warrants further investigation to elucidate the potential benefit versus harm of this treatment modality for this patient population.

If our suspicions, which are grounded in the patient's presentation, are correct, it would substantially adjust future patient care. We emphasize the importance of genotyping patients with TS [24] as well as TS patients with psoriasis receiving closer observation and more aggressive management. As such, this report will bring awareness to this type of presentation, allowing practitioners to further confirm or disconfirm our suspicions.

Acknowledgments

The authors thank Emmett Egger for carefully editing the manuscript.

References

[1] J. M. Gelfand and H. Yeung, "Metabolic syndrome in patients with psoriatic disease," *The Journal of Rheumatology Supplement*, vol. 89, pp. 24–28, 2012.

[2] H.-N. Kim, K. Han, Y.-G. Park, and J. H. Lee, "Metabolic syndrome is associated with an increased risk of psoriasis: a nationwide population-based study," *Metabolism*, vol. 99, pp. 19–24, 2019.

[3] P. Rosina, G. Segalla, M. Magnanini, C. Chieregato, and A. Barba, "Turner's syndrome associated with psoriasis and alopecia areata," *Journal of the European Academy of Dermatology and Venereology*, vol. 17, no. 1, pp. 50–52, 2003.

[4] D. Kurgansky and J. W. Burnett, "Widespread lichen planus in association with Turner's syndrome and multiple endocrinopathies," *Cutis*, vol. 54, no. 2, pp. 108–110, 1994.

[5] W. S. Lee and M. S. Yoo, "Alopecia areata in a patient with Turner's syndrome," *British Journal of Dermatology*, vol. 135, no. 6, p. 1013, 1996.

[6] C. H. Gravholt, S. Juul, R. W. Naeraa, and J. Hansen, "Morbidity in Turner syndrome," *Journal of Clinical Epidemiology*, vol. 51, no. 2, pp. 147–158, 1998.

[7] N. Oiso, T. Ota, S. Kawara, and A. Kawada, "Pustular psoriasis and vitiligo in a patient with Turner syndrome," *The Journal of Dermatology*, vol. 34, no. 10, pp. 727–729, 2007.

[8] S. M. Davis and M. E. Geffner, "Cardiometabolic health in Turner syndrome," *American Journal of Medical Genetics Part C: Seminars in Medical Genetics*, vol. 181, pp. 52–58, 2019.

[9] A. M. Bowcock and J. G. Krueger, "Getting under the skin: the immunogenetics of psoriasis," *Nature Reviews Immunology*, vol. 5, no. 9, pp. 699–711, 2005.

[10] P. Gisondi, A. C. Fostini, I. Fossà, G. Girolomoni, and G. Targher, "Psoriasis and the metabolic syndrome," *Clinics in Dermatology*, vol. 36, no. 1, pp. 21–28, 2018.

[11] M. B. Ranke and P. Saenger, "Turner's syndrome," *The Lancet*, vol. 358, no. 9278, pp. 309–314, 2001.

[12] V. Calcaterra, P. Brambilla, G. C. Maffè et al., "Metabolic syndrome in Turner syndrome and relation between body composition and clinical, genetic, and ultrasonographic characteristics," *Metabolic Syndrome and Related Disorders*, vol. 12, no. 3, pp. 159–164, 2014.

[13] P. L. Van, V. K. Bakalov, and C. A. Bondy, "Monosomy for the X-chromosome is associated with an atherogenic lipid profile," *The Journal of Clinical Endocrinology & Metabolism*, vol. 91, no. 8, pp. 2867–2870, 2006.

[14] V. K. Bakalov, C. Cheng, J. Zhou, and C. A. Bondy, "X-chromosome gene dosage and the risk of diabetes in Turner syndrome," *The Journal of Clinical Endocrinology & Metabolism*, vol. 94, no. 9, pp. 3289–3296, 2009.

[15] Y. Lebenthal, S. Levy, E. Sofrin-Drucker et al., "The natural history of metabolic comorbidities in Turner syndrome from childhood to early adulthood: comparison between 45,X monosomy and other karyotypes," *Front Endocrinol (Lausanne)*, vol. 9, p. 27, 2018.

[16] M. El-Mansoury, M.-L. Barrenäs, I. Bryman et al., "Chromosomal mosaicism mitigates stigmata and cardiovascular risk factors in Turner syndrome," *Clinical Endocrinology*, vol. 66, no. 5, pp. 744–751, 2007.

[17] D. Ibarra-Gasparini, P. Altieri, E. Scarano et al., "New insights on diabetes in Turner syndrome: results from an observational

study in adulthood," *Endocrine*, vol. 59, no. 3, pp. 651–660, 2018.

[18] M. Ito, Y. Maejima, S. Okazaki, M. Isobe, and H. Saeki, "Generalized pustular psoriasis associated with Turner syndrome and dilated cardiomyopathy," *The Journal of Dermatology*, vol. 43, no. 7, pp. 829-830, 2016.

[19] M. L. Davenport, "Approach to the patient with Turner syndrome," *The Journal of Clinical Endocrinology & Metabolism*, vol. 95, no. 4, pp. 1487–1495, 2010.

[20] C. S. O'Gorman, C. Syme, J. Lang, T. J. Bradley, G. D. Wells, and J. K. Hamilton, "An evaluation of early cardiometabolic risk factors in children and adolescents with Turner syndrome," *Clinical Endocrinology*, vol. 78, no. 6, pp. 907–913, 2013.

[21] C. H. Gravholt, N. H. Andersen, G. S. Conway et al., "Clinical practice guidelines for the care of girls and women with Turner syndrome: proceedings from the 2016 Cincinnati International Turner Syndrome Meeting," *European Journal of Endocrinology*, vol. 177, no. 3, pp. G1–G70, 2017.

[22] R. E. Kalb, B. Strober, G. Weinstein, and M. Lebwohl, "Methotrexate and psoriasis: 2009 National Psoriasis Foundation consensus conference," *Journal of the American Academy of Dermatology*, vol. 60, no. 5, pp. 824–837, 2009.

[23] L. Miele, S. Vallone, C. Cefalo et al., "Prevalence, characteristics and severity of non-alcoholic fatty liver disease in patients with chronic plaque psoriasis," *Journal of Hepatology*, vol. 51, no. 4, pp. 778–786, 2009.

[24] A. Cameron-Pimblett, C. La Rosa, T. F. J. King, M. C. Davies, and G. S. Conway, "The Turner syndrome life course project: karyotype-phenotype analyses across the lifespan," *Clinical Endocrinology*, vol. 87, no. 5, pp. 532–538, 2017.

30

Cytophagic Histiocytic Panniculitis (CHP) in a Patient with SLE Found after Autopsy: When a Rash is "Complicated!"

Hafsa Abbas,[1] Ahsan Aslam,[2] Muhammad Saad,[3] Masooma Niazi,[4] and Sridhar Chilimuri[3]

[1]*Department of Medicine, Division of Gastroenterology, Bronxcare Hospital Center, Bronx, NY 10457, USA*
[2]*Department of Medicine, IU Health University Hospital, Indianapolis, IN 46202, USA*
[3]*Department of Medicine, Bronxcare Hospital Center, Bronx, NY 10457, USA*
[4]*Department of Pathology, Bronxcare Hospital Center, Bronx, NY 10457, USA*

Correspondence should be addressed to Hafsa Abbas; hafsaabbas20@gmail.com

Academic Editor: Kowichi Jimbow

Introduction. Cytophagic histolytic panniculitis (CHP) is a clinical disorder characterized by nodular panniculitis of the subcutaneous adipose tissue. It was first described in 1980 by Winkelmann. Histologically it is described as an infiltration of the adipose tissue by T- lymphocytes and phagocytic macrophages (also known as "bean bag cells"). Most of the cases are reported under the age of 50 and is a rare cause of panniculitis. We report a case of CHP in a young patient who presented to our emergency room (ER). *Case Summary.* A 39-year-old African American woman who presented to our hospital with lethargy, progressive confusion, and generalized rash involving both lower extremities of 1 week duration. She had a history of pancytopenia and focal proliferative and membranous lupus nephritis classes 3 and 5. Her physical examination was remarkable for bilateral lower extremity pitting edema and a desquamating rash on both of her legs. The Nicolsky sign was positive. She was noted to be hypotensive and was started on intravenous fluids and broad spectrum antibiotics. Routine laboratory tests revealed severe pancytopenia, with a hemoglobin of 3.9 g/dl, white blood cell count 600/ul, and platelet count of 11000/ul. Within an hour of arrival to the ER she developed acute respiratory failure. She was intubated and placed on mechanical ventilation. She developed shock requiring vasopressors. No imaging could be done due to her unstable condition. Four hours after her initial presentation she developed asystole and expired. Postmortem histopathology of the adipose tissue revealed CHP. *Conclusion.* CHP can be rapidly fatal. The treatment involves high dose of intravenous steroids and immunosuppressants such as cyclosporine.

1. Introduction

Cytophagic histiocytic panniculitis (CHP) is a rare clinical disorder, characterized by nodular panniculitis of the subcutaneous adipose tissue [1]. It was first described in 1980 by Winkelmann, as an infiltration of the subcutaneous adipose tissue by T lymphocytes and phagocytic histiocytes (also known as the "bean bag cells") [2]. It is a rare cause of aseptic panniculitis [2–4] that is seen in association with viral infections (HSV, EBV) [5], hematopoietic disorders (malignant lymphoma), hemophagocytic lymphohistiocytosis (HLH), acute leukemias (acute lymphoid leukemia, acute myeloid leukemia), Hodgkin's and non-Hodgkin's lymphoma, rhabdomyosarcoma, neuroblastoma, and Langerhans cell histiocytosis [6, 7]. Reports of CHP after H1N1 vaccination are available in the literature [8]. Its association with autoimmune diseases like systemic lupus erythematosus (SLE) is also reported and has a high mortality rate [9–12]. However, only a few such cases confirming the association between SLE and CHP are available. We report one such case of CHP in a patient with SLE that ultimately resulted in the demise of the patient.

2. Case Report

A 39-year-old African American woman was brought to our emergency room (ER) with lethargy, progressive confusion, and generalized rash involving both lower extremities of 1-week duration. Two months ago, the patient had presented

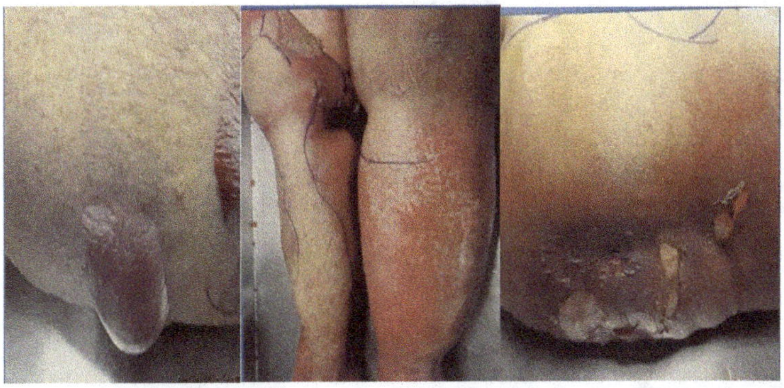

FIGURE 1: Rash on the back with bullae, rash on the posterior aspect of legs, and desquamating rash on the back.

to our hospital with left lower quadrant pain and nonbloody diarrhea and dizziness. A Computed Tomography (CT) of the abdomen and pelvis had revealed pancolitis and she was treated with antibiotics. At that time she was also found to have proteinuria, pedal edema and photosensitive rash on her face. The proteinuria was attributed to glomerular disease of unclear etiology. Autoimmune work-up revealed positive ANA, anti-Smith Ab, and anti-RNP. Parvovirus IgG was also positive. She was found to have pancytopenia and the diagnosis of aplastic anemia was considered and she was transferred to another tertiary care hospital. There, she underwent a renal biopsy that revealed focal proliferative and membranous lupus nephritis classes 3 and 5. She was discharged on prednisone, mycophenolate, and hydroxychloroquine. Now she had presented with the current complains.

In the ER she was found to be lethargic. On physical examination, her temperature was 97.5°F, pulse was 102 beats per minute, the initial blood pressure was 136/79 mm of Hg, and respiratory rate was 22 breaths per minute. There was no scleral icterus. Oral mucosa was dry without visible lesions. The neck was supple. Skin was warm and had desquamating rash on both lower extremities from hip down (Figure 1). The rash was nonblanching and erythematous, and Nicolsky sign was positive. The abdomen was soft but mild tenderness was noted in the epigastric region without any guarding or rebound tenderness. There was no organomegaly and the bowel sounds were sluggish. There was bilateral pitting pedal edema. The patient was arousable with verbal and tactile stimulation and was moving all extremities spontaneously. Rest of the physical examination was unremarkable.

Later she developed hypotension and was given on intravenous fluids. Sepsis was suspected and broad spectrum antibiotics were initiated. The early differential diagnosis included Steven Johnson syndrome vs. necrotizing fasciitis causing sepsis. Her labs revealed severe pancytopenia and severe metabolic acidosis. Detailed results of the laboratory parameters are given in Table 1.

She was transfused 2 units of packed red blood cells and 6 units of platelets. Within an hour of arrival to the ER she developed acute respiratory failure and was intubated and placed on mechanical ventilation. She developed septic shock requiring vasopressors. She was deemed too unstable for imaging studies but a portable chest X-ray revealed right basilar atelectasis and portable X-ray of the lower extremities showed soft tissue edema. Four

TABLE 1: Initial laboratory workup.

Parameter	Initial laboratory results	Reference range
Hemoglobin (g/dl)	3.9	12-16
White blood cell count (per mm^3)	0.6	4.8-10.8
Platelet count (k/ul)	11	150-400
Sodium (mEq/L)	129	135-145
Potassium (mEq/L)	7.1	3.5-5.0
HCO3 (mEq/L)	11	24-30
Ph	6.9	7.35-7.45
BUN (mg/dl)	52	6- 20
Creatinine (mg/dl)	3	0.5 -1.5
Glucose (mg/dl)	376	70-120
Lactic acid (mmoles/L)	6.7	0.5-1.6
AST (mg/dl)	50	9-48
ALT (mg/dl)	20	5 -40
Total bilirubin/direct (mg/dl)	0.2	0.2-1.2
Alkaline phosphatase U/L	20	53-141
Albumin (g/dl)	0.4	3.2-4.8
Urine toxicology screen	negative	negative
Blood culture	Serratia marcescens positive	negative

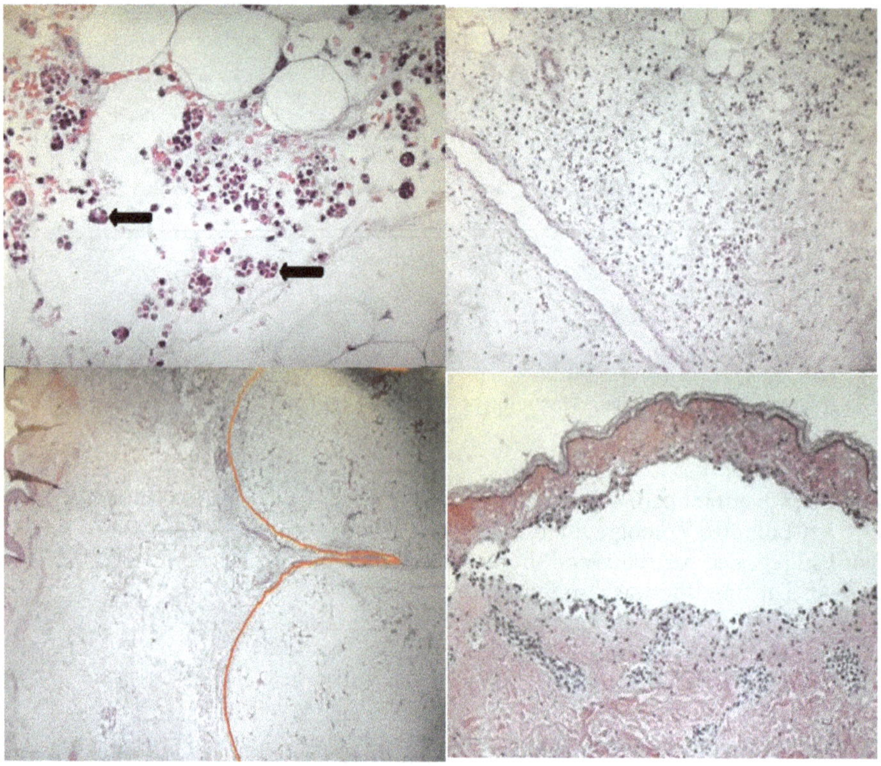

FIGURE 2: (a) The arrows indicate macrophages engulfing mostly the red blood cells (bean bag cells), (b) this is lobular panniculitis comprised of cellular infiltrate of lymphocytes, macrophages, and plasma cells, (c) septal panniculitis (highlighted), and (d) subepidermal bullous lesion.

hours after the initial presentation she developed asystole and expired after failed resuscitative measures. An autopsy was done that revealed CHP (Figure 2), Libman Sacks endocarditis, bilateral pleural effusion, proliferative and membranous lupus glomerular nephropathy, and bilateral adrenal hemorrhage. Blood culture postmortem grew serratia marcescens.

3. Discussion

CHP has an elaborate spectrum of clinical presentations. It can present with a wide array of symptoms ranging from local skin lesions to a life threatening systemic illness as associated with hemophagocytic syndrome (HLH) [12]. It can present with recurrent fever, subcutaneous nodules, hepatosplenomegaly, abnormal liver function tests, pancytopenia, polyserositis, and hemorrhagic diathesis [2, 13].

Its clinical course is variable depends on degree of severity. Some patients developed chronicity having recurring bouts over the course of their illness and surviving for years [14–16]. In others, it can rapidly progress resulting in the demise of the patients from sepsis and multiorgan failure [2, 13, 17]. Diagnosis is particularly challenging as it is a rare disorder and limited literature is available for guiding the management of this disease. The differential diagnosis is wide, including tuberculosis and histiocytosis. The diagnosis requires a skin biopsy, which shows characteristic histologic findings; "bean bag cells" are pathognomonic.

The current treatment options include high dose of steroids and immunosuppressants such as cyclosporine A as the first line agents [9, 18]. Recently other treatment modalities like chemotherapy have also been used successfully, CHOP (cyclophosphamide, doxorubicin, vincristine, and prednisolone) being the most commonly used chemotherapy regimen. In treatment refractory cases the use of azathioprine, cyclophosphamide, tacrolimus, plasmapheresis, and autologous peripheral blood stem cell transplantation has also been reported [19].

CHP has a poor prognosis and a high mortality up to 70% in severe cases, while other cases are successfully treated with immunosuppressive agents like cyclosporine [9, 15, 18, 19]. CHP in patients with SLE is a rare combination and to date only a handful such cases have been reported in medical literature. Fever, lymphadenopathy, and pancytopenia are some of the clinical features that indicate poor prognosis in such patients [9]. Our patient had pancytopenia and had a rapidly progressive decline in clinical picture that is characteristic of this disorder in severe cases as mentioned earlier. Unfortunately our patient expired in a very short period of presentation to the ER and diagnosis was made postmortem with autopsy. Clinicians should be aware of this uncommon disorder as the delay in treatment can be rapidly fatal.

References

[1] W. Liao, S. Xiao, J. Yong et al., "Bilateral ptosis as first presentation of cytophagic histiocytic panniculitis: A case report," *BMC Ophthalmology*, vol. 17, no. 1, 2017.

[2] R. K. Winkelmann and E. J. Bowie, "Hemorrhagic diathesis associated with benign histiocytic, cytophagic panniculitis and systemic histiocytosis," *Archives of Internal Medicine*, vol. 140, no. 11, pp. 1460–1463, 1980.

[3] V. A. Alegre and R. K. Winkelmann, "Histiocytic cytophagic panniculitis," *Journal of the American Academy of Dermatology*, vol. 20, no. 2, pp. 177–185, 1989.

[4] A. J. Craig, H. Cualing, G. Thomas, C. Lamerson, and R. Smith, "Cytophagic histiocytic panniculitis—a syndrome associated with benign and malignant panniculitis: Case comparison and review of the literature," *Journal of the American Academy of Dermatology*, vol. 39, no. 5, pp. 721–736, 1998.

[5] N. R. Maakaroun, A. Moanna, J. T. Jacob, and H. Albrecht, "Viral infections associated with haemophagocytic syndrome," *Reviews in Medical Virology*, vol. 20, no. 2, pp. 93–105, 2010.

[6] A. H. Filipovich, "Hemophagocytic lymphohistiocytosis and other hemophagocytic disorders," *Immunology and Allergy Clinics of North America*, vol. 28, no. 2, pp. 293–313, 2008.

[7] T. Celkan, S. Berrak, E. Kazanci et al., "Malignancy-associated hemophagocytic lymphohistiocytosis in pediatric cases: a multicenter study from Turkey," *The Turkish Journal of Pediatrics*, vol. 51, no. 3, pp. 207–213, 2009.

[8] C. Pauwels, C. Bulai Livideanu, A. Maza, L. Lamant, and C. Paul, "Cytophagic histiocytic panniculitis after H1N1 vaccination: a case report and review of the cutaneous side effects of influenza vaccines," *Dermatology*, vol. 222, no. 3, pp. 217–220, 2011.

[9] H. Hasegawa, F. Mizoguchi, H. Kohsaka, and N. Miyasaka, "Systemic lupus erythematosus with cytophagic histiocytic panniculitis successfully treated with high-dose glucocorticoids and cyclosporine A," *Lupus*, vol. 22, no. 3, pp. 316–319, 2013.

[10] T. Tsukahara, A. Fujioka, Y. Horiuchi et al., "A case of cytophagic histiocytic panniculitis with sicca symptoms and lupus nephritis," *The Journal of Dermatology*, vol. 19, no. 9, pp. 563–569, 1992.

[11] T. Tsukahara, Y. Horiuchi, and K. Iidaka, "Cytophagic histiocytic panniculitis in systemic lupus erythematosus.," *Hiroshima Journal of Medical Sciences*, vol. 44, no. 1, pp. 13–16, 1995.

[12] Y. Mori, T. Sugiyama, R. Chiba et al., "A case of systemic lupus erythematosus with hemophagocytic syndrome with cytophagic histiocytic panniculitis," *Ryūmachi*, vol. 41, no. 1, pp. 31–36, 2001.

[13] R. K. Winkelmann, "Panniculitis with cellular phagocytosis. Chronic form of histiocytic panniculitis with fever, pancytopenia, polyserositis and lethal hemorrhagic diathesis," *Hautarzt*, vol. 31, no. 11, pp. 588–594, 1980.

[14] C. Pasqualini, M. Jorini, I. Carloni et al., "Cytophagic histiocytic panniculitis, hemophagocytic lymphohistiocytosis and undetermined autoimmune disorder: Reconciling the puzzle," *Italian Journal of Pediatrics*, vol. 40, no. 1, 2014.

[15] J. W. White and R. K. Winkelmann, "Cytophagic histiocytic panniculitis is not always fatal," *Journal of Cutaneous Pathology*, vol. 16, no. 3, pp. 137–144, 1989.

[16] D. R. Barron, B. R. Davis, J. R. Pomeranz, J. D. Hines, and C. H. Park, "Cytophagic histiocytic panniculitis. A variant of malignant histiocytosis," *Cancer*, vol. 55, no. 11, pp. 2538–2542, 1985.

[17] G. Secmeer, H. Sakalli, F. Gok, S. Ozen, A. Kara, A. B. Cengiz et al., "Fatal cytophagic histiocytic panniculitis," *Pediatric Dermatology*, vol. 21, no. 3, pp. 246–249, 2004.

[18] B. E. Ostrov, B. H. Athreya, A. H. Eichenfield, and D. P. Goldsmith, "Successful treatment of severe cytophagic histiocytic panniculitis with cyclosporine A," *Seminars in Arthritis and Rheumatism*, vol. 25, no. 6, pp. 404–413, 1996.

[19] M. Ito, H. Ohira, M. Miyata, T. Suzuki, Y. Sato, S. Kaise et al., "Cytophagic histiocytic panniculitis improved by combined chop and cyclosporin a treatment," *Internal Medicine*, vol. 38, no. 3, pp. 296–301, 1999.

31

Nasolabial Ulcerated Placard Revealing a Primary Cutaneous Aggressive Epidermotropic CD8+ T-cell Lymphoma

J. B. Ntihebuwayo,[1] **F. Hali,**[1] **A. Kerouach,**[1] **H. Rachadi,**[1] **S. Chiheb,**[1] **and F. Marnissi**[2]

[1]*Dermatology and Venereology Department, Ibn Rochd University Hospital-Casablanca, Casablanca, Morocco*
[2]*Laboratory of Pathological Anatomy, Ibn Rochd University Hospital-Casablanca, Casablanca, Morocco*

Correspondence should be addressed to J. B. Ntihebuwayo; ntiheba@gmail.com

Academic Editor: Alireza Firooz

Primary cutaneous aggressive epidermotropic CD8+ T-cell lymphoma is a rare entity representing less than 1% of cutaneous lymphomas. It has an aggressive clinical manifestation with a poor prognosis. It is characterized by cytotoxic and epidermotropic CD8+ proliferation. It also expresses the TIA-1 marker. We report a new case for its display and aggressive character, diagnostic difficulty, and good therapeutic response to chemotherapy. This is a 62-year-old female patient admitted to the hospital for a nasolabial ulcerated placard evolving for two years. Clinical examination revealed submandibular lymph nodes. The specimen analysis associated with anatomoclinical manifestation was concluded for a primary cutaneous aggressive epidermotropic CD8+ T-cell lymphoma. Tumor extent assessment did not show any secondary localization. The blood tests and serology were unremarkable. The patient had benefited from a CHOEP-type multidrug therapy protocol with complete healing of the lesion after three courses of chemotherapy.

1. Introduction

Primary cutaneous aggressive epidermotropic CD8+ T-cell lymphoma is a rare and provisional entity according to the 2017 revised WHO classification. It represents less than 1% of all cutaneous lymphomas. It is characterized by the proliferation of epidermotropic CD8+ cytotoxic T cells with TIA-1 marker expression. It is an aggressive tumor with a poor prognosis. It affects adults, without gender predominance and without predisposing factors [1, 2]. Slowly and localized progression forms are rarely described, while diffuse forms are the most frequent [1–3]. We report an atypical case of primary cutaneous aggressive epidermotropic CD8+ T-cell lymphoma of nasal localization with a good response to chemotherapy.

2. Observation

A 62-year-old female patient was hospitalized with an erythematous and pruritic papular lesion of the right upper lip that had been evolving for two years. The lesion was infiltrated at the base with ulceration in its center and destruction of the right wing of the nose (Figure 1).

The clinical examination found two submandibular nodes with altered general condition. There was no nasal obstruction or discharge. Biopsy of the lesion showed diffuse lymphoid cell proliferation in layers occupying the entire dermis and hypodermis with epidermotropism and skin ulceration. The cells were of medium size with reduced cytoplasm and rounded or cleaved nuclei with 6 mitoses/10 HPF (Figure 2).

Immunohistochemistry showed a lymphoid infiltrate expressing CD3, CD8, and granzyme B. The cytotoxic marker T1A1 was positive. Ki67, a proliferative index, was estimated at 50% (Figure 3). CD4, CD5, CD 20, PAX5, EBV, CD30, CD56, CD10, CD23, BCL6, and MUMI were negative.

After anatomic and clinical confrontation, the diagnosis of a primary cutaneous aggressive epidermotropic CD8+ T-cell lymphoma was retained.

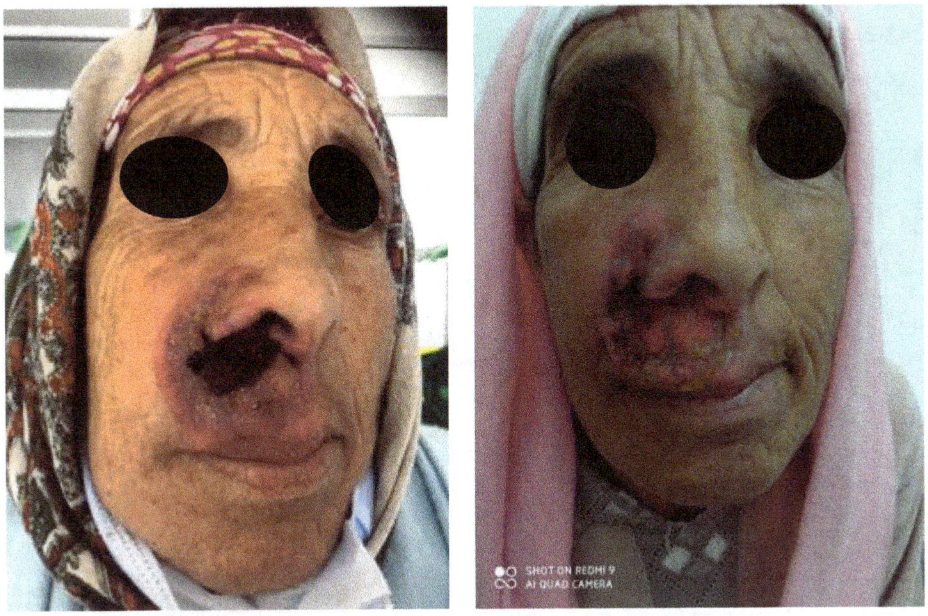

(a) (b)

Figure 1: (a) Ulcerated and necrotic right nasolabial plaque with destruction of the right nasal wing on day 1 of the consultation. (b) Ulcerated and necrotic nasolabial plaque with significant loss of substance one month later after the first day of consultation.

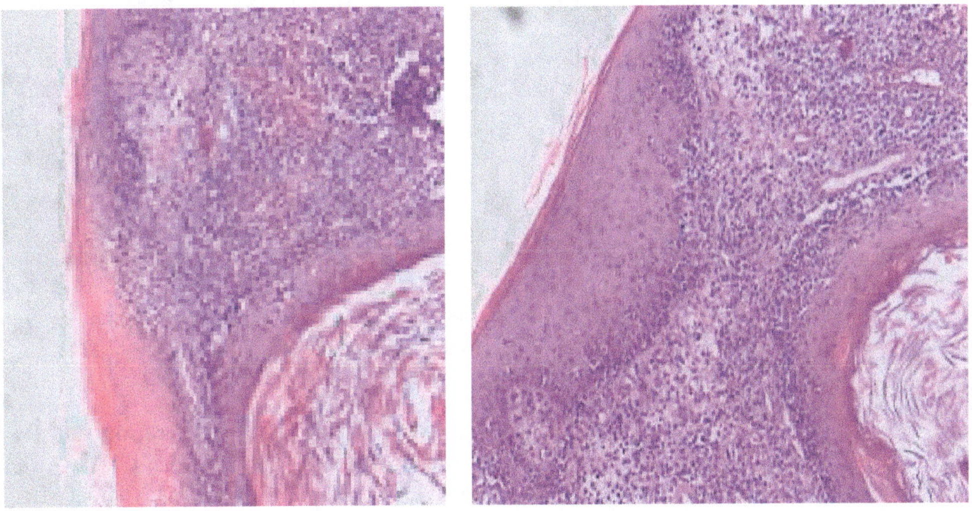

(a) (b)

Figure 2: (a) Diffuse lymphoid infiltrate of the dermis and hypodermis epidermotropism, (b) diffuse lymphoid infiltrate of the dermis and hypodermis epidermotropism.

The biological tests did not show any inflammatory or infectious disease, and the viral and syphilitic tests were negative (Table 1).

The cervico-cranio-facial CT scan showed a tumor process invading the right nostril and the vestibule without maxillary bone or sinus invasion. The thoraco abdominopelvic CT scan did not show any tumor localization. Aggressive multidrug therapy (CHOEP protocol) was initiated (Endoxan, doxorubicin, vincristine, onset, etoposide, and Isone). After three doses of multidrug therapy, the lesion was completely healed (Figure 4). The patient has been in complete remission for 7 months after the last chemotherapy treatment.

3. Discussion

The particularity of our case is its rarity, clinical presentation, and evolution but also therapeutic which lies on chemotherapy. Clinically, primary cutaneous aggressive epidermotropic CD8 + T-cell lymphoma is characterized by the sudden and generalized appearance of extensive and ulcerated papules, placards, or tumors, with or without mucosal and/or visceral involvement [1, 3].

Localized forms, especially facial, of slower evolution have been rarely reported in the literature [1, 2].

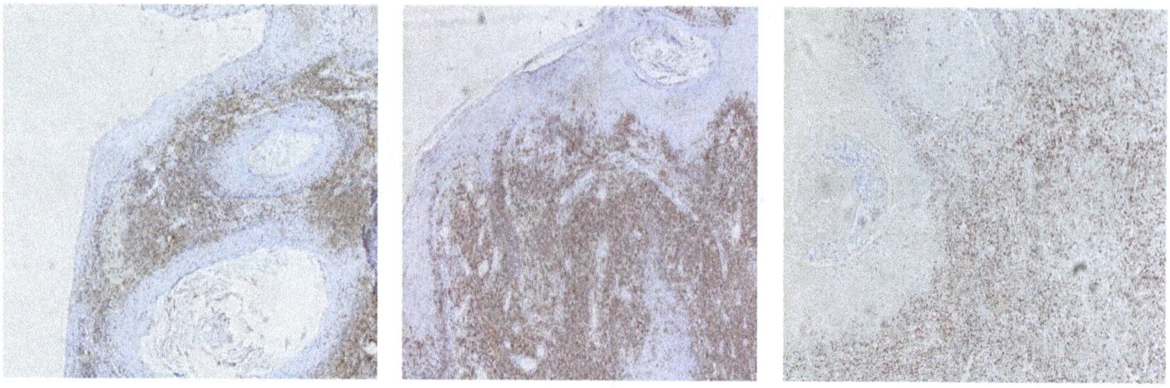

(a) (b) (c)

FIGURE 3: Immunohistochemistry had shown a lymphoid infiltrate expressing (a) CD3 +: positive, (b) CD8 + positive, and (c) KI67: proliferative index estimated at 50%.

TABLE 1: Biological workup performed.

Realized balance sheet	Value recovered	Usual value
Hb	11, 2	12–16 g/dl
Lymphocytes	1170	1000–5000 cells/μL
VS	21	<20 mm in young women
CRP	1, 7	1–4 mg/L
LDH	174	125–220 UI/L
ASAT	17	5–34 UI/L
ALAT	13	0–55 UI/L
Urea	0, 27	0, 13–0, 43 g/L
Creatinine	6, 1	5, 7–11, 1 mg/L
TPHA	Negative	
VDRL	Negative	
EBV	Negative	
Anti-HIV 1-2 combined	Negative	
Anti HTLV 1 antibodies	Negative	

Hb: hemoglobin, ASAT: aspartate aminotransferase, ALAT: alanine aminotransferase, LDH: lactate dehydrogenase, CRP: C-reactive protein, VS: sedimentation rate, TPHA: *Treponema pallidum* hemagglutination assay, VDRL: venereal disease research laboratory, anti-HIV 1-2 combined: human immunodeficiency virus, EBV: Epstein–Barr virus, HTLV-1: human T-lymphotropic virus.

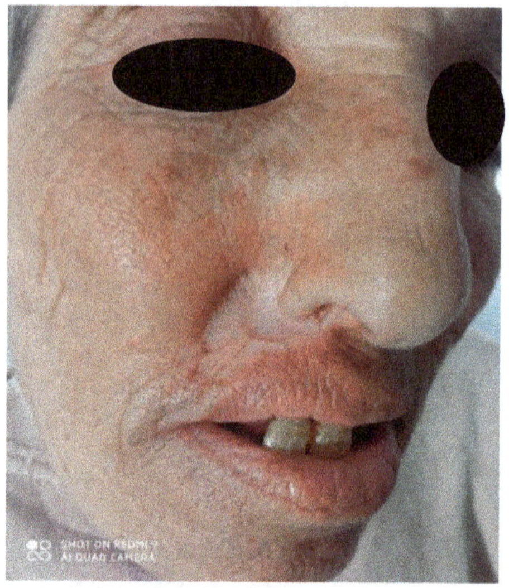

FIGURE 4: Complete healing of the lesion three months after the last chemotherapy treatment.

Our patient presented with a localized facial involvement with an initially slow then rapidly aggressive evolution posing a problem of differential diagnosis with a nasal-type T/NK lymphoma.

The positive diagnosis requires an anatomoclinical confrontation. Histologically, the lymphoid infiltrate is nodular or diffuse dermohypodermal with a pagetoid or lichenoid epidermotropism. The cells are small to large with irregular hyperchromatic nuclei and pleomorphic cytology. The presence of keratinocyte necrosis indicates the cytotoxic nature of the tumor cells [2, 4–6]. Immunohistochemically, the CD3+, CD8+, CD4-, CD45RA+, CD45RO−, granzyme B+, perforin+, TIA-1+, and beta-F1+ phenotype is constant. The CD56, CD2, CD7, CD5, CD15, BCL2 and βF1+, and MIB-1 phenotype is variable. Loss of CD2/CD5 antigens would reflect rapid progression, and CD2+/CD7—phenotype would favor indolent progression. MIB-1 shows a high proliferation index with Ki67 > 75%. The CD4, CD5, CD15, CD25, CD1a, ALK1, CD56, CD57, CD45RO, EBV/EBER, EBNA2, and LMP1 phenotypes are negative. Rare cases have been reported with the CD30 phenotype. Molecular biology shows clonal rearrangement of TCR genes and cytogenetics shows haploinsufficiency for TP53 [1, 2, 4, 6].

Our patient had a lymphoid infiltrate expressing CD3, CD8, and granzyme B with a positive TIA1 and a high proliferation index of 50%. The main differential diagnosis in our case was extranodal nasal-type T/NK cell lymphoma. It combines upper respiratory tract involvement and skin involvement with ulcerated nodules or tumors. The evolution is rapidly progressive. The phenotypes EBV and EBR and CD3+ and CD56+ are positive. It has a very poor prognosis [2, 4, 7].

Other differential diagnoses are primary cutaneous anaplastic large cell lymphoma, lymphomatoid papulosis, pagetoid T-cell lymphoma, primary cutaneous acral CD8+ T-cell lymphoma, Ketron-Goodman disease, and primary cutaneous $\gamma\delta$ T-cell lymphoma [1, 4, 6, 8]. Treatment is not well codified and is based on multidrug therapy with different protocols: CHOP (Endoxan, doxorubicin, vincristine, onset, and Isone), CHOEP (Endoxan, doxorubicin, vincristine, onset, etoposide, and Isone), hyper CVAD (Endoxan, vincristine, Adriamycin, and dexamethasone). The response is unsatisfactory and usually partial [1, 9]. Partial or complete responses have been reported in the literature with electron therapy [9, 10]. Stem cell transplantation with or without chemotherapy or anti-CD 52 monoclonal antibody has been reported in the literature with partial efficacy [1, 3, 10]. Despite the poor therapeutic response reported in the literature, our patient responded well to multidrug therapy. The prognosis is unfavorable with an aggressive clinical course. Survival at 5 years is estimated between 18 and 32% with a median survival of 12–32 months. Diagnosis at the tumor lesion stage is associated with a poor prognosis [1, 3, 8, 10, 11].

4. Conclusion

Primary cutaneous aggressive epidermotropic CD8+ T-cell lymphoma is a rare entity with a poor prognosis. Its clinical manifestation and history are unusual. The presentation and clinical history of our patient are unusual and constitute a diagnostic challenge, hence the interest of anatomical and clinical confrontation to confirm the diagnosis. Despite the poor therapeutic response reported in the literature, our patient responded well to chemotherapy, hence the interest of monitoring. Early diagnosis and management could improve patient survival.

References

[1] J. Guitart, M. E. Martinez-Escala, A. Subtil et al., "Primary cutaneous aggressive epidermotropic cytotoxic T-cell lymphomas: reappraisal of a provisional entity in the 2016 WHO classification of cutaneous lymphomas," *Modern Pathology*, vol. 30, pp. 761–772, 2017.

[2] M. Rolland, M. Dinulescu, C. Saillard et al., "Nodules ulcérés du visage révélant un lymphome T cutané épidermotrope CD8+ cytotoxique agressif," *Annales de Dermatologie et de Venereologie*, vol. 147, pp. 764–768, 2020.

[3] A. Nofal, M. Y. Abdel-Mawla, M. Assaf, and E. Salah, "Primary cutaneous aggressive epidermotropic CD8+ T-cell lymphoma: proposed diagnostic criteria and therapeutic evaluation," *Journal of the American Academy of Dermatology*, vol. 67, no. 4, pp. 748–759, 2012.

[4] P. Combemale and T. Petrella, *Lymphome T Cutané Épidermotrope Agressif CD8 +. Lymphomes Cutanés*, Springer Paris, Paris, France, 2013.

[5] L. L. Wessman, K. J. Gaddis, and D. R. Pearson, "Rapidly evolving necrotic plaques and nodules in a middle-aged woman," *JAMA Dermatol*, vol. 156, no. 4, p. 455, 2020.

[6] E. Gardette, P. Moguelet, S. Barete, C. Frances, and P. Senet, "Unusual course of CD8+ epidermotropic cutaneous T-cell lymphoma," *Annales de Dermatologie et de Vénéréologie*, vol. 143, no. 12, pp. 846–851, 2016.

[7] S. Geller, P. L. Myskowski, and M. Pulitzer, "NK/T-cell lymphoma, nasal type, $\gamma\delta$ T-cell lymphoma, and CD8-positive epidermotropic T-cell lymphoma—clinical and histopathologic features, differential diagnosis, and treatment," *Seminars in Cutaneous Medicine and Surgery*, vol. 37, no. 1, pp. 30–38, 2018.

[8] W.-S. Kim, J. Lee, Y. Yang, J.-I. Kim, and J.-H. Park, "Primary cutaneous aggressive epidermotropic CD8 + T-cell lymphoma on upper eyelid," *Indian Journal of Ophthalmology*, vol. 63, no. 1, p. 81, 2015.

[9] B. M. Intriago, O. C. Peña, H. A. M. Gray, C. M. E. Cabrera, and C. V. Martínez, "Linfoma primario cutáneo agresivo epidermotrópico de células T citotóxicas CD8 positivo: caso clínico," *Revista Medica de Chile*, vol. 140, no. 3, pp. 368–372, 2012.

[10] R. H. Gormley, S. D. Hess, D. Anand, J. Junkins-Hopkins, A. H. Rook, and E. J. Kim, "Primary cutaneous aggressive epidermotropic CD8+ T-cell lymphoma," *Journal of the American Academy of Dermatology*, vol. 62, no. 2, pp. 300–307, 2010.

[11] A. M. Corazón-Monzón, L. M. Juárez-Salcedo, and S. Dalia, "Primary cutaneous CD8 aggressive epidermotropic cytotoxic T cell lymphoma," *Atlas of Genetics and Cytogenetics in Oncology and Haematology*, no. 8, 2020.

Multibacillary Leprosy Presenting as Anetoderma in a Young Teenager

Niraj Parajuli,[1] Shraddha Shrestha,[1] Laila Lama,[1] Rushma Shrestha,[1] Sumida Tiwari,[2] and Anupama Karki[1]

[1]*Department of Dermatology & Venereology, National Academy of Medical Sciences, Bir Hospital, Kathmandu, Nepal*
[2]*Department of Pathology, National Academy of Medical Sciences, Bir Hospital, Kathmandu, Nepal*

Correspondence should be addressed to Niraj Parajuli; drnirajparajuli@gmail.com

Academic Editor: Jacek Cezary Szepietowski

Anetoderma presents as a circumscribed area of slack skin. It can present as either primary or secondary, if associated with other conditions. Leprosy is one of the causes of secondary anetoderma, but it is not commonly reported, especially in multibacillary leprosy. Here, we report a case of a 16-year-old young girl who presented with fever, joint pain, and only three anetodermic plaques. A slit skin smear from the lesion showed multiple acid-fast bacilli with a bacillary index of 3+, thus confirming the diagnosis of leprosy. This case is unique since multibacillary leprosy presented with only few anetoderma lesions in a young teenager girl from a leprosy-eliminated country.

1. Introduction

Anetoderma refers to a circumscribed area of slack skin associated with a loss of dermal substance on palpation and a loss of elastic tissue on histological examination [1]. Anetoderma is an elastolytic disorder characterized by localized areas of flaccid skin, which may be depressed, macular, or papular [2]. "Primary" anetoderma is associated with no localized underlying cutaneous disease, whereas "secondary" anetoderma can be attributed to some associated condition like leprosy, tuberculosis, urticaria pigmentosa, pityriasis versicolor, granuloma annulare, and others [1].

Here, we report a case of multibacillary leprosy presenting as anetoderma in a young teenager girl during the post-elimination era.

2. Case Report

A 16-year-old female from the Terai region presented to the emergency department with complaints of high-grade fever for 5 days. She was being managed empirically with parenteral antibiotics. An opinion was sought from the dermatological team regarding few asymptomatic, skin-colored lesions over the extremities. The soft plaques were first noticed over the left lower leg and, then, over the right arm within a period of 6 months. There was no significant past and family history.

On general examination, an ill-looking young female with fever, bilateral pedal pitting edema, and diffuse swelling of the face was observed. Vital signs were all within normal limits. On skin examination, few round-to-oval plaques with an atrophic, wrinkled surface of approximate $1 \times 1\,cm^2$ were present over the right arm, forearm, and left lower leg. On stretching, atrophic plaques became flat (Figure 1(a)), and on leaving the skin lax, the plaques returned to initial texture (Figure 1(b)).Similar plaques were also present over the left lower thigh (Figure 2). All the plaques had decreased sensation to cold and touch. Bilateral ulnar nerves and the left common peroneal nerve were enlarged and tender. No motor deficit or deformity was noted during the examination. A slit skin smear with Ziehl–Neelsen stain was performed, revealing multiple acid-fast bacilli with a bacillary index (BI) of 3+. Excisional biopsy and histopathological examination of atrophic plaques from the

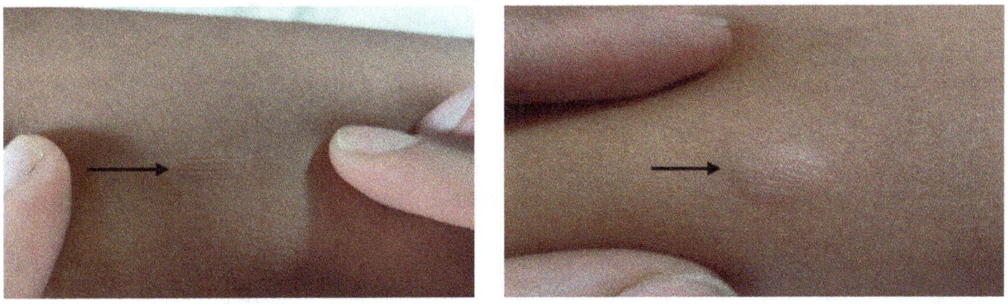

(a) (b)

FIGURE 1: (a) Skin-colored atrophic plaques which became flat on stretching. (b) the skin becoming lax after release, returning to the initial wrinkly texture.

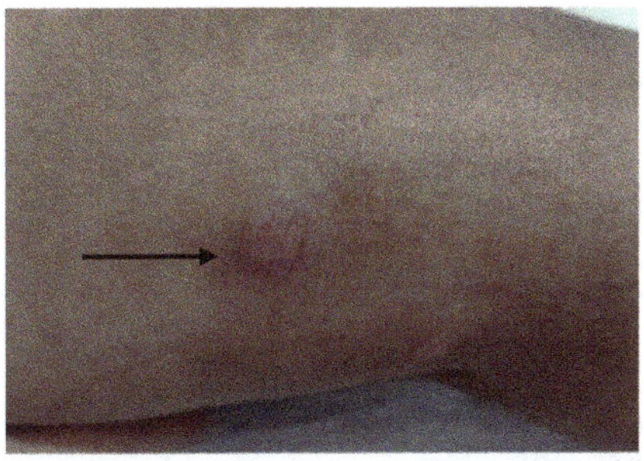

FIGURE 2: Atrophic wrinkled plaques over the left lower thigh.

right arm revealed multiple well-formed granulomas consisting of epithelioid cells with peripheral rimming of lymphocytes in the upper dermis and perineural and periadnexal lymphocytic infiltrates along with few multinucleated giant cells (Figures 3(a) and 3(b)).

Venereal disease research laboratory (VDRL) tests and serologies for HIV and hepatitis B and C were negative. The antinuclear antibodies test was negative as well.

The patient was diagnosed as a case of multibacillary leprosy with Type 1 reaction. Treatment was started on multidrug therapy-multibacillary type (MDT-MB) along with oral prednisolone 40 mg/day on a tapering dose. The patient and the parents were counselled regarding the nature of the disease and were advised for regular follow-up.

Contact examination in immediate family members did not show any features of leprosy.

3. Discussion

Anetoderma, first described by Jadassohn, is characterized by localized areas of loss of substance and elastic tissue with flaccid skin and often leads to a herniation phenomenon [3]. Usually, it presents as crops of round or oval pink macules or plaques 0.5–1 cm in diameter seen mostly over the trunk, thighs, and upper arms [1]. The skin lesion fades and flattens from the center outwards, leaving wrinkled, atrophic macules which yield on pressure [4].

Primary anetoderma occurs idiopathically from normal skin and is strongly associated with antiphospholipid syndrome. Secondary anetoderma is reported with tuberculosis, leprosy, lupus, syphilis, granuloma annulare, B- and T-cell lymphomas, and other conditions [5]. The exact etiology of anetoderma is unknown, but the condition is associated with an increase in elastolysis [6]. The loss of elastic fibers can be due to several factors including a decrease in elastolytic enzyme inhibitors, increased production of elastolytic enzymes, or autoimmune-mediated destruction of fibers [7].

Special staining methods such as Verhoeff-Van Gieson are required for the confirmatory diagnosis of the condition, which identify the elastic fibers, elastolysis, and elastorrhexis that affect both the papillary and reticular dermis [6]. This staining was not performed due to lack of its availability in our institute.

There are a few case reports of leprosy presenting as secondary anetoderma. Anetoderma is a rare form of presentation of Hansen's disease [6, 7].

This case is being reported due to the unusual and rare presentation of leprosy. Our patient presented with a multibacillary type of leprosy but with only few atrophic wrinkled plaques with a BI of 3+ and without any family history of leprosy. This case suggests that there is still ongoing transmission in the community. Nepal has been able to maintain its status of leprosy elimination till date, but this rare form of leprosy in the community poses a big threat to this status due to the delay in diagnosis. Leprosy presents with varied morphology, so people from endemic areas should be screened for leprosy even on a slightest of suspicion. Active case finding should be intensified to find the hidden cases for early detection and treatment. This case also emphasizes the role of more strong leprosy programs to provide early diagnosis and prompt treatment, as well as the role of clinician for prompt diagnosis of the rare forms of

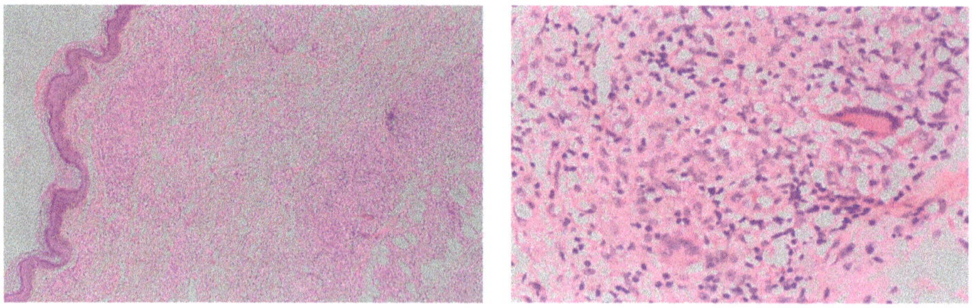

(a) (b)

Figure 3: (a) Histopathological examination showing dermal granuloma with epithelioid cell aggregates and few giant cells (H&E stain 40x magnification). (b) Histopathological examination in higher magnification showing epitheloid cell granulomas with few multinucleated giant cells (H&E stain 100x magnification).

leprosy. Physicians should suspect and rule out leprosy in any unusual dermatological presentations despite the leprosy elimination status of the country.

References

[1] C. Griffiths, J. Barker, T. Bleiker, R. Chalmers, and D. Creamer, "Anetoderma," in *Rook's Textbook of Dermatology*, Blackwell Science Ltd Oxford, Oxford, UK, 9th edition, 2016.

[2] C. Maari and J. Powell, "Anetoderma and other atrophic disorders of the skin," in *Fitzpatrick's Dermatology*, S. Kang, M. Amagai, A. L. Bruckner et al., Eds., McGraw-Hill Education, New York, NY, USA, 9th edition, 2019.

[3] S. Aghaei, M. Sodaifi, F. S. Aslani, and N. Mazharinia, "An unusual presentation of anetoderma: a case report," *BMC Dermatology*, vol. 4, no. 1, p. 9, 2004.

[4] N. Jain, B. S. Rathore, A. Bhardwaj, and R. Bansal, "Primary anetoderma in a young male involving palms, soles and the scalp: rarest of the rare," *Indian Journal of Dermatology*, vol. 60, no. 2, p. 215, 2015.

[5] J. E. Kim, K. M. Sohn, Y. J. Woo et al., "A clinicoimmunohistopathologic study of anetoderma: is protruding type more advanced in stage than indented type?" *Journal of Immunology Research*, vol. 2016, Article ID 4325463, 10 pages, 2016.

[6] T. D. S. R. Neto, F. R. De Oliveira Carneiro, and C. Dos Santos Lima, "Anetoderma secondary to borderline leprosy," *Skin*, vol. 09, Article ID 1330352000, 2009.

[7] D. P. Kineston, Y. Xia, and G. W. Turiansky, "Anetoderma: a case report and review of the literature," *Cutis*, vol. 81, no. 6, p. 501, 2008.

33

Atypical Presentation of Post-Kala-Azar Dermal Leishmaniasis in Bhutan

Ambika Pradhan,[1] Tashi Tobgay,[2] Sithar Dorjee,[2] Tenzin Wangdi,[3] Guofa Zhou,[4] and Nadira D. Karunaweera[5]

[1]*Jigmi Dorji Wangchuck National Referral Hospital, Thimphu, Bhutan*
[2]*Khesar Gyalpo University of Medical Sciences of Bhutan, Thimphu, Bhutan*
[3]*Vector-borne Disease Control Programme, Ministry of Health, Thimphu, Bhutan*
[4]*Program in Public Health, University of California, Irvine, CA, USA*
[5]*Department of Parasitology, Faculty of Medicine, University of Colombo, Colombo, Sri Lanka*

Correspondence should be addressed to Nadira D. Karunaweera; nadira@parasit.cmb.ac.lk

Academic Editor: Ravi Krishnan

This article describes an atypical case of post-kala-azar dermal leishmaniasis associated with complications due to delayed diagnosis and poor case management. The grave consequences of the prolonged disease process that continued for over 2 decades with eventual healing included facial disfigurement, visual impairment, and mental distress both to the patient and the family. The persistent infection within the skin over a lengthy period with likely increased risk of infection spread in the community highlights its potential negative impact on the ongoing leishmaniasis elimination program in the Indian subcontinent. Bhutan is a member of the leishmaniasis elimination network in Asia, and the government continues to invest in maintenance of the national healthcare system. The case study reveals the gaps in the healthcare system with hardships faced by a patient to access quality healthcare and poor patient outcome used as proxy indicators. It also points to the need to enhance access to healthcare to ensure early diagnosis and effective treatment for leishmaniasis patients including those who live in remote areas, in order to achieve the planned disease elimination targets. It also points towards the key challenges faced by a resource poor nation such as Bhutan in achieving universal health coverage and reaching the set goals for disease elimination. The findings underscore the need for a careful review of the national health care system and to address the deficiencies.

1. Introduction

Bhutan plans to achieve universal health coverage (UHC) early [1] and to eliminate leishmaniasis by 2020. However, leishmaniasis surveys have not been conducted since 2006 [2]. Therefore, the existing VL incidence data [3] are unreliable and are based on clinical suspicion alone. Furthermore, the actual cases may go unrecorded due to the dearth of healthcare professionals. The causative agent of VL in Bhutan is *Leishmania donovani*, closely related to the Indian subtype with several *Phlebotomus* spp. identified as probable vector(s) [4].

This article reports the first case of post-kala-azar dermal leishmaniasis (PKDL) from Bhutan with an atypical presentation. Its complex nature, prolonged history, and resultant complications underscore the need for careful review of the healthcare delivery system in Bhutan, with a focus on successful control of neglected tropical diseases (NTDs). This case adds to the evidence that, unless diagnosed early and treated effectively, leishmaniasis may result in considerable debility with devastating socioeconomic consequences and, therefore, pose a formidable challenge to achieve UHC in Bhutan.

2. Methodology

Patient consent was sought as per study protocol and ethics approval granted by the Research Ethic Board of Health, Bhutan. We collected information through review of medical records, laboratory reports, prescriptions maintained since 1999, and patient and family member interviews.

2.1. Case Description. We present the case of a 37-year-old female, a mother of three children from the eastern part of Bhutan, seen by a dermatologist in 2014 at Jigme Dorji Wangchuck National Referral Hospital (JDWNRH). The patient presented with extensive erythematous plaques on forehead, central face, perioral, and cheeks that extended to both ears (Figure 1(a)). The left eye was damaged, and marked swelling was observed in the right eyelid with lid scarring and lagophthalmos. There were plaques extending to the nasal mucosa without intraoral involvement. Other skin and system examinations were apparently normal. Blood investigations showed hemoglobin of 11.7 g/dl, total leukocyte count of 6390 mm^3, lymphocyte 28%, monocyte 4%, neutrophil 62%, eosinophils 5%, platelet count 191,000 mm^3, ESR 39 mm/1st hour, SGOT 35 units/L, SGPT 68 units/L, serum bilirubin 1 mg/dl, urea 21 mg/dl, creatinine 0.8 mg/dl, and fasting blood sugar 80 mg/dl. Tests for HIV, hepatitis B and C, and syphilis were negative. Chest radiograph, ECG, and ultrasound scan of the abdomen were normal. Slit-skin smear (SSS) stained with Giemsa showed numerous Leishman-Donovan (LD) bodies. The kala azar dip stick test (rK-39) was positive. Skin biopsy was done, which showed granulomatous inflammation with predominant infiltration of lymphocytes, a few histiocytes, and LD bodies (Figure 2).

She was treated with intramuscular injections of sodium stibogluconate (SSG) 20 mg/kg/day, given on alternate days with a total of 28 doses. Her lesions markedly improved but with residual scarring (Figure 1(b)). She again presented in 2017 with new dermal plaques over old healed lesions (Figure 1(c)). Both SSS and skin biopsy were positive for LD bodies. She responded to liposomal amphotericin B injections 2 mg/kg/day given for 28 days.

Her clinical history dated back to February 1999 when she presented at a medical clinic with fever, weight loss, and anemia. She was 4 months pregnant and had low hemoglobin (6.5 mg/dl), total leukocyte count of 3500 mm^3, with 57% polymorphs and 43% lymphocytes, ESR 43 mm/1st hour, and elevated liver enzymes. The aldehyde test was positive. Ultrasound scan of the abdomen showed hepatomegaly. Bone marrow aspirate report was unavailable. She was diagnosed as VL and treated with SSG injections 850 mg/day for 20 days. She also received 4 units of blood, and her condition improved. Seven months later, erythematous lesions appeared on her forehead that spread over the face. She was seen by a dermatologist in 2002 who recorded papules and plaques over her cheeks, periorbital, and perioral areas that were suspected as chronic dermatitis or cutaneous lupus erythematosus. She was initially treated with corticosteroids topical therapy, but subsequently, the steroids were given intralesionally and orally. In 2007, she was seen by a WHO consultant for kala azar who suspected PKDL. By this time, she had lid edema with left corneal scarring. The aldehyde test was positive, and ultrasound scan of the abdomen was normal. She was again treated with SSG 850 mg/day for 20 days. Her lesions improved only transiently. Skin biopsies in 2006, 2010, and 2013 failed to confirm leishmaniasis; therefore, no firm diagnosis was recorded. Her eye lesions progressed with the development of phthisis bulbi on the left side with swelling and scarring of the right eye lid.

She again visited the JDWNRH for follow-up in February 2019. New plaques were seen on the nostrils and chin with marked perioral scarring limiting the mouth movements (Figure 1(d)). SSS was negative for *Leishmania* parasites, and skin biopsy showed dense granulomatous inflammation in dermis with lymphocytes, histiocytes, and multinucleated giant cells with histiocytes containing small particles suggestive of LD bodies. PKDL was diagnosed, and oral miltefosine 100 mg/day was started but reduced to 50 mg/day after a month due to severe nausea and elevated liver enzymes (transaminases). Treatment continued with the reduced dosage for further 2 months with clinical improvement (Figure 1(e)) or apparent healing of lesions. No major side effects were noted.

2.2. Socioeconomic Aspects. The patient lives with her children and parents in a remote village of Kalapang. Her husband is a cook and lives away from home in another district. The family lives by subsistence farming. A narrow path leads to the village. Residents walk for 4-5 hours to reach the nearest town to hire a taxi to reach Mongar where the eastern regional referral hospital is located. It takes a further two-day bus ride to reach Thimphu, the capital city to access services of the dermatologist. Over a period of 20 years (1999–2019), she has visited multiple health centers incurring a considerable cost that the family could barely afford. Chronic and debilitating form of disease has had devastating impact on her and her family in terms of economic, social stigmatization, and isolation.

3. Discussion

PKDL that manifests as painless macular and/or papulonodular skin lesions may be a rich source of parasites, promoting transmission. Therefore, early patient management with appropriate drugs is critical to contain the infection spread [5]. Its pathophysiology is obscure and associated risk factors remain debatable [6, 7]. As per records, 10–20% in the Indian subcontinent [6, 8] and almost 50% in Sudan are affected [9] months to years after apparent drug cure of VL or as a sequel of asymptomatic infections [6]. Mucosal involvement rarely occurs [10–12]. Blepheroconjuctivitis and uveitis as sequelae are known with organisms demonstrated in extraocular/intraocular and adnexal muscles [13]. Associated eye inflammation may have grave consequences (aptly demonstrated through this

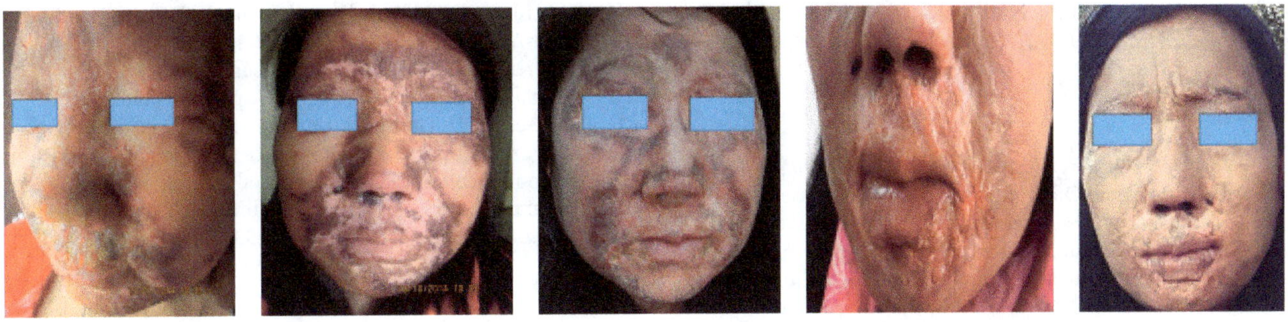

(a) (b) (c) (d) (e)

FIGURE 1: Lesion and/or residual scarring after treatment at different time points. (a) First presentation in 2014 with erythematous plaques with crusting and loss of the left eye. (b) Marked improvement after 28 doses of sodium stibogluconate (SSG) in 2014. (c) In 2017, reappearance of plaques over old healed areas. (d) In 2019, relapsed and diagnosed (and subsequently treated) as post-kala-azar dermal leishmaniasis. (e) In 2019, after treatment with miltefosine.

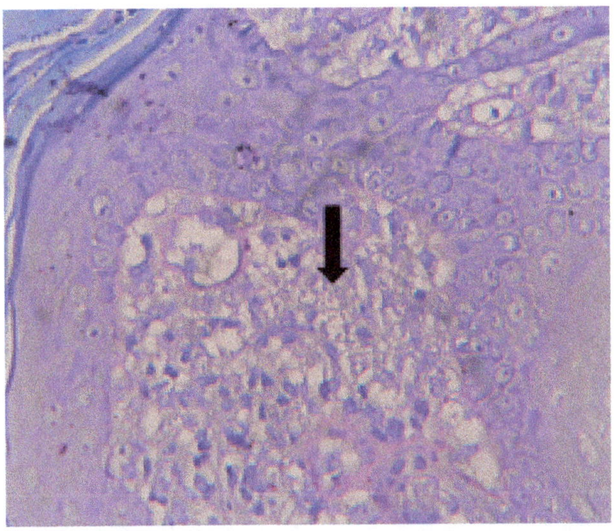

FIGURE 2: Microscopic image (×1000) of the punch biopsy tissue section stained with hematoxylin and eosin (H&E). Arrow points to Leishman-Donovan parasite bodies.

case study). Diagnosis of PKDL is frequently based on clinical picture and epidemiological pattern, since the confirmation through parasite isolation has low sensitivity [14] and, nevertheless, can be improved with the use of molecular techniques [6]. Serological diagnosis (rK-39 or ELISA) is useful to detect exposure to infection, although interpretation of a positive result may be difficult due to persistence of post-VL antibodies. Poor response to anti-leishmanial agents and drug-resistance is widely known in PKDL with the causative agents demonstrating lower in vitro susceptibility to drugs when compared to those of VL [15]. The unacceptable treatment regimens used over the years may have led to the prolonged persistence of infection and recurrences with poor overall patient outcome described. It highlights the need for standard treatment guidelines and availability of effective treatment options in endemic areas to minimize both the resultant morbidity due to PKDL and the risk of further community spread. The latter is due to its potential to act as a reservoir for VL and trigger the emergence of infection in nonendemic areas or its reemergence in areas that have successfully eliminated the disease. PKDL is, therefore, of considerable public health significance in the region [16].

4. Conclusion

This case portrays the challenges faced by patients and clinicians in PKDL management, in Bhutan, which may also be applicable to other resource poor settings where the disease is generally prevalent. It highlights areas that need attention within the healthcare system of Bhutan, including the need for national level guidelines for leishmaniasis treatment and more effective disease awareness programs for public as well as healthcare personnel. Active case detection studies to assess the true burden of leishmaniasis (including PKDL) will also help to understand the magnitude of the problem. The apparent hurdles to achieve UHC in Bhutan highlight the need for remodeling of services based on primary healthcare principles to ensure equality in access to quality healthcare.

Disclosure

The content is solely the responsibility of the authors and does not necessarily represent the official views of the funders.

Authors' Contributions

Ambika Pradhan and Tashi Tobgay contributed equally.

Acknowledgments

Richard Carter, formerly from the University of Edinburgh, United Kingdom, is gratefully acknowledged for editing and review of the manuscript. The study was supported through funds awarded by the National Institute of Allergy and

Infectious Diseases of the National Institutes of Health, USA, under award number U01AI136033.

References

[1] World Health Organization, *Health SDG Profile: Bhutan*, WHO Regional Office for South-East Asia, Geneva, Switzerland, 2019, https://apps.who.int/iris/handle/10665/327755.

[2] S. K. Bhattacharya, N. Rinzin, P. Chusak et al., "Occurrence and significance of kala-azar in Bhutan," *Indian Journal of Medical Research*, vol. 132, no. 9, pp. 337-338, 2010.

[3] Ministry of Health, *Annual Health Bulletin 2017. Policy & Planning Division, Ministry of Health*, Royal Government of Bhutan, Thimphu, Bhutan, 2017, http://www.health.gov.bt/wp-content/uploads/ftps/annual-health-bulletins/Annual%20Health%20Bulletin-2017.pdf.

[4] T. Yangzom, J. Alvar, D. Argaw et al., "Endemic transmission of visceral leishmaniasis in Bhutan," *The American Journal of Tropical Medicine and Hygiene*, vol. 87, no. 6, pp. 1028–1037, 2012.

[5] World Health Organization, "Post-kala-azar dermal leishmaniasis," in *Proceedings of the A Manual for Case Management and Control: Report of a WHO Consultative Meeting*, Kolkata, India, July 2012, https://www.who.int/neglected_diseases/resources/9789241505215/en/.

[6] E. E. Zijlstra, F. Alves, S. Rijal, B. Arana, and J. Alvar, "Post-kala-azar dermal leishmaniasis in the Indian subcontinent: a threat to the south-east Asia region kala-azar elimination programme," *PLoS Neglected Tropical Diseases*, vol. 11, no. 11, Article ID e0005877, 2017.

[7] S. Das, R. Mandal, V. N. Rabidas et al., "Chronic arsenic exposure and risk of post kala-azar dermal leishmaniasis development in India: a retrospective cohort study," *PLoS Neglected Tropical Diseases*, vol. 10, no. 10, Article ID e0005060, 2016.

[8] S. Uranw, B. Ostyn, A. Rijal et al., "Post-Kala-azar dermal leishmaniasis in Nepal: a retrospective cohort study (2000–2010)," *PLoS Neglected Tropical Diseases*, vol. 5, no. 12, p. e1433, 2011.

[9] E. E. Zijlstra, E. A. G. Khalil, P. A. Kager, and A. M. El-Hassan, "Post-kala-azar dermal leishmaniasis in the Sudan: clinical presentation and differential diagnosis," *British Journal of Dermatology*, vol. 143, no. 1, pp. 136–143, 2000.

[10] M. A. Salam, M. A. Siddiqui, S. G. Nabi, K. R. H. Bhaskar, and D. Mondal, "Post-kala-azar dermal leishmaniasis with mucosal involvement: an unusual case presentation including successful treatment with miltefosine," *Journal of Health, Population and Nutrition*, vol. 31, no. 2, pp. 294–297, 2013.

[11] V. Ramesh, H. Kaushal, A. K. Mishra, R. Singh, and P. Salotra, "Clinico-epidemiological analysis of Post kala-azar dermal leishmaniasis (PKDL) cases in India over last two decades: a hospital based retrospective study Infectious Disease epidemiology," *BMC Public Health*, vol. 15, p. 1092, 2015.

[12] S. K. Rathi, R. K. Pandhi, N. Khanna, and P. Chopra, "Mucosal and peri-orificial involvement in post-kala-azar dermal leishmaniasis," *Indian Journal of Dermatology, Venereology and Leprology*, vol. 70, no. 5, pp. 280–282, 2004.

[13] E. A. G. Khalil, A. M. Musa, B. M. Younis, M. E. E. Elfaki, E. E. Zijlstra, and A. M. Elhassan, "Blindness following visceral leishmaniasis: a neglected post-kala-azar complication," *Tropical Doctor*, vol. 41, no. 3, pp. 139-140, 2011.

[14] E. E. Zijlstra, "Biomarkers in post-kala-azar dermal leishmaniasis," *Frontiers in Cellular and Infection Microbiology*, vol. 9, p. 228, 2019.

[15] J. Mishra, R. Madhubala, and S. Singh, "Visceral and post-Kala-Azar dermal leishmaniasis isolates show significant difference in their in vitro drug susceptibility pattern," *Parasitology Research*, vol. 112, no. 3, pp. 1001–1009, 2013.

[16] R. Molina, D. Ghosh, E. Carrillo et al., "Infectivity of post-kala-azar dermal leishmaniasis patients to sand flies: revisiting a proof of concept in the context of the kala-azar elimination program in the Indian Subcontinent," *Clinical Infectious Diseases*, vol. 65, no. 1, pp. 150–153, 2017.

A Multimodal Hair-Loss Treatment Strategy using a New Topical Phytoactive Formulation: A Report of Five Cases

Sanusi Umar[1,2,3] **and Marissa J. Carter**[4]

[1]*Department of Medicine, Dermatology Division, University of California at Los Angeles, Los Angeles, CA, USA*
[2]*Division of Dermatology, Harbor-UCLA Medical Center, Torrance, CA, USA*
[3]*Dr. U Hair and Skin Clinic, Manhattan Beach, CA, USA*
[4]*Strategic Solutions, Inc., Bozeman, MT, USA*

Correspondence should be addressed to Sanusi Umar; drumar@dru.com

Academic Editor: Jacek Cezary Szepietowski

Introduction. Current approved medications for hair loss, such as topical minoxidil and oral finasteride, may have suboptimal efficacy or side effects precluding continued use in some patients. Thus, we report an evaluation of the efficacy, safety, and tolerability of a new topical botanical formulation -GASHEE containing over 12 phytoactive ingredients that affect multiple targets in the cascade of pathophysiologic events that cause hair loss. Five patients with various hair-loss conditions, including cases of previous treatment failures, are presented. *Case Presentation.* This is a case series of four women and one man with hair loss due to various causes, four of whom had failed minoxidil treatment for over a year. All patients used the topical treatment as a sole therapy for at least 3 months before the documentation of outcomes, which involved interval changes noted through each patient's account, direct observation, and photography. *Discussion.* In all patients, we observed significant improvements in hair regrowth in the nape, crown, vertex, and temple areas after 3–15 months of treatment. All patients were highly satisfied with their results and reported no adverse events. Although the use of botanicals in the treatment of hair loss is in an infant stage, the new formulation used in this study demonstrated a good efficacy related to hair growth, warranting further evaluation.

1. Introduction

Androgenetic alopecia (AGA, also called male and female pattern alopecia) is the most common cause of hair loss and is estimated to affect 30–58% of men by age 50 and 12–40% of women depending on age and race [1–4]. It is characterized by progressive hair follicular miniaturization caused by the actions of androgens on epithelial cells of genetically susceptible hair follicles in androgen-dependent areas [5]. While complex genetic inheritance and age of the individual are major risk factors in AGA development, on a cellular level, the initiation of an inflammatory condition in the follicle microenvironment is considered the central event, with contributory mechanisms, including abnormal signal transduction (the wingless-type integration site pathway), high levels of apoptosis, and oxidative stress [6–11]. This supports the need for a multifaceted approach for the treatment of AGA, managing central causes, such as 5-dihydrotestosterone (DHT), oxidative stress, and inflammation, as well as downstream factors that precipitate hair loss by adversely affecting hair stem cells and hair cycles (Figure 1). For instance, DHT, a major factor causing hair loss in AGA, has been found to act downstream by inducing the production of interleukin- (IL-) 6 and transforming growth factor- (TGF-) $\beta 2$ by dermal papilla cells (DPCs), thus suppressing hair growth and premature onset of the catagen phase [12, 13].

To date, there is no permanent cure for AGA, which often precipitates anxiety and depression in affected patients [14]. Two drugs, topical minoxidil and oral finasteride, have been approved by the United States Food and Drug Administration for AGA, with finasteride restricted to men

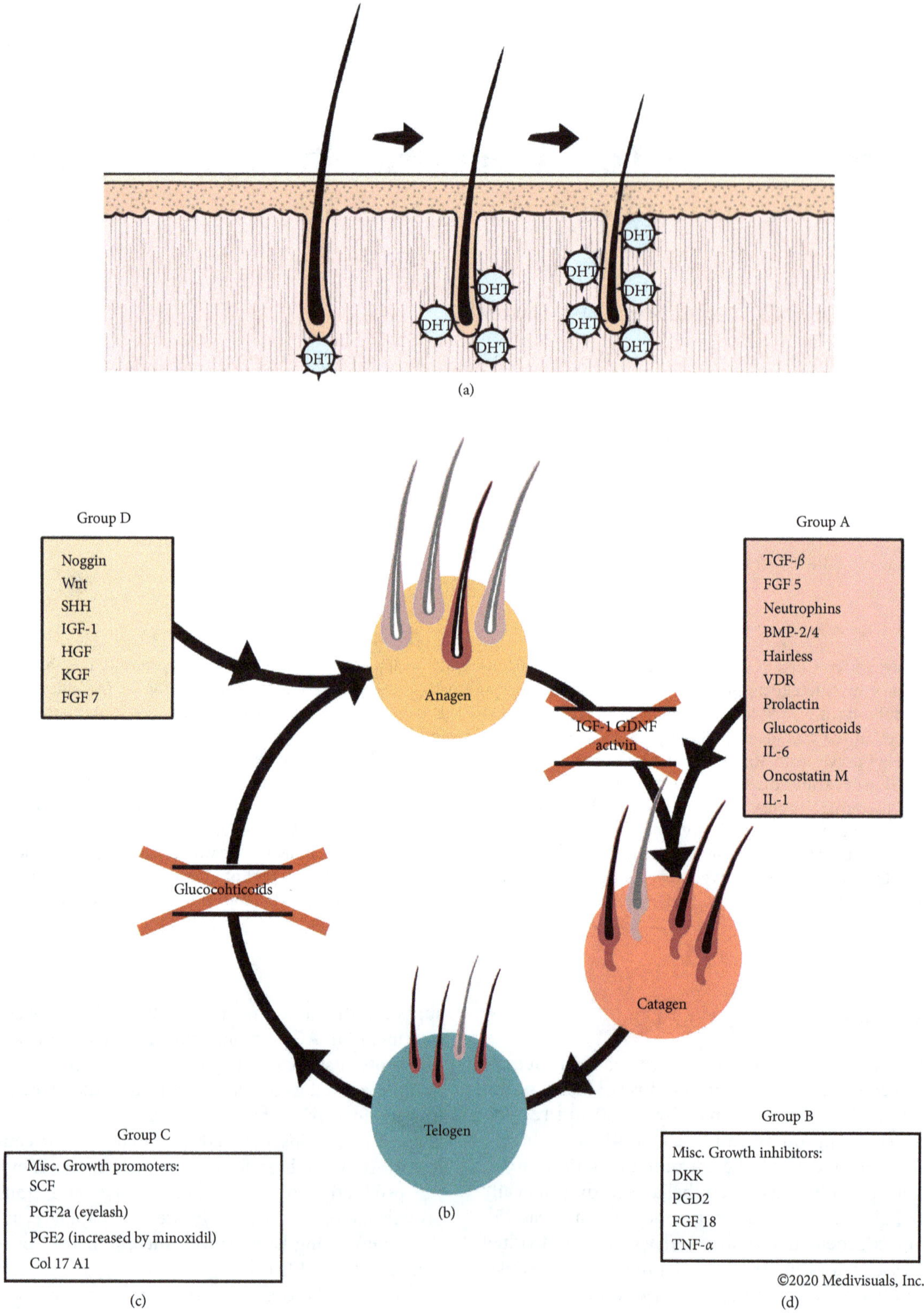

FIGURE 1: The hair follicle cycle showing the effects of various cytokines, growth promoters, and growth inhibitors regarding different stage transitions. BDNF, brain-derived neurotrophic factor; BMP-2/4, bone morphogenetic protein-2/4; col 17 A1, collagen-type XVII α 1 chain; DKK, Dickkopf-related protein; FGF5/7/18, fibroblast growth factor 5/7; GDNF, glial cell line-derived neurotrophic factor; HGF, hepatocyte growth factor; IGF-1, insulin-like growth factor-1; IL-1/6, interleukin-6; KGF, keratinocyte growth factor; PG D2/E2/F2a, prostaglandin D2/E2/F2a; SCF, stem cell factor; SHH, sonic hedgehog; TGF, transforming growth factor; TNF-α, tumor necrosis factor α; VDR = vitamin D receptor; WNT, wingless-type integration site.

because of teratogenicity in women of child-bearing age and poor effects in postmenopausal women. While their mechanism of action is not fully understood, minoxidil is believed to shorten the telogen phase, accelerate the telogen-exogen phase, initiate premature entry of resting hair follicles into the anagen phase, and increase hair follicle size [15]; in contrast, finasteride is a type II 5-α reductase that inhibits the final conversion step of testosterone to its active form, DHT [16]. Both drugs can curtail progressive hair loss and stimulate new hair growth. However, their efficacy is suboptimal. Studies have shown that, after 1 year and 4 months of administering oral finasteride and 5% topical minoxidil, respectively, only 48% and 38.6% of the subjects, respectively, experienced hair growth [17, 18]. Additionally, a study revealed that finasteride was ineffective in treating hair loss in postmenopausal women [19]. Furthermore, finasteride is contraindicated in women of childbearing age because of teratogenicity concerns (Propecia (U.S. package insert) 2013 Merck: Whitehouse Station, NJ), while some men would experience sexual dysfunction from its use. Scalp irritation may occur due to topical minoxidil, which, in addition to instances of suboptimal efficacy, has been cited by some patients as a reason for seeking botanical alternatives to pharmaceuticals [20, 21]. Therefore, there is an unsatisfied need for additional safe and effective therapies for AGA.

Another cause of hair loss is traction alopecia (TA), which results from continuous and prolonged tension to the hair. It is most commonly observed in Black/African American women and children who wear hairstyles that pull excessively at the frontotemporal hairline [22]. TA typically affects the frontal and temporal scalp, as well as anterior and superior to the ears. Hairstyles reported by patients with TA include tight braids, weaves, cornrows, ponytails, chignons, or religious head coverings. It should be noted that traction applied to chemically treated hair (i.e., relaxers and dyes) can further increase the risk of TA [23]. The finding of retained hairs along the frontal and/or temporal hairline ("fringe sign") can help in making a clinical diagnosis of TA [24]. Apart from avoiding all the practices that lead to TA, treatment options have included intralesional corticosteroids directed at the periphery of hair loss to suppress perifollicular inflammation [25], antibiotics used early in the disease for their anti-inflammatory effect [26], minoxidil [27], and hair transplantation.

Central centrifugal cicatricial alopecia (CCCA) is another common cause of alopecia in African American women, perhaps only exceeded in frequency of hair loss by TA, with a likely prevalence of 3–7%, although its true prevalence in various populations is unknown [28]. A genetic basis involving mutations in *PAD13*, which encodes a protein that is essential for proper hair-shaft formation, has been associated with CCCA [29]. Harsh hair grooming practices may precipitate CCCA in genetically predisposed individuals. The scarring alopecia that results from CCCA occurs mainly on the vertex of the scalp with symmetric spread in a centrifugal pattern, hence the name of the disease. The presence of a peripilar white halo as a feature found under dermoscopy, along with other findings, suggests CCCA in an African American patient with mild central thinning. Medical treatments similar to those used for TA have been used, as well as hydroxychloroquine and doxycycline, although all are inadequate and mostly ineffective.

Lastly, there is diffused thinning in postmenopausal women, likely due to the decline in estrogen, which protects hair in women, which would have succumbed to hair loss from androgenic pattern hair loss [30]. Men manifest hair loss from androgenic alopecia early in life because they lack estrogen which protects women from the same problem. However, during and after menopause, the protective effect of estrogen is lost. This accounts for the onset of hair loss, which typically manifests as diffuse hair thinning. Estrogen supplementation is generally not an option because of the inherent dangers of increased risk of breast cancer, as well as other complications of estrogen treatment. As a result, minoxidil is used but is often not effective.

Botanical extracts are obtained from whole plants or specific plant parts, such as the flower, stem, leaves, bark, root, or fruit, and are delivered topically or as dietary supplements. Extracts are typically complex mixtures consisting of numerous individual phytochemical constituents and potential contaminants. Their use as therapeutics has expanded enormously in the last few decades. This approach is attractive, as its wide availability and low cost will allow many different formulations to be devised to address specific disease-related problems. However, a few botanicals are subject to regulation or rigorous research, as they are not labeled for a specific disease [31]. Consequently, their effectiveness or safety is often unclear.

We report the treatment outcomes of five patients treated with a new topical lotion consisting of over 12 phytoactive botanical ingredients and discuss the possible mechanisms of action using published literature.

2. Case Presentation

2.1. Evaluation of Dr. UGro Gashee® Efficacy and Safety. The study was conducted in accordance with the Declaration of Helsinki (1964). All patients signed informed consent forms.

A diverse group of five patients (in terms of age, sex, race, and cause of hair loss) who exclusively used Dr. UGro Gashee® (GASHEE) for their hair treatment is reported. They all reported a high satisfaction level and safety profile after using the topical cosmeceutical.

2.2. Case 1. A 68-year-old Caucasian woman had AGA with significant hairline recession and thinning of the front, top, and crown. She desired to stop her hair loss, as well as stimulate hair growth in the affected areas, and therefore began applying 2% topical minoxidil solution to the affected area as well as taking oral hair- and nail-growth supplements. After over 1 year of using minoxidil without noticeable results, she discontinued both treatments (Figures 2(a) and 3(a)). She began applying the GASHEE lotion formulation to her scalp once at night for 3 months.

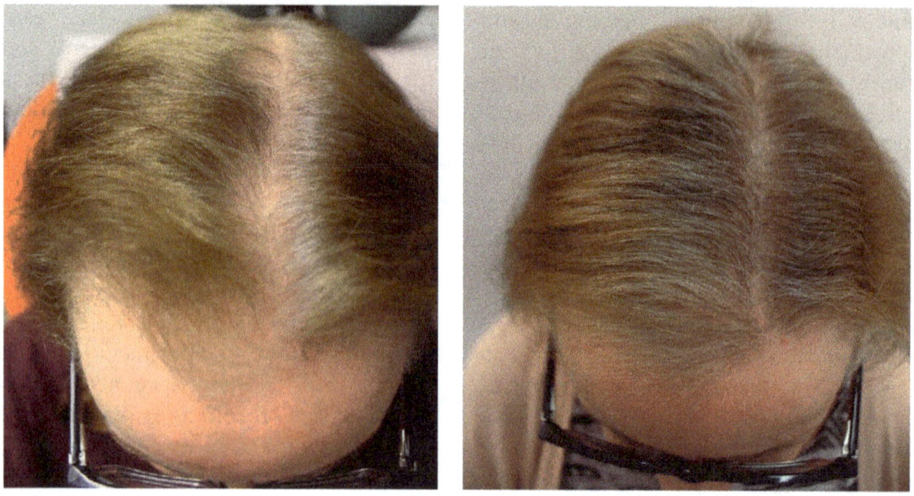

(a) (b)

FIGURE 2: Patient 1: a 68-year-old Caucasian woman. Top of the head before (a) and after (b) 3 months of treatment.

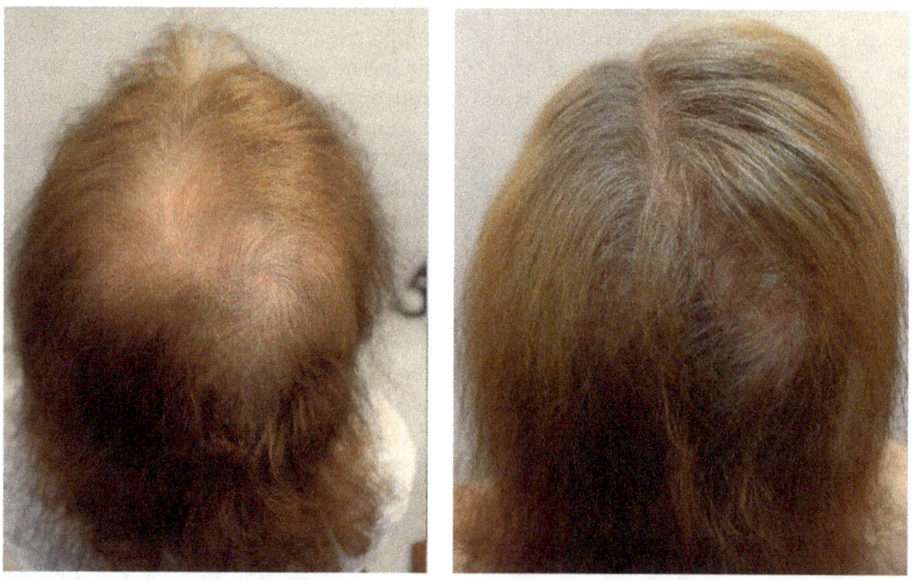

(a) (b)

FIGURE 3: Patient 1: back of the head before (a) and after (b) 3 months of treatment.

After leaving the lotion on her scalp throughout the night, she washed her scalp each morning. In between washings, she noted a reduction in the rate of hair shedding. After 3 months, new hair growth in the affected area was observable, and her hair loss completely stopped (Figures 2(b) and 3(b)). Trichograms (Dino-Lite 1.3MP, AnMo Electronics Co., New Taipei City) of a tattooed spot in the hair path line area of the midscale, performed at 2, 3, and 15 months, revealed progressive interval improvement in hair density and caliber (Figures 4(a)–4(c)). She reported no adverse effects.

2.3. Case 2. A 48-year-old, premenopausal, Chinese woman with hair loss caused by female-pattern hair loss (Figure 5(a)) had a family history of advanced female- and male-pattern hair loss, specifically in her mother and brother. She washed her hair three to five times a week and typically kept her hairstyle natural. She did not want to use pharmaceuticals or any oral treatments and began applying GASHEE lotion to her hair and scalp every night. After 3 months of using the product, she reported hair growth in the areas where the spray lotion was applied to her scalp (Figure 5(b)), and no adverse effects were reported.

2.4. Case 3. A 35-year-old African American male patient with hair loss used minoxidil and finasteride for 12 years with minimal benefits (Figure 6(a)). He applied GASHEE lotion to his hair and entire scalp twice a day. After 4 months of using the product, he reported decreased scarring and

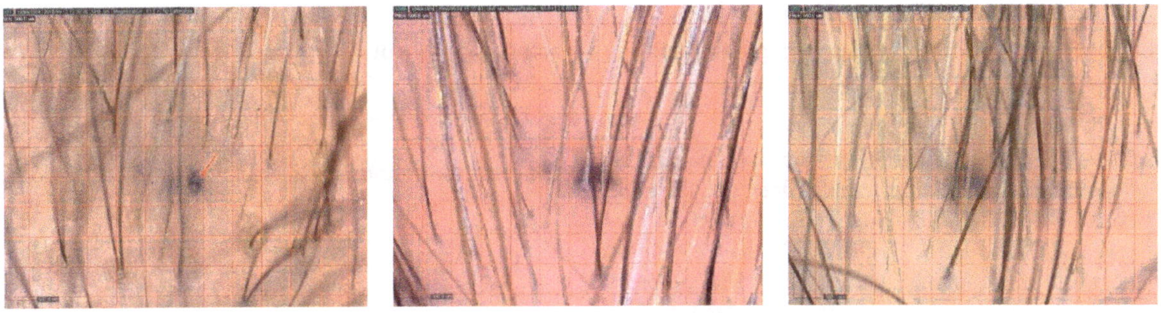

(a) (b) (c)

FIGURE 4: Trichograms of a tattooed spot in the hair path line area of the midscale from patient 1, performed at 2, 3, and 15 months ((a), (b), and (c), respectively). A progressive interval improvement in hair density and caliber was noted.

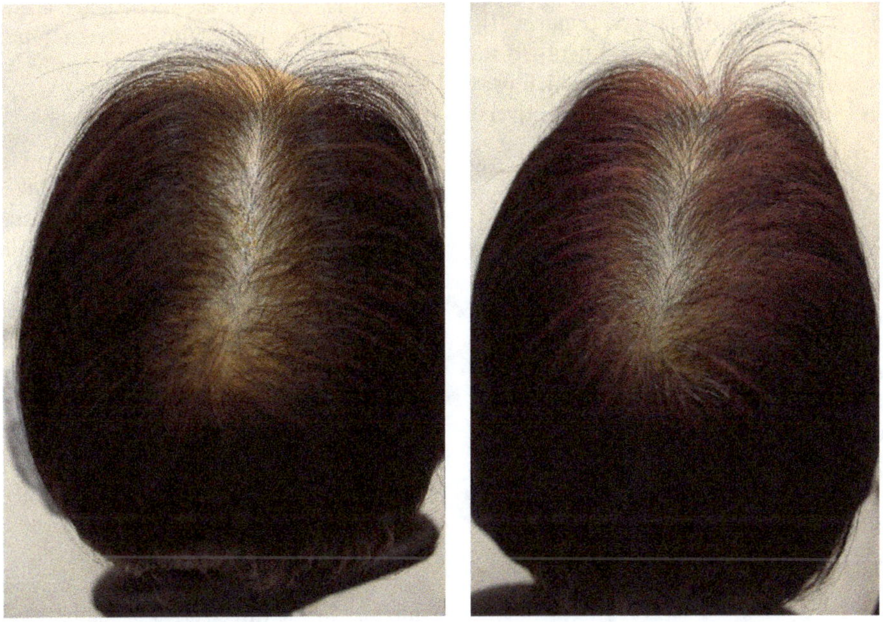

(a) (b)

FIGURE 5: Patient 2: a 48-year-old Chinese woman. Top of the head before (a) and after 3 months of treatment (b).

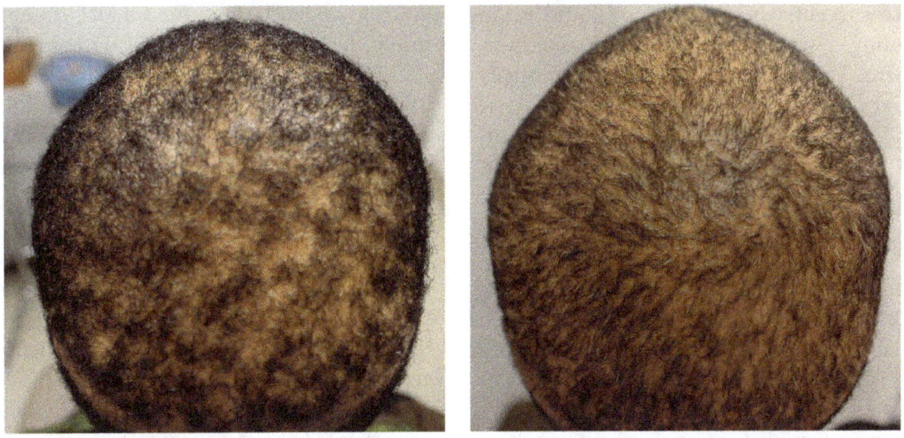

(a) (b)

FIGURE 6: Patient 3: a 35-year-old African American man. Crown before (a) and after 3 months of treatment (b).

inflammation of his scalp and increased hair density in areas where he applied the lotion formulation (Figures 6(b)). He reported no adverse effects.

2.5. Case 4. A 50-year-old African American woman had a history of hair loss in her hairline, temple edges, and the nape area, all consistent with a clinical diagnosis of traction alopecia (Figures 7(a) and 8(a)). Similarly, she had a biopsy-proven diagnosis of central centrifugal cicatricial alopecia involving the vertex (Figure 9(a)). She had used topical minoxidil for over 1 year on all areas of hair loss, as well as intralesional steroid injections, albeit with minimal benefits. After discontinuing all treatments, she began applying the GASHEE lotion twice a day. At 3 months, she reported significant improvement of hair fullness in the hairline, temples, and her nape areas of traction alopecia (Figures 7(b) and 8(b)). She equally observed some improvements in the vertex, with the exception of shiny scarred areas which were devoid of hair follicles (Figure 9(b)). She reported no adverse effects.

2.6. Case 5. A 56-year-old, postmenopausal, Hispanic woman completed chemotherapy for breast cancer and developed hair loss. When it regrew, she had generalized thinness with marked appearance in the crown, top, and frontal areas. She similarly reported a global loss of volume and inability to grow her hair long. Treatment with minoxidil for over 1 year showed no improvement. Within 6 weeks of initiating GASHEE lotion application, she noticed improvement in her global hair volume. Improvement was sustained through 18 months of documentation. She reported no adverse effects. Figures 10(a) and 10(b) depict the crown before and after 9 months of treatment.

3. Discussion

3.1. Dr. UGro Gashee®. Dr. UGro Gashee® (FineTouch Laboratories: Manhattan Beach, CA) is a novel, proprietary topical formulation consisting of over 12 different botanicals, vitamins, and cosmeceuticals, available as a liquid lotion or pomade, containing a similar amount of phytoactives. Each of its components has been incorporated to potentially apply a multifaceted approach to the treatment of AGA (Table 1). Similarly, the formulation contains methylsulfomethane, designed to aid penetration of the active topical ingredients [32]. Since it is used as a topical formulation, it minimizes adverse or toxic effects that are sometimes experienced after the ingestion of botanical extracts. The ingredients are derived by either cold pressing or using natural solvents, thus keeping in alignment with a holistic approach to cosmeceuticals and health care. In addition, the preparation of many topical botanical solutions involves the use of high temperatures to attain a desired texture or achieve maximum dissolution and emulsification. However, such an approach may destabilize or deactivate heat-sensitive phytochemicals, thus defeating the purpose of their use. Using ingredients obtained by implementing methods based on close-to-ambient temperatures and a formulation process that avoids heat, the biochemical or biological activity of active components is optimally retained.

Furthermore, GASHEE formulation favors using whole extracts as opposed to compounds isolated from plants. There is evidence suggesting that, at comparable doses and concentrations, industrially isolated compounds do not have as much activity as the unrefined plant due to the absence of interacting substances present in the extract [52].

Finally, one issue that has made many topical botanicals commercially nonviable is the inability to preserve them such that their shelf life is optimal without resorting to harsh chemical preservatives. GASHEE overcomes this challenge owing to its heat-free proprietary formulation process and blend of ingredients, as well as the naturally derived sustainable preservatives it contains. All of these factors are aimed at the increasing number of people who are reluctant to consume pharmaceuticals and oral medications and prefer topical natural solutions that are safer.

3.2. Dr. UGro Gashee® Ingredients and the Hair Follicle Cycle. Human hair follicles are in a constant state of cycling throughout their biological life. The cycle (Figure 1) consists of a growth phase (anagen) during which the follicle elongates and is at its thickest in caliber; a degeneration phase (catagen) which marks the end of anagen and is characterized by apoptotic changes involving the sections that extend from and include the hair bulb where DPCs reside to the bulge area where the hair stem cells live; and a resting phase (telogen) during which follicle miniaturizes and may shed (exogen). Resumption of anagen is marked by regeneration of the hair bulb and the hair follicle sections leading up to the follicle bulge area.

Several genes encode proteins that act as activators or inhibitors in the three stages of the hair follicle cycle (Figure 1). Understanding the mechanism underlying the influence of various components of the GASHEE formulation on many of these proteins will elucidate how it can be of benefit against hair loss. For example, one of the primary active constituents of green tea, epigallocatechin, is a DHT inhibitor, which prevents insulin-like growth factor- (IGF-) 1 levels from being depressed. IGF-1 prevents hair follicles from transitioning from anagen to catagen while encouraging the telogen to anagen transition [47]. *Eclipta alba* extract includes substances that can downregulate TGF-1β, a cytokine that encourages the hair follicle to transfer to the catagen phase, although the exact regulation pathway by which this occurs remains unknown [50]. Fenugreek extract can counteract the effects of proinflammatory cytokines, such as IL-6 and tumor necrosis factor- (TNF-) α, thus positively intervening in anagen-to-catagen and catagen-to-telogen stages of the hair cycle [53]. An abnormally functioning vitamin D receptor and inadequate vitamin D3 levels are known to disrupt the normal hair follicle cycle [51, 54]. Extracts of Gotu kola have been shown to be angiogenic. The angiogenesis marker, vascular endothelial growth factor, can mitigate androgen-induced apoptosis through the phosphoinositide-3-kinase-protein kinase B (Akt) pathway, which could affect the progression of anagen to catagen [55, 56].

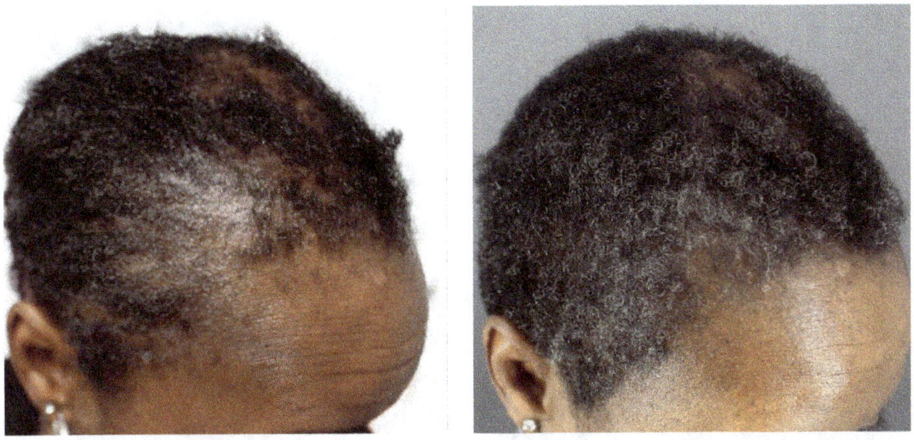

(a) (b)

FIGURE 7: Patient 4: a 50-year-old African American woman diagnosed with central centrifugal cicatricial alopecia in the vertex and midscalp and traction alopecia in the temple, hairline, and nape areas. Right temple before (a) and after (b) 3 months of lotion use.

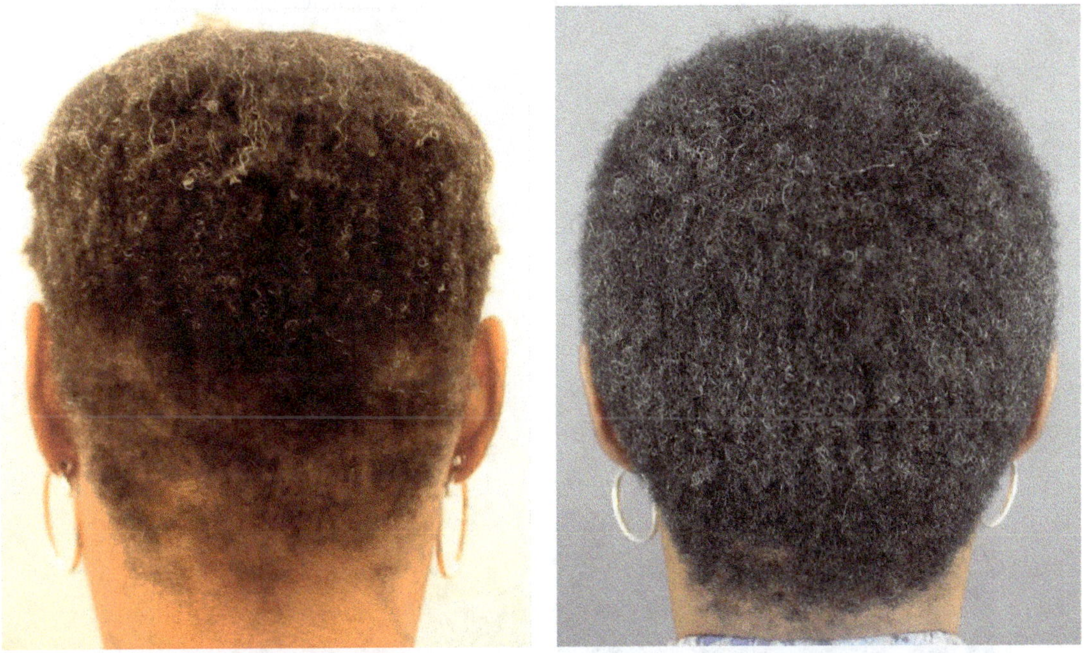

(a) (b)

FIGURE 8: Patient 4: back of the head before (a) and after (b) 3 months of lotion use.

3.3. Main Dr. UGro Gashee® Ingredients in Detail

3.3.1. Gotu Kola. Gotu kola (*Centella asiatica* (*C. asiatica*)) is an herb used for thousands of years in the Ayurvedic Indian tradition, the activities of which have been attributed to several saponin moieties [57, 58]. Extracts of this herb have demonstrated antioxidant activity, as evidenced by several murine studies. For example, administration of Gotu extracts resulted in a significant oxidative defense in an Alzheimer's disease model [59]. In a neuroprotective model, *C. asiatica* mitigated the neurotoxic effects of 3-nitropropionic acid on oxidative stress in the cytosol and mitochondria and prevented the significant depletion of glutathione, total thiols, and other enzymic antioxidant systems [59, 60]. Finally, a significant decrease in malondialdehyde and an increase in glutathione and catalase levels were observed in male Wistar rats treated with 200 and 300 mg/kg of *C. asiatica* [33]. Notably, *C. asiatica* extracts were demonstrated to activate the hair-inductive capacity in cultured human DPCs [61].

3.3.2. Green Tea Extract. Green tea extract is made from leaves of the plant, *Camellia sinensis* L. (Theaceae), in which enzymatic oxidation has been minimized. It is one of the most extensively studied botanicals due to its antioxidant, metal-chelating,

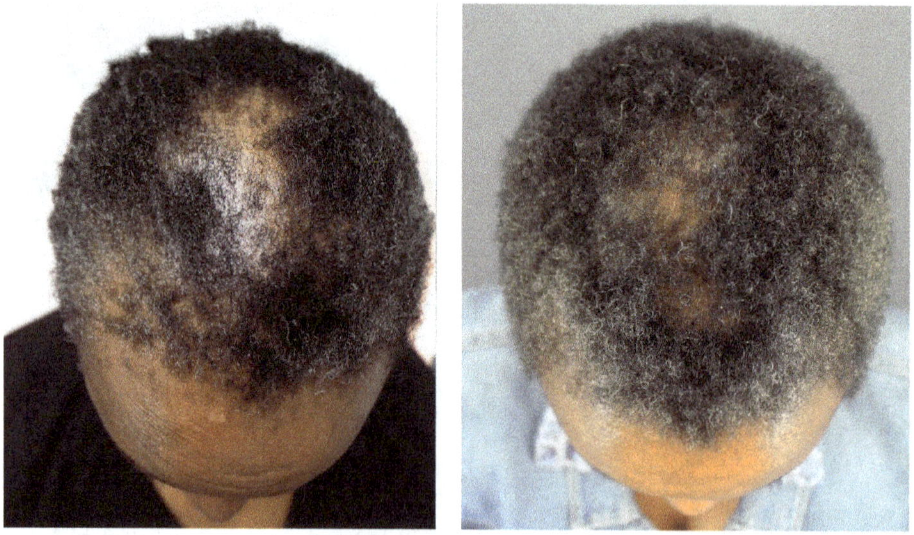

(a) (b)

Figure 9: Patient 4: top of the head before (a) and after (b) 3 months of lotion use.

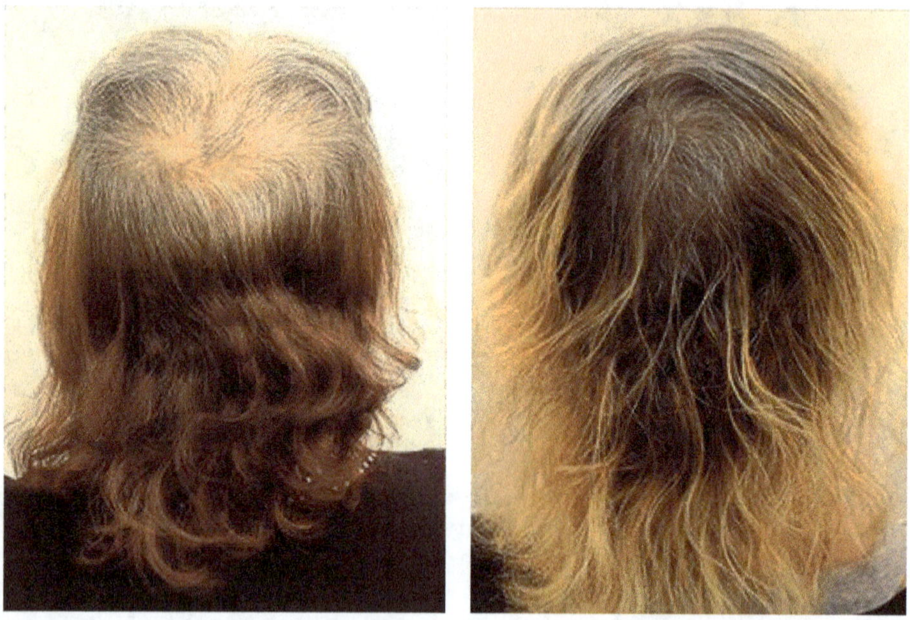

(a) (b)

Figure 10: Patient 5: a 56-year-old, postmenopausal, Hispanic woman with marked thinning in the crown area, global loss of volume, and inability to grow hair long. Crown and back of head before (a) and after (b) 9 months of treatment.

anticarcinogenic, anti- and proapoptotic, and anti-inflammatory properties, originating from constituent catechins, 50–80% of which consist of epigallocatechin gallate (EGCG) [62]. An early study used BALB/black mice devoid of hair on the head, neck, and dorsal areas and randomly assigned them to an experimental group treated with 50% fraction of polyphenol extract from dehydrated green tea in their drinking water for six months and a control group given plain water. The authors showed that one-third of the mice in the experimental group had significant hair regrowth ($p = 0.014$) compared to that in the control group [63]. Similarly, further investigation revealed that EGCG promotes hair growth in an *ex vivo* culture of hair follicles and the proliferation of cultured DPCs [64]. The authors suggested that growth stimulation of DPCs by EGCG *in vitro* was mediated by the upregulation of phosphorylated extracellular signal-regulated kinases and Akt, which are important for regulating cell growth, proliferation, survival, mobility, and invasion, as well as by the increased B-cell lymphoma 2/bcl-2-like protein 4 ratio, functioning like a rheostat to determine cell susceptibility to apoptosis. Notably, similar results were also obtained *in vivo* in dermal papillae of human scalps [64].

Table 1: Components of Dr. UGro Gashee®.

Generic name	INCI name	Properties
Gotu kola	*Centella asiatica*	Activates hair-inductive capacity in three-dimensional spheroid cultured dermal papilla cells [33]
Aloe barbadensis extract	*Aloe barbadensis* extract	Immunomodulatory and anti-inflammatory properties [34]
Red (Asian) ginseng extract	Panax root ginseng extract	May reduce hair loss despite the presence of DKK-1, a strong catagen inducer via apoptosis [35]
Polygonum fo-ti extract	Polygonum multiflorum root extract	Increases the proliferation of dermal papillary cells [36]
Cysteine/N-acetyl-cysteine	Cysteine/N-acetyl cysteine	Androgen-inducible TGF-β1 promotes androgenetic alopecia; however, it is significantly suppressed by the ROS scavenger, N-acetyl cysteine [37]
Turmeric	*Curcuma longa*	Scavenger of reactive oxygen species, anti-inflammatory agent, and immunomodulator [38, 39]; anti-androgen [40] inhibits androgenic induction of TGF-β, which induces catagen and inhibits hair growth and perifollicular fibrosis [41–43]
Horsetail extract	*Equisetum arvense* extract	5α-reductase inhibitor [44]
Fenugreek oil	*Trigonella foenum-graecum* oil	Anti-inflammatory, antioxidant, antifungal, and antibacterial properties [45]
Tall oil fatty acids	Tall oil fatty acid	β-Sitosterol component may be an effective 5-alpha reductase inhibitor [46]
Green tea extract with 95% EGCG	*Camellia sinensis* leaf extract	Phytoconstituent epigallocatechin 3-gallate is a 5-α reductase inhibitor [47]
Saw palmetto	*Serenoa serrulata*	Inhibits both isoforms of 5-α reductase, preventing conversion of testosterone to its active form, DHT, and also promotes hair follicle vascularization [48, 49]
Eclipta alba oil	*Eclipta alba* (bhringraj oil)	Stimulates follicular keratinocyte proliferation and delays terminal differentiation by downregulating TGF-β1 expression [50]
Vitamin D3	Vitamin D3	Animal studies show that vitamin D3 analogs stimulate hair regrowth [51]

DHT: 5-dihydrotestosterone; DKK-1: Dickkopf WNT signaling pathway inhibitor 1; EGCG: epigallocatechin gallate; IGF-1: insulin growth factor 1; INCI: International Nomenclature of Cosmetic Ingredients; ROS: reactive oxygen species; TGF: transforming growth factor.

Finally, researchers used a micro-RNA (miRNA) microarray to identify miRNA expression levels in DPCs and determine the influence of this expression on the protective effects of EGCG against DHT-induced cell death, growth arrest, intracellular reactive oxygen species (ROS) levels, and senescence [65]. The experiments demonstrated that EGCG does protect against the effects of DHT by altering the miRNA expression profile in human DPCs, attenuating DHT-mediated cell death and growth arrest and decreasing intracellular ROS levels and senescence.

3.3.3. Fenugreek. Fenugreek (*Trigonella foenum-graecum*) is a traditional medicinal herb commonly used in India, China, Thailand, and South-East Asian countries [66]. Bioactive molecules identified in extracts include saponins, flavonoids, coumarins, and alkaloids, targeting several molecules involved in inflammation and cancer cell proliferation, invasion, migration, angiogenesis, and metastasis [66, 67].

The antioxidative and anti-inflammatory properties of fenugreek have been noted in several studies [68–73]. It demonstrated a significant acute anti-inflammatory activity relative to water (control) and sodium diclofenac (standard) in mice with carrageenan-induced rat paw edema [68]. Diosgenin, the major steroidal sapogenin in the fenugreek seed, has demonstrated various anti-inflammatory functions, such as reducing the production of several inflammatory mediators, including nitric oxidase, IL-1, and IL-6, in murine macrophages [69, 70]. Similarly, it has been shown to inhibit superoxide generation in bone marrow-activated mouse neutrophils along with blocking cyclic adenosine monophosphate, protein kinase A, cytosolic phospholipase A2, p21-activated kinase, Akt, and mitogen-activated protein kinase (MAPK) signaling pathways [71]. This eventually leads to a reduction in the adhesive capacity of vascular smooth muscle cells (VSMCs) and TNF-α-mediated induction of intercellular adhesion molecule 1 and vascular cell adhesion molecule 1 in VSMCs by inhibiting the MAPK/Akt/nuclear factor-κB signaling pathway and ROS production [72]. Additionally, it has been demonstrated to alleviate oxidative stress and inflammatory and apoptotic markers induced by monocrotaline [73].

In conclusion, the results reported here in five patients with hair loss show that meaningful improvement with a high safety profile was attainable using a topical botanical formulation that focuses on multiple targets of pathophysiologic hair-loss pathways. This formulation may present an alternative for people who wish to avoid the use of pharmaceuticals either due to concerns of adverse effects or suboptimal efficacy. A large randomized, double-blind, placebo-controlled study would be necessary to define the safety and efficacy of this formulation.

References

[1] J. B. Hamilton, "Patterned loss of hair in man: types and incidence," *Annals of the New York Academy of Sciences*, vol. 53, no. 3, pp. 708–728, 1951.

[2] K. S. Shankar, M. Chakravarthi, and R. Shilpakar, "Male androgenetic alopecia: population-based study in 1005 subjects," *International Journal of Trichology*, vol. 1, no. 2, pp. 131–133, 2009.

[3] M. P. Birch, J. F. Messenger, and A. G. Messenger, "Hair density, hair diameter and the prevalence of female pattern hair loss," *British Journal of Dermatology*, vol. 144, no. 2, pp. 297–304, 2001.

[4] O. T. Norwood, "Incidence of female androgenetic alopecia (female pattern alopecia)," *Dermatologic Surgery*, vol. 27, no. 1, pp. 53-54, 2001.

[5] F. Lolli, F. Pallotti, A. Rossi et al., "Androgenetic alopecia: a review," *Endocrine*, vol. 57, no. 1, pp. 9–17, 2017.

[6] Y. F. Mahé, J.-F. Michelet, N. Billoni et al., "Androgenetic alopecia and microinflammation," *International Journal of Dermatology*, vol. 39, no. 8, pp. 576–584, 2000.

[7] C. M. Magro, A. Rossi, J. Poe, S. Manhas-Bhutani, and N. Sadick, "The role of inflammation and immunity in the pathogenesis of androgenetic alopecia," *Journal of Drugs in Dermatology*, vol. 10, no. 12, pp. 1404–1411, 2011.

[8] L. Martinez-Jacobo, C. I. Ancer-Arellano, R. Ortiz-Lopez et al., "Evaluation of the expression of genes associated with inflammation and apoptosis in androgenetic alopecia by targeted RNA-seq," *Skin Appendage Disorders*, vol. 4, no. 4, pp. 268–273, 2018.

[9] R. Dey-Rao and A. A. Sinha, "A genomic approach to susceptibility and pathogenesis leads to identifying potential novel therapeutic targets in androgenetic alopecia," *Genomics*, vol. 109, no. 3-4, pp. 165–176, 2017.

[10] J. H. Upton, R. F. Hannen, A. W. Bahta, N. Farjo, B. Farjo, and M. P. Philpott, "Oxidative stress-associated senescence in dermal papilla cells of men with androgenetic alopecia," *Journal of Investigative Dermatology*, vol. 135, no. 5, pp. 1244–1252, 2015.

[11] B. E. Prie, L. Iosif, I. Tivig et al., "Oxidative stress in androgenetic alopecia," *Journal of Medicine and Life*, vol. 9, pp. 79–83, 2016.

[12] T. Hibino and T. Nishiyama, "Role of TGF-β2 in the human hair cycle," *Journal of Dermatological Science*, vol. 35, no. 1, pp. 9–18, 2004.

[13] M. H. Kwack, J. S. Ahn, M. K. Kim, J. C. Kim, and Y. K. Sung, "Dihydrotestosterone-inducible IL-6 inhibits elongation of human hair shafts by suppressing matrix cell proliferation and promotes regression of hair follicles in mice," *Journal of Investigative Dermatology*, vol. 132, no. 1, pp. 43–49, 2012.

[14] G. Titeca, L. Goudetsidis, B. Francq et al., "'The psychosocial burden of alopecia areata and androgenetica': a cross-sectional multicentre study among dermatological out-patients in 13 European countries," *Journal of the European Academy of Dermatology and Venereology*, vol. 34, no. 2, pp. 406–411, 2020.

[15] M. Barbareschi, "The use of minoxidil in the treatment of male and female androgenetic alopecia: a story of more than 30 years," *Giornale Italiano di Dermatologia e Venereologia: Organo Ufficiale, Societa Italiana di Dermatologia e Sifilografia*, vol. 153, no. 1, pp. 102–106, 2018.

[16] S. W. Lee, M. Juhasz, P. Mobasher, C. Ekelem, and N. A. Mesinkovska, "A systematic review of topical finasteride in the treatment of androgenetic alopecia in men and women," *Journal of Drugs in Dermatology*, vol. 17, no. 4, pp. 457–463, 2018.

[17] K. D. Kaufman, E. A. Olsen, D. Whiting et al., "Finasteride in the treatment of men with androgenetic alopecia," *Journal of the American Academy of Dermatology*, vol. 39, no. 4, pp. 578–589, 1998.

[18] E. A. Olsen, D. Whiting, W. Bergfeld et al., "A multicenter, randomized, placebo-controlled, double-blind clinical trial of a novel formulation of 5% minoxidil topical foam versus placebo in the treatment of androgenetic alopecia in men," *Journal of the American Academy of Dermatology*, vol. 57, no. 5, pp. 767–774, 2007.

[19] V. H. Price, J. L. Roberts, M. Hordinsky et al., "Lack of efficacy of finasteride in postmenopausal women with androgenetic alopecia," *Journal of the American Academy of Dermatology*, vol. 43, no. 5, pp. 768–776, 2000.

[20] D. A. Whiting, E. A. Olsen, R. Savin et al., "Efficacy and tolerability of finasteride 1mg in men aged 41 to 60 years with male pattern hair loss," *European Journal of Dermatology*, vol. 13, pp. 150–160, 2003.

[21] E. S. Friedman, P. M. Friedman, D. E. Cohen, and K. Washenik, "Allergic contact dermatitis to topical minoxidil solution: etiology and treatment," *Journal of the American Academy of Dermatology*, vol. 46, no. 2, pp. 309–312, 2002.

[22] C. N. Lawson, J. Hollinger, S. Sethi et al., "Updates in the understanding and treatments of skin & hair disorders in women of color," *International Journal of Women's Dermatology*, vol. 3, no. 1, pp. S21–S37, 2017.

[23] N. P. Khumalo, S. Jessop, F. Gumedze, and R. Ehrlich, "Hairdressing and the prevalence of scalp disease in African adults," *British Journal of Dermatology*, vol. 157, no. 5, pp. 981–988, 2007.

[24] A. Samrao, V. H. Price, D. Zedek, and P. Mirmirani, "The "Fringe Sign"-a useful clinical finding in traction alopecia of the marginal hair line," *Dermatology Online Journal*, vol. 17, p. 1, 2011.

[25] L. Uwakwe, B. De Souza, A. Tovar-Garza, and A. McMichael, "Intralesional triamcinolone acetonide in the treatment of traction alopecia," *Journal of Drugs in Dermatology*, vol. 19, no. 2, pp. 128–130, 2020.

[26] V. D. Callender, A. J. McMichael, and G. F. Cohen, "Medical and surgical therapies for alopecias in black women," *Dermatologic Therapy*, vol. 17, no. 2, pp. 164–176, 2004.

[27] N. P. Khumalo and R. M. Ngwanya, "Traction alopecia: 2% topical minoxidil shows promise. Report of two cases," *Journal of the European Academy of Dermatology and Venereology*, vol. 21, no. 3, pp. 433-434, 2007.

[28] T. A. Ogunleye, A. McMichael, and E. A. Olsen, "Central centrifugal cicatricial alopecia," *Dermatologic Clinics*, vol. 32, no. 2, pp. 173–181, 2014.

[29] L. Malki, O. Sarig, M.-T. Romano et al., "Variant *PADI3* in central centrifugal cicatricial alopecia," *New England Journal of Medicine*, vol. 380, no. 9, pp. 833–841, 2019.

[30] Q. Q. Dinh and R. Sinclair, "Female pattern hair loss: current treatment concepts," *Clinical Interventions in Aging*, vol. 2, no. 2, pp. 189–199, 2007.

[31] A. L. Roe, D. A. McMillan, and C. Mahony, "A tiered approach for the evaluation of the safety of botanicals used as dietary supplements: an industry strategy," *Clinical Pharmacology & Therapeutics*, vol. 104, no. 3, pp. 446–457, 2018.

[32] S. Shanmugam, R. Baskaran, S. Nagayya-Sriraman et al., "The effect of methylsulfonylmethane on hair growth promotion of magnesium ascorbyl phosphate for the treatment of alopecia," *Biomolecules and Therapeutics*, vol. 17, no. 3, pp. 241–248, 2009.

[33] M. Veerendra Kumar and Y. Gupta, "Effect of *Centella asiatica* on cognition and oxidative stress in an intra-

cerebroventricular streptozotocin model of Alzheimer's disease in rats," *Clinical and Experimental Pharmacology and Physiology*, vol. 30, no. 5-6, pp. 336–342, 2003.

[34] B. J. Balan, M. Niemcewicz, J. Kocik et al., "Oral administration of aloe vera gel, anti-microbial and anti-inflammatory herbal remedy, stimulates cell-mediated immunity and antibody production in a mouse model," *Central European Journal of Immunology*, vol. 39, pp. 125–130, 2014.

[35] Y. Lee, S. N. Kim, Y. D. Hong, B. C. Park, and Y. Na, "Panax ginseng extract antagonizes the effect of DKK-1-induced catagen-ike changes of hair follicles," *International Journal of Molecular Medicine*, vol. 40, no. 4, pp. 1194–1200, 2017.

[36] Y. N. Sun, L. Cui, W. Li et al., "Promotion effect of constituents from the root of Polygonum multiflorum on hair growth," *Bioorganic & Medicinal Chemistry Letters*, vol. 23, no. 17, pp. 4801–4805, 2013.

[37] H. Shin, H. G. Yoo, S. Inui et al., "Induction of transforming growth factor-beta 1 by androgen is mediated by reactive oxygen species in hair follicle dermal papilla cells," *BMB Reports*, vol. 46, no. 9, pp. 460–464, 2013.

[38] A. Rahmani, M. Alsahli, S. Aly, M. Khan, and Y. Aldebasi, "Role of curcumin in disease prevention and treatment," *Advanced Biomedical Research*, vol. 7, no. 1, p. 38, 2018.

[39] M. C. L. C. Fadus and L. H. Bikhchandi, "Curcumin: an age-old anti-inflammatory and anti-neoplastic agent," *Journal of Traditional and Complementary Medicine*, vol. 7, pp. 339–346, 2016.

[40] G. Pumthong, P. Asawanonda, S. Varothai et al., "Curcuma aeruginosa, a novel botanically derived 5α-reductase inhibitor in the treatment of male-pattern baldness: a multicenter, randomized, double-blind, placebo-controlled study," *Journal of Dermatological Treatment*, vol. 23, no. 5, pp. 385–392, 2012.

[41] S. Shishodia, "Molecular mechanisms of curcumin action: gene expression," *Biofactors*, vol. 39, no. 1, pp. 37–55, 2013.

[42] S. C. Gupta, S. Patchva, and B. B. Aggarwal, "Therapeutic roles of curcumin: lessons learned from clinical trials," *The AAPS Journal*, vol. 15, no. 1, pp. 195–218, 2013.

[43] S. Huh, J. Lee, E. Jung et al., "A cell-based system for screening hair growth-promoting agents," *Archives of Dermatological Research*, vol. 301, no. 5, pp. 381–385, 2009.

[44] W. Chaiyana, C. Punyoyai, S. Somwongin et al., "Inhibition of 5α-reductase, IL-6 secretion, and oxidation process of equisetum debile Roxb. Ex vaucher extract as functional food and nutraceuticals ingredients," *Nutrients*, vol. 9, no. 10, p. 1105, 2017.

[45] K. C. Nagulapalli-Venkata, A. Swaroop, D. Bagchi et al., "A small plant with big benefits: fenugreek (*Trigonella foenum-graecum* Linn.) for disease prevention and health promotion," *Molecular Nutrition & Food Research*, vol. 61, 2017.

[46] N. Prager, K. Bickett, N. French, and G. Marcovici, "A randomized, double-blind, placebo-controlled trial to determine the effectiveness of botanically derived inhibitors of 5-α-Reductase in the treatment of androgenetic alopecia," *The Journal of Alternative and Complementary Medicine*, vol. 8, no. 2, pp. 143–152, 2002.

[47] O. Parisi, L. Scrivano, F. Amone et al., "Interconnected PolymerS TeChnology (IPSTiC): an effective approach for the modulation of 5α-reductase activity in hair loss conditions," *Journal of Functional Biomaterials*, vol. 9, no. 3, p. 44, 2018.

[48] S. L. Ooi and S. C. Pak, "*Serenoa repens* for lower urinary tract symptoms/benign prostatic hyperplasia: current evidence and its clinical implications in naturopathic medicine," *The Journal of Alternative and Complementary Medicine*, vol. 23, no. 8, pp. 599–606, 2017.

[49] H. L. Zhu, Y. H. Gao, J. Q. Yang, J. B. Li, and J. Gao, "Serenoa repens extracts promote hair regeneration and repair of hair loss mouse models by activating TGF-β and mitochondrial signaling pathway," *European Review for Medical and Pharmacological Sciences*, vol. 22, no. 12, pp. 4000–4008, 2018.

[50] S. Begum, M. R. Lee, L. J. Gu, J. Hossain, and C. K. Sung, "Exogenous stimulation with Eclipta alba promotes hair matrix keratinocyte proliferation and downregulates TGF-β1 expression in nude mice," *International Journal of Molecular Medicine*, vol. 35, no. 2, pp. 496–502, 2015.

[51] K. T. Amor, R. M. Rashid, and P. Mirmirani, "Does D matter? the role of vitamin D in hair disorders and hair follicle cycling," *Dermatology Online Journal*, vol. 16, p. 3, 2010.

[52] H. Wagner and G. Ulrich-Merzenich, "Synergy research: approaching a new generation of phytopharmaceuticals," *Phytomedicine*, vol. 16, no. 2-3, pp. 97–110, 2009.

[53] A. A. Chowdhury, N. B. Gawali, R. Munshi, and A. R. Juvekar, "Trigonelline insulates against oxidative stress, proinflammatory cytokines and restores BDNF levels in lipopolysaccharide induced cognitive impairment in adult mice," *Metabolic Brain Disease*, vol. 33, no. 3, pp. 681–691, 2018.

[54] S. M. Lee and J. W. Pike, "The vitamin D receptor functions as a transcription regulator in the absence of 1,25-dihydroxyvitamin D3," *The Journal of Steroid Biochemistry and Molecular Biology*, vol. 164, pp. 265–270, 2016.

[55] X. Nie, H. Zhang, X. Shi et al., "Asiaticoside nitric oxide gel accelerates diabetic cutaneous ulcers healing by activating Wnt/β-catenin signaling pathway," *International Immunopharmacology*, vol. 79, Article ID 106109, 2020.

[56] X. Zhang, D. Zhou, T. Ma, and Q. Liu, "Vascular endothelial growth factor protects CD200-rich and CD34-positive hair follicle stem cells against androgen-induced apoptosis through the phosphoinositide 3-kinase/Akt pathway in patients with androgenic alopecia," *Dermatologic Surgery*, vol. 46, no. 3, pp. 358–368, 2020.

[57] K. Gohil, J. Patel, and A. Gajjar, "Pharmacological review on *Centella asiatica*: a potential herbal cure-all," *Indian Journal of Pharmaceutical Sciences*, vol. 72, no. 5, pp. 546–556, 2010.

[58] B. Singh and R. P. Rastogi, "A reinvestigation of the triterpenes of *Centella asiatica*," *Phytochemistry*, vol. 8, no. 5, pp. 917–921, 1969.

[59] G. K. Shinomol and Muralidhara, "Prophylactic neuroprotective property of *Centella asiatica* against 3-nitropropionic acid induced oxidative stress and mitochondrial dysfunctions in brain regions of prepubertal mice," *Neurotoxicology*, vol. 29, no. 6, pp. 948–957, 2008.

[60] G. K. Shinomol, H. Ravikumar, and Muralidhara, "Prophylaxis with *Centella asiatica* confers protection to prepubertal mice against 3-nitropropionic-acid-induced oxidative stress in brain," *Phytotherapy Research*, vol. 24, no. 6, pp. 885–892, 2010.

[61] Y. M. Choi, S. An, J. Lee et al., "Titrated extract of *Centella asiatica* increases hair inductive property through inhibition of STAT signaling pathway in three-dimensional spheroid cultured human dermal papilla cells," *Bioscience, Biotechnology, and Biochemistry*, vol. 81, no. 12, pp. 2323–2329, 2017.

[62] M. Pervin, K. Unno, A. Takagaki, M. Isemura, and Y. Nakamura, "Function of green tea catechins in the brain: epigallocatechin gallate and its metabolites," *International Journal of Molecular Sciences*, vol. 20, no. 15, p. 3630, 2019.

[63] A. Esfandiari and A. P. Kelly, "The effects of tea polyphenolic compounds on hair loss among rodents," *Journal of the National Medical Association*, vol. 97, no. 8, pp. 1165–1169, 2005.

[64] O. S. Kwon, J. H. Han, H. G. Yoo et al., "Human hair growth enhancement in vitro by green tea epigallocatechin-3-gallate (EGCG)," *Phytomedicine*, vol. 14, no. 7-8, pp. 551–555, 2007.
[65] S. Shin, K. Kim, M. J. Lee et al., "Epigallocatechin gallate-mediated alteration of the MicroRNA expression profile in 5α-dihydrotestosterone-treated human dermal papilla cells," *Annals of Dermatology*, vol. 28, no. 3, pp. 327–334, 2016.
[66] G. Sethi, M. Shanmugam, S. Warrier et al., "Pro-apoptotic and anti-cancer properties of diosgenin: a comprehensive and critical review," *Nutrients*, vol. 10, no. 5, p. 645, 2018.
[67] S. A. Wani and P. Kumar, "Fenugreek: a review on its nutraceutical properties and utilization in various food products," *Journal of the Saudi Society of Agricultural Sciences*, vol. 17, no. 2, pp. 97–106, 2018.
[68] S. Vyas, R. P. Agrawal, P. Solanki, and P. Trivedi, "Analgesic and anti-inflammatory activities of Trigonella foenum-graecum (seed) extract," *Acta Poloniae Pharmaceutica*, vol. 65, pp. 473–476, 2008.
[69] M. Jesus, A. P. Martins, E. Gallardo, and S. Silvestre, "Recent highlights on pharmacology and analytical methodology," *Journal of Analytical Methods in Chemistry*, vol. 2016, Article ID 4156293, 2016.
[70] D.-H. Jung, H.-J. Park, H.-E. Byun et al., "Diosgenin inhibits macrophage-derived inflammatory mediators through downregulation of CK2, JNK, NF-κB and AP-1 activation," *International Immunopharmacology*, vol. 10, no. 9, pp. 1047–1054, 2010.
[71] Y. Lin, R. Jia, Y. Liu et al., "Diosgenin inhibits superoxide generation in FMLP-activated mouse neutrophils via multiple pathways," *Free Radical Research*, vol. 48, no. 12, pp. 1485–1493, 2014.
[72] K.-W. Choi, H.-J. Park, D. H. Jung et al., "Inhibition of TNF-α-induced adhesion molecule expression by diosgenin in mouse vascular smooth muscle cells via downregulation of the MAPK, Akt and NF-κB signaling pathways," *Vascular Pharmacology*, vol. 53, no. 5-6, pp. 273–280, 2010.
[73] L. A. Ahmed, A. A. Z. Obaid, H. F. Zaki, and A. M. Agha, "Role of oxidative stress, inflammation, nitric oxide and transforming growth factor-beta in the protective effect of diosgenin in monocrotaline-induced pulmonary hypertension in rats," *European Journal of Pharmacology*, vol. 740, pp. 379–387, 2014.

An Unusual TEN-Like Presentation of Juvenile Bullous Pemphigoid: A Diagnostic Challenge

Zahra Nikyar,[1,2] Parvaneh Hatami,[1] Zeinab Aryanian,[1,3] Soheila Sotoudeh,[4] Vahid Ziaee,[5,6] and Azadeh Goodarzi[7,8]

[1]*Autoimmune Bullous Diseases Research Center, Tehran University of Medical Sciences, Tehran, Iran*
[2]*Department of Dermatology, Skin Diseases and Leishmaniasis Research Center, School of Medicine, Isfahan University of Medical Sciences, Isfahan, Iran*
[3]*Department of Dermatology, Babol University of Medical Sciences, Babol, Iran*
[4]*Department of Dermatology, Children's Medical Center, Center of Excellence, Tehran University of Medical Sciences, Tehran, Iran*
[5]*Pediatric Rheumatology Research Goroup, Rheumatology Research Center, Tehran University of Medical Sciences, Tehran, Iran*
[6]*Department of Pediatrics, Tehran University of Medical Sciences, Tehran, Iran*
[7]*Department of Dermatology, Rasool Akram Medical Complex Clinical Research Development Center, School of Medicine, Iran University of Medical Sciences, Tehran, Iran*
[8]*Skin and Stem Cell Research Center, Tehran University of Medical Sciences, Tehran, Iran*

Correspondence should be addressed to Parvaneh Hatami; p_hatami2001@yahoo.com and Zeinab Aryanian; z_aryanian@yahoo.com

Academic Editor: Alireza Firooz

Bullous pemphigoid (BP) is an acquired autoimmune bullous disorder rarely seen in the pediatric population. It usually presents as large and tense bullae, predominantly distributed in the acral areas. Herein, we describe a case of childhood BP with an atypical presentation mimicking toxic epidermal necrolysis (TEN). This case shows us that juvenile BP should be considered in the differential diagnosis of TEN in children, particularly if there are unusual features and an intractable course.

1. Introduction

Bullous pemphigoid (BP) is an acquired autoimmune bullous disorder rarely seen in the pediatric population [1]. BP is characterized by linear deposition of autoantibodies and C3 along the dermoepidermal junction (DEJ), leading to a subepidermal bullae formation. It usually presents as large and tense bullae with a predominant acral involvement [2]. The exact etiopathogenesis of BP is not fully understood, but some infections, medications, and vaccines, along with genetic susceptibility, have been shown to play a role [3–6].

Here, we present a 3-year-old patient with an atypical presentation of BP whose clinical features were perplexing and provided a distinct diagnostic challenge.

2. Case Presentation

A 3-year-old girl presented to a general clinic with generalized vesiculobullous lesions. Her parents reported that symptoms began as pruritic, red, and scaly lesions on her feet which were initially diagnosed as eczema and treated with emollients and topical steroids. However, despite the treatment, the lesions progressed and extended to the abdomen and upper extremities within one month. Extension of the lesions raised suspicion of a scabies infestation. Permethrin cream 5% was prescribed which was not effective. Parents also reported the use of an unknown herbal remedy for a week which led to the appearance of some new vesiculobullous and erosive lesions.

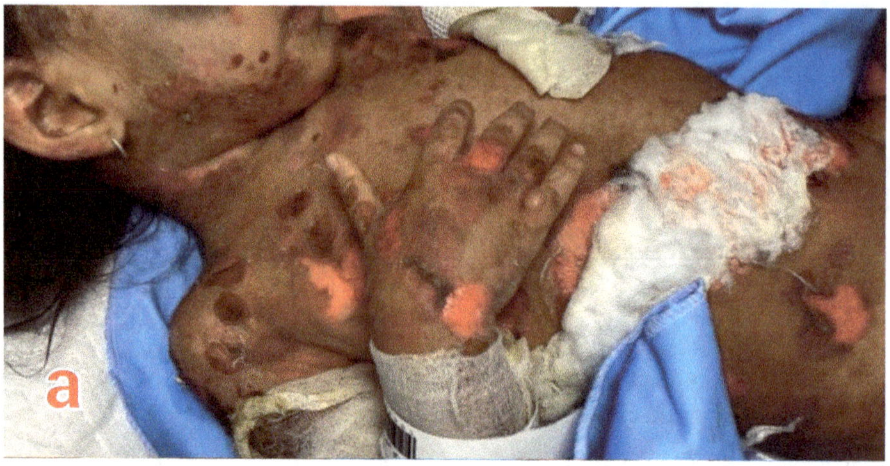

(a)

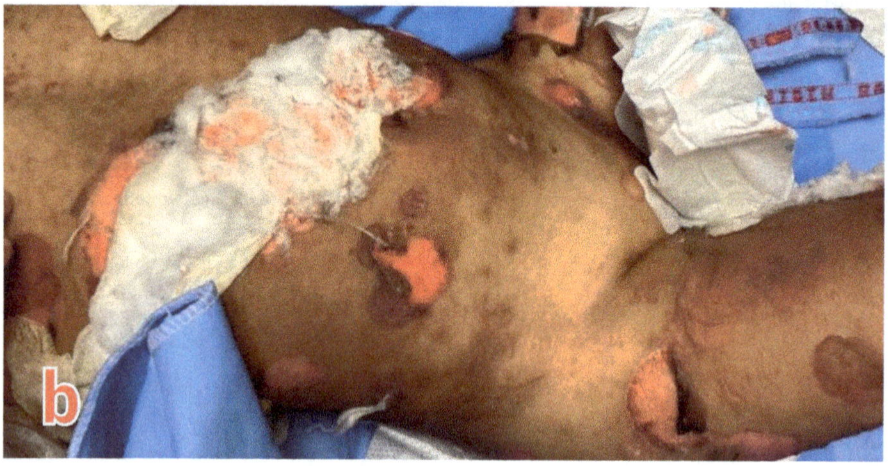

(b)

FIGURE 1: Generalized erosions and flaccid bullae (a, b).

The patient was referred to our hospital, Markaz e Tebi Atfal, Tehran University of Medical Sciences (TUMS), Tehran, Iran, at February 2021, when she was ill with generalized erythematous patches, plaques, and flaccid bullae filled with clear fluid, along with some erosions, distributed all over her body (Figure 1). Nikolsky's sign was positive.

Mucosal examination revealed erosive lesions in the buccal area, with minor erythema on the vaginal mucosa; the ocular mucosa was normal.

No positive family history of any dermatosis was noted.

Lab tests: WBC, 17900 (cell/mcL); lymph, 4300 (cell/mcL); poly, 12800 (cell/mcL); mono, 1350 (cell/mcL); Hb, 14 (g/dL); RBC, 5.38 (millions); MCV, 77.9 (fL); Plt, 686000 (cell/mcL); FANA, negative; CRP, 67 (mg/L); ESR, 9 (mm/h); IgG,1466 (mg/dL); IgM, 29 (mg/dL); IgA, 54 (mg/dL). Smear and cultures taken from intact bullae were negative. Blood culture was positive for *S. aureus*.

Initially, based on the extensive bullous and erosive lesions, positive Nikolsky's sign, and mucosal involvement, it was assumed to be a case of toxic epidermal necrolysis (TEN) possibly caused by the unknown herbal remedies. However, several points did not support this diagnosis; there was no history of any systemic medication; the course of presentation was subacute; erythema in the vaginal mucosa was considered to be normal by the pediatric dermatologist; and oral lesions were less severe than normally seen in TEN. Other differential diagnoses considered were staphylococcal scalded skin syndrome (SSSS), pemphigus vulgaris, bullous pemphigoid, and bullous impetigo.

A 4 mm punch biopsy was taken from one of the new lesions for a histopathologic assessment and another from a perilesional skin for a direct immunofluorescence (DIF) evaluation.

Histopathology showed distinct subepidermal bulla and dermal infiltration of lymphocytes with numerous eosinophils compatible with the diagnosis of BP (Figure 2).

DIF also revealed a linear pattern of C3 and IgG deposition at DEJ and confirmed the diagnosis of BP (Figure 3).

Initially, treatment had been started with IVIG (1 g/kg/day for three days) due to the involvement of >90% of the surface area of the body. However, the lesions were resistant to 3 cycles of IVIG, and new bullous lesions continued to appear; therefore, cyclosporine (3 mg/kg/day) was added to the treatment. After the diagnosis of BP was approved,

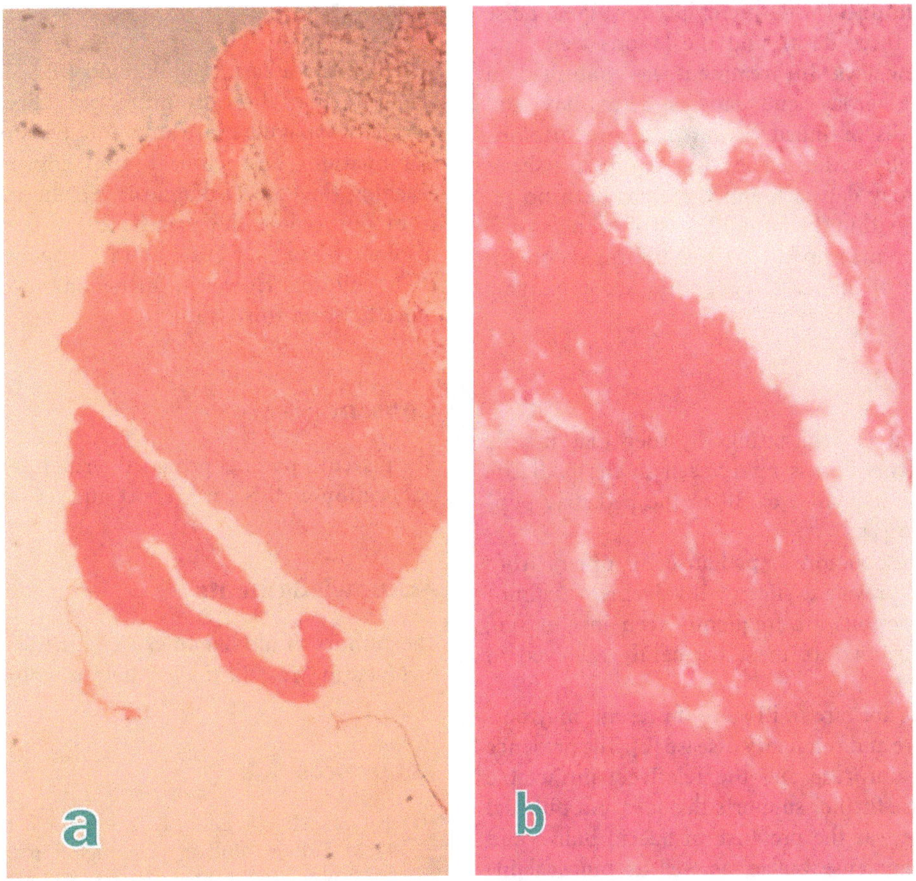

(a) (b)

Figure 2: Distinct subepidermal bulla (H&E, x40) (a). Dermal infiltration of lymphocytes with numerous eosinophils compatible with the diagnosis of BP (H&E, x100) (b).

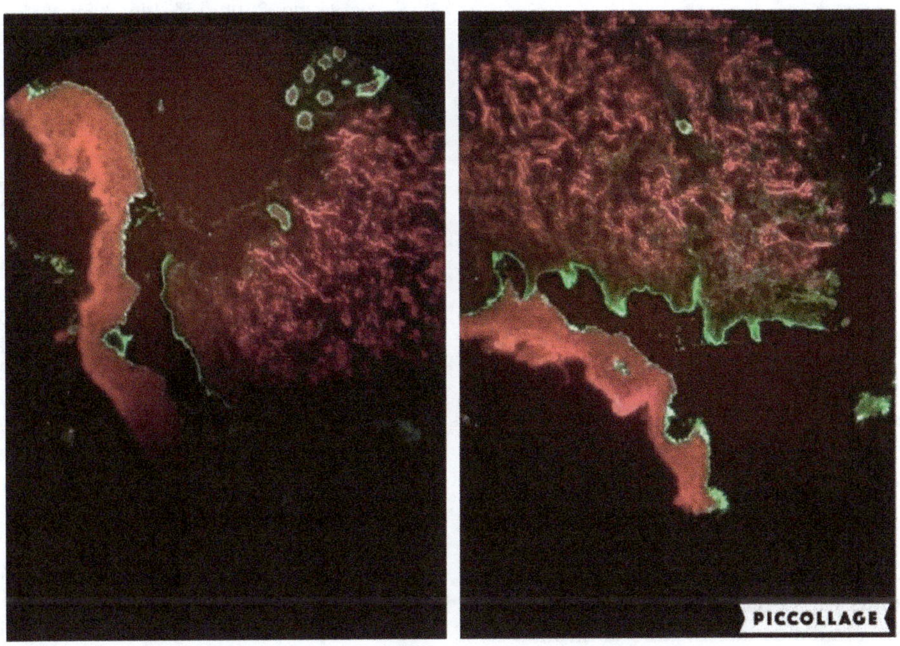

Figure 3: Linear deposition of IgG and C3 at DEJ.

treatment was continued with methylprednisolone pulse (30 mg/kg/day for three days), and the lesions went into remission after a few days. The treatment was continued on prednisolone (2 mg/kg/day) and dapsone 25 mg/day, and cyclosporine was discontinued. Eventually, prednisolone was tapered gradually within 3 months. At present, she is taking only 25 mg/day dapsone, and there has been no recurrence of lesions within the 5-month period of follow-up.

The patient's parents provided written informed consent for the publication of this case report and accompanying images.

3. Discussion

Bullous pemphigoid is a blistering disorder that mainly affects elderly patients and is rarely seen in the pediatric population [1]. The incidence of BP in the pediatric population is unknown [1].

The clinical presentation of pediatric BP differs from adults in terms of prevalent sites of involvement: palmoplantar and facial lesions are frequently seen in children, whereas flexural regions are most frequently involved in adults [2, 3].

Mucosal lesions are rare in BP, and if present, may be a sign of a more severe and refractory disease [7]. The presence of oral lesions in our case and the relatively intractable course of the disease further supports this idea. An unusual feature of this case was the presence of flaccid bullae and erosions rather than tense bullae, as well as mucosal involvement, which could mislead the clinician.

Moreover, lack of the positive history of any triggering factor, including infection, medication, or recent vaccination, along with the severe and intractable course of the disorder, made it even more challenging to diagnose before histopathologic evaluation. However, the final diagnosis in our case was made based on histopathologic and DIF data, and an indirect immunofluorescence (IIF) study was not performed for further confirmation of the diagnosis which should be considered as a limitation of this report.

TEN-like presentation of BP has been rarely reported in adults [8], but to the best of our knowledge, no similar article has been published regarding this issue in pediatric population.

Initial BP treatment is potent topical steroid ointments and systemic prednisolone [9]. According to a systematic review on 81 infants suffering from BP, prednisolone and dapsone were the most common monotherapies in pediatric BP [4].

However, due to the severity of the condition in our patient and the initial diagnosis of TEN, we had to consider more potent options, including IVIG (1 mg/kg/day for three days), cyclosporine (3 mg/kg/day), and methylprednisolone pulse to control the disease. After initial remission, dapsone (2 mg/kg) was added as a steroid-sparing agent, but it was reduced to 0.5 mg/kg due to the development of hemolytic anemia. Dapsone was well-tolerated by the patient, so prednisolone could be tapered successfully within 3 months. This result corresponds with a recent report of a refractory case of childhood BP that was successfully controlled by dapsone and systemic steroids [10].

4. Conclusion

We reported a case of childhood BP with an unusual presentation that clinically mimicked TEN to emphasize the necessity of paying more attention to history taking, physical examination, and clinical suspicion as key factors to reaching the correct diagnosis. Furthermore, one can infer from our report the priority of prescribing methylprednisolone pulse over IVIG and cyclosporine in hard-to-treat BP in children. However, further studies are needed to shed more light on this issue.

Consent

The patient's parents provided written informed consent to publication of this case report and accompanying images.

Acknowledgments

The authors would like to express their deepest appreciation to Maryam Moslehi for her help in editing this article.

References

[1] E. G. D. M. Reis-Filho, T. D. A. Silva, L. H. D. L. Aguirre, and C. M. S. Reis, "Bullous pemphigoid in a 3-month-old infant: case report and literature review of this dermatosis in childhood," *Anais Brasileiros de Dermatologia*, vol. 88, no. 6, pp. 961–965, 2013.

[2] O. Waisbourd-Zinman, D. Ben-Amitai, A. D. Cohen et al., "Bullous pemphigoid in infancy: clinical and epidemiologic characteristics," *Journal of the American Academy of Dermatology*, vol. 58, no. 1, pp. 41–48, 2008.

[3] D. Miyamoto, C. G. Santi, V. Aoki, and C. W. Maruta, "Bullous pemphigoid," *Anais Brasileiros de Dermatologia*, vol. 94, no. 2, pp. 133–146, 2019.

[4] A. T. Lopez, T. Khanna, N. Antonov, C. Audrey-Bayan, and L. Geskin, "A review of bullous pemphigoid associated with PD-1 and PD-L1 inhibitors," *International Journal of Dermatology*, vol. 57, no. 6, pp. 664–669, 2018.

[5] K. Tasanen, O. Varpuluoma, and W. Nishie, "Dipeptidyl peptidase-4 inhibitor-associated bullous pemphigoid," *Frontiers in Immunology*, vol. 10, p. 1238, 2019.

[6] Y. Wang, X. Mao, Y. Liu, Y. Yang, H. Jin, and L. Li, "IL-13 genetic susceptibility to bullous pemphigoid: a potential target for treatment and a prognostic marker," *Frontiers in Immunology*, vol. 13, Article ID 824110, 2022.

[7] X. Chen, W. Zhao, H. Jin, and L. Li, "Risk factors for mucosal involvement in bullous pemphigoid and the possible mechanism: a review," *Frontiers in Medicine*, vol. 8, Article ID 680871, 2021.

[8] C. Qiu, A. Shevchenko, and S. Hsu, "Bullous pemphigoid secondary to pembrolizumab mimicking toxic epidermal necrolysis," *JAAD Case Reports*, vol. 6, no. 5, pp. 400–402, 2020.

[9] V. A. Venning, K. Taghipour, M. F. Mohd Mustapa et al., "British association of dermatologists' guidelines for the management of bullous pemphigoid 2012," *British Journal of Dermatology*, vol. 167, no. 6, pp. 1200–1214, 2012.

[10] K. Thomsen, M. Deleuran, C. Vestergaard, M. Holm, R. Riber-Hansen, and R. Bech, "Severe infantile bullous pemphigoid treated with dapsone after bridging with systemic glucocorticoid," *Case Reports in Dermatology*, vol. 11, no. 2, pp. 187–193, 2019.

36

Neutrophilic Dermatosis of the Dorsal Hands: Report of a Case and Review of the Literature

Narciss Mobini,[1,2,3] **Kaviyon Sadrolashrafi**,[4] **and Susun Michaels**[5,6]

[1] *University of Nevada, School of Medicine, Reno and Las Vegas, NV, USA*
[2] *Director of Dermatopathology, Associated Pathologists, Chartered, Las Vegas, NV, USA*
[3] *4230 Burnham Ave., Las Vegas, NV, 89119, USA*
[4] *University of California, Los Angeles (UCLA), Department of Life Sciences, Los Angeles, CA, USA*
[5] *Touro College of Osteopathic Medicine, Las Vegas, NV, USA*
[6] *Las Vegas Skin and Cancer Clinics, Las Vegas, NV, USA*

Correspondence should be addressed to Narciss Mobini; mscons@aol.com

Academic Editor: Thomas Berger

Neutrophilic dermatosis of the dorsal hands is an underrecognized entity, which is a distributional variant of Sweet's syndrome. It is often clinically misdiagnosed as an infectious process in overwhelming majority of the cases and the treatment is therefore delayed. Also, its association with underlying systemic and neoplastic disorders makes the need for an accurate diagnosis more crucial. We present a 45-year-old Caucasian woman who was initially diagnosed as having a hand infection with unsuccessful courses of antibiotic therapy. A later biopsy revealed a diffuse dermal infiltrate of neutrophils with leukocytoclasis, vasculopathic changes, and marked papillary dermal edema. Patient responded rapidly to oral prednisone treatment. By sharing a new case and comprehensive review of available published literature, we intend to raise awareness of this underreported entity and emphasize the role of timely biopsy of the lesions that will not only lead to an accurate diagnosis, but also avoid unnecessary antibiotic treatments, potentially aggressive management strategies such as surgical debridement or amputation, and referrals to wound care centers. More importantly, it will prompt a search to exclude any possible association, particularly hematopoietic malignancies.

1. Introduction

Pustular vasculitis of the hands was first introduced by Strutton et al. in 1995, to describe an eruption on the dorsal hands resembling Sweet's syndrome, but showing leukocytoclastic vasculitis histologically [1]. Later, clinically similar cases were reported with no vasculitis [2–4]. Neutrophilic dermatosis of the dorsal hands (NDDH), proposed by Galaria et al. in 2000 is currently the widely accepted term for this clinicopathologic entity [4]. We present a new case of NDDH in a woman who was originally misdiagnosed as having an infection.

2. Case Report

A 45-year-old Caucasian obese woman presented with small painful ulcers on the back of her hands and fingers that had started three weeks prior to her visit. She first noticed small red flat discolored areas which gradually worsened by developing pain, swelling, and ulcers within two weeks. She did not recall a prior trauma. She had a history of previous laparoscopic gastric sleeve surgery for morbid obesity and a vague diagnosis of mild diabetes for which she was not on any medication. She denied taking a new drug. With the clinical diagnosis of an infectious process, bacterial culture and sensitivity were performed and she was given oral and topical antibiotics (Bactrim and mupirocin, respectively) along with wound care instructions. The patient started developing fever with malaise and was admitted to the emergency room, where she was placed on intravenous antibiotic (vancomycin) due to suspicion of sepsis, originating from her "hand infection". After a few days, she returned to our clinic. Compared to the original visit, the condition appeared worse with development of erythematous ulcerated nodules and

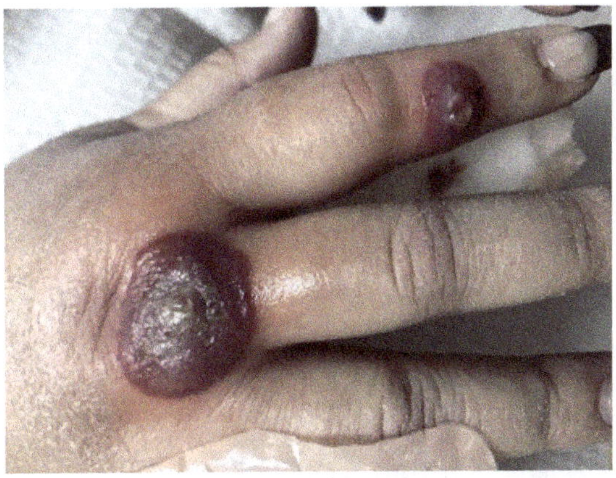

FIGURE 1: Centrally ulcerated edematous nodules with violaceous borders on the dorsal aspects of right index finger and proximal metacarpophalangeal joint of mainly third finger. Note the bulbous edema of the affected digits.

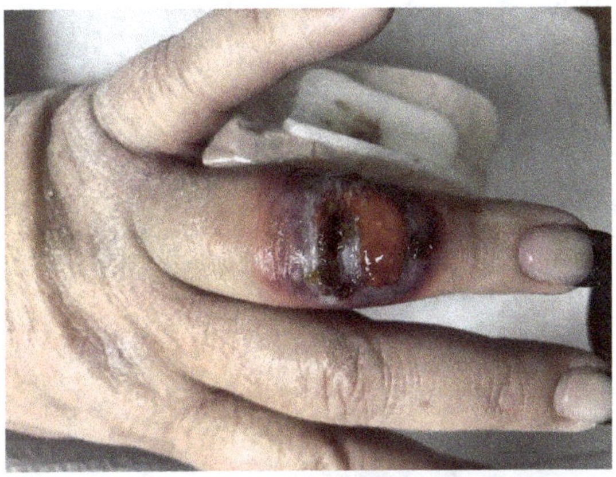

FIGURE 2: Large ulcerated oozing plaque on the dorsum of left ring finger with purulent-appearing exudate.

plaques, violaceous borders, and marked surrounding edema, present on the dorsal aspects of right index and left ring fingers along with proximal metacarpophalangeal joint of third digit. The fingers in the nonulcerated areas displayed a fusiform swelling (Figures 1 and 2). She also developed tender indurated erythematous plaques on the dorsum of the right wrist. Examination of the rest of the body, including the mucosal surfaces, failed to show any involvement. Based on the clinical progression and lack of response to antibiotics, biopsy was obtained to rule out atypical pyoderma gangrenosum (PG), deep fungal or mycobacterial infection, or other possibilities. Histopathologic examination revealed marked subepidermal edema associated with a superficial and deep perivascular, interstitial, and diffuse infiltrate of neutrophils, many of which were present within the vessel walls, associated with leukocytoclasia and extravasation of erythrocytes. Despite vasculopathic changes, there was no evidence of true vasculitis (Figures 3(a), 3(b), 3(c) and 3(d)). Although the histopathologic differential diagnosis was most consistent with Sweet's syndrome, based on the clinical presentation, NDDH was the rendered diagnosis. She was immediately started on oral prednisone 80mg per day. In the meantime, a systemic workup was carried out. After a week, the ulcers were already healing and the swelling was subsiding. Tissue cultures yielded negative results and systemic workup was normal. We started to taper down the prednisone at this point. One week later, there was continued flattening of the lesions. After one month, there was mild residual erythema at the previous sites (Figures 4(a) and 4(b)). We continued to taper down her prednisone and prescribed a potent topical corticosteroid in case of local recurrence. She reported complete clearing of the lesions. Seven months later, she presented with a mildly erythematous patch on the dorsum of right third digit. An intralesional steroid injection was performed followed by topical steroids for two weeks. She has not had any recurrence, after one year from the original incidence.

3. Discussion

The term neutrophilic dermatosis of the dorsal hands (NDDH) was first proposed by Galaria et al. in 2000, who considered it to be a subset of Sweet's syndrome [4]. A thorough review of the literature reveals that only close to 100 cases have so far been reported [5–10]. Today, NDDH is most widely accepted to represent a 'distributional or localized variant' of Sweet's syndrome which belongs to the spectrum of neutrophilic dermatoses, rather than a primary vasculitis and that any vasculitis seen histologically is a secondary phenomenon [11, 12]. It is likely that the timing of the biopsy during the evolutionary phases of the lesions may result in different findings with regard to presence or absence of vasculitis. Clinically, the lesions are characterized by painful erythematous and violaceous papules, plaques, nodules, pustules, and hemorrhagic bullae. These may eventually ulcerate in 50% of the cases. The most common sites of eruption are the dorsal aspect of both hands. Also, back of fingers or wrists can be affected with rare involvement of the palms. There may be concurrent or subsequent lesions elsewhere, such as back, lips, legs, and forehead [5, 8, 13–16]. Women are affected more than men, comprising 70% of the cases [7]. In one series, up to 65% of cases reported a proceeding trauma, which may be misleading [10]. Fever is mentioned in 33% of the reports [7]. The most common clinical differential diagnosis is an infection, for which the patients receive antibiotics, with no success. Deep fungal, atypical mycobacterial, parasitic, and viral infections may also be considered clinically. In the noninfectious category, atypical PG, bullous Sweet's or Sweet's-like syndrome, bullous erythema multiforme, or a pustular drug reaction are in the differential diagnosis [6]. Although rather deep ulceration with undermining edges is common in classic PG, a superficial ulcer with hemorrhagic bullae is more commonly seen in atypical PG or bullous Sweet's syndrome. On the other hand, ulceration is uncommon in typical Sweet's syndrome and, if present, is suggestive of an underlying hematologic malignancy. It is suggested that many cases diagnosed as atypical Sweet syndrome, atypical PG, or PG-Sweet overlap, in fact represent NDDH, when manifesting in this distinctive anatomic distribution [7, 17]. Histologically, there is prominent papillary dermal edema, superficial and

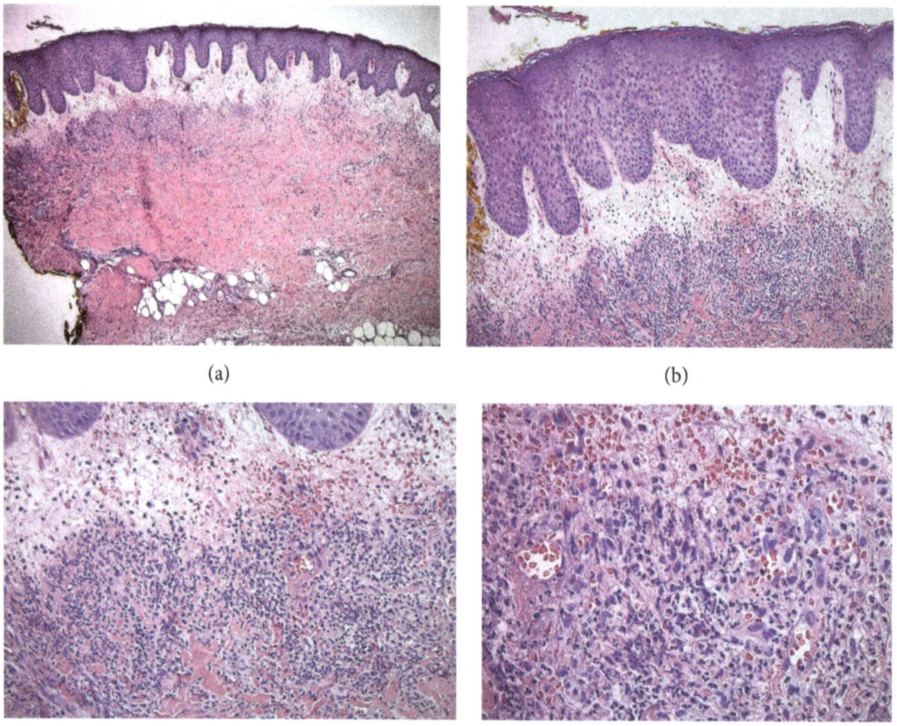

(a) (b) (c) (d)

Figure 3: (a,b,c,d) Marked papillary dermal edema, superficial and deep perivascular, interstitial, and diffuse infiltrate of neutrophils with leukocytoclasia, extravasation of erythrocytes, vasculopathic changes, and absence of true vasculitis (hematoxylin-eosin 4X, 10X, 20X, and 40X, respectively).

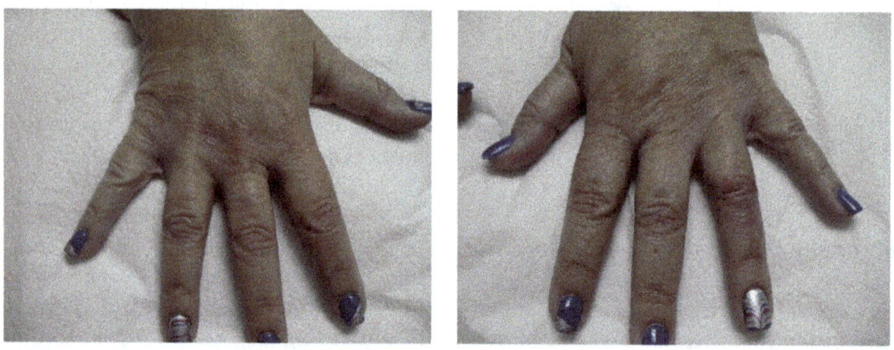

(a) (b)

Figure 4: (a,b) Healed lesions with subtle residual erythematous patches, four weeks after treatment with oral prednisone.

deep perivascular, and diffuse infiltrate of neutrophils with leukocytoclasia, extravasated erythrocytes, and no vasculitis. Admixed lymphocytes and occasional eosinophils can also be seen. It appears that any vasculitis observed, is of secondary type rather than a primary phenomenon, similar to PG or Sweet's. Occasionally one may see epidermal changes such as spongiosis, neutrophilic microabscesses, or pseudoepitheliomatous hyperplasia [5, 9, 10]. The most important associations with NDDH are neoplastic disorders in 27% of cases, where it may represent a paraneoplastic phenomenon. The most common are hematologic disorders, such as myelodysplastic syndrome, acute leukemia, lymphoma, or other diseases in 21% of cases [7, 17–19]. In addition, solid neoplasms can be seen such as cancers of breast, kidney, colon, stomach, lung, and hypopharynx [1, 2, 7, 19–22]. Associated nonneoplastic disorders include inflammatory bowel disease, in approximately 15% of cases [7, 17, 22]. Diverticulosis, diverticulitis, acute proctitis, and history of small bowel obstruction or bypass have also been reported [5]. In bowel-associated dermatosis-arthritis syndrome, the skin lesions develop in patients with prior bowel bypass surgeries and other bowel disorders; however, the cutaneous eruption is more widespread, involving the upper extremities and trunk. Classic PG is seen with increased incidence of inflammatory bowel disorders as well; however, the distribution of lesions is different. Our patient had a history of laparoscopic sleeve gastrectomy for morbid obesity in the past. Other conditions reported in NDDH include diabetes mellitus, peripheral ulcerative keratitis, erythema nodosum, sarcoidosis, chronic hepatitis C, urinary tract infection, streptococcal tonsillitis, and chronic glomerulonephritis [5, 6, 23–26]. There is a report of NDDH after exposure to a chemical fertilizer containing ammonium nitrate and calcium salts [27]. An insect bite has been proposed as possible culprit of NDDH through a pathergic reaction, which occurred in a unilateral distribution [28]. Among drug-induced cases, thalidomide and its analogue lenalidomide are the main reported agents [29, 30]. NDDH occurring after chemotherapy for AML has also been reported [31]. There are many occasions that no underlying cause can be found [12, 32]. The mainstay of treatment is oral corticosteroids, with strikingly rapid response. Some have included dapsone, colchicine, minocycline, or pentoxifylline [4, 5, 7, 17, 25, 32]. There may be recurrences as high as 10% [20]. In our patient, after complete healing of the lesions, there was a mild recurrence seven months later, treated with an intralesional injection of Kenalog, followed by topical steroids for two weeks. No further recurrence has been noted in about a year from her original visit.

4. Conclusion

NDDH is best regarded as a distributional variant of Sweet's syndrome, where the lesions occur on the dorsal aspects of both hands in its typical presentation. In the majority of cases, the initial clinical diagnosis is an infectious process. In addition, patients are referred to wound care centers due to nonhealing wounds. Therefore, unsuccessful antibiotic treatments, failed surgical debridements, and even amputations could follow. By presenting a new case of NDDH and review of the existing published data, we intend to raise awareness of this clinicopathologic entity for dermatology practitioners and dermatopathologists. NDDH should be strongly considered in lesions occurring on the dorsal hands, particularly if suspicious of infection, and timely biopsy be performed. In addition, recognizing this disease should prompt the clinician for a thorough investigation to rule out any associated malignancy or systemic disorder.

References

[1] G. Strutton, D. Weedon, and I. Robertson, "Pustular vasculitis of the hand," *Journal of the American Academy of Dermatology*, vol. 32, pp. 192–198, 1995.

[2] N. Curcó, X. Pagerols, X. Tarroch, and P. Vives, "Pustular vasculitis of the hands. Report of two men," *Dermatology*, vol. 196, no. 3, pp. 346-347, 1998.

[3] A. P. Hall, R. J. Goudge, H. J. Ireton, and L. M. Burrell, "Pustular vasculitis of the hands," *Australasian Journal of Dermatology*, vol. 40, no. 4, pp. 204–207, 1999.

[4] N. A. Galaria, J. M. Junkins-Hopkins, D. Kligman, and W. D. James, "Neutrophilic dermatosis of the dorsal hands: Pustular vasculitis revisited," *Journal of the American Academy of Dermatology*, vol. 43, no. 5, pp. 870–874, 2000.

[5] D. J. DiCaudo and S. M. Connolly, "Neutrophilic dermatosis (pustular vasculitis) of the dorsal hands: A report of 7 cases and review of the literature," *Archives of Dermatology*, vol. 138, no. 3, pp. 361-365, 2002.

[6] H. Larsen, A. Danielsen, D. Krustrup, and K. Weismann, "Neutrophil dermatosis of the dorsal hands," *Journal of the European Academy of Dermatology and Venereology*, vol. 19, no. 5, pp. 634–637, 2005.

[7] H. W. Walling, C. J. Snipes, P. Gerami, and W. W. Piette, "The relationship between neutrophilic dermatosis of the dorsal hands and Sweet syndrome: Report of 9 cases and comparison to atypical pyoderma gangrenosum," *JAMA Dermatology*, vol. 142, no. 1, pp. 57–63, 2006.

[8] J. Del Pozo, F. Sacristán, W. Martínez, S. Paradela, B. Fernández-Jorge, and E. Fonseca, "Neutrophilic dermatosis of the hands: Presentation of eight cases and review of the literature," *The Journal of Dermatology*, vol. 34, no. 4, pp. 243–247, 2007.

[9] P. P. Paparone, P. A. Paparone, and R. Y. Senyatso, "Neutrophilic dermatosis of the dorsal hand," *Wounds*, vol. 25, no. 6, pp. 148–152, 2013.

[10] A. M. Cheng, H. S. Cheng, B. J. Smith, and D. A. Stewart, "Neutrophilic Dermatosis of the Hands: A Review of 17 Cases," *The Journal of Hand Surgery*, vol. 43, no. 2, pp. 185.e1–185.e5, 2018.

[11] D. Wallach, "Neutrophilic dermatoses: An overview," *Clinics in Dermatology*, vol. 18, no. 3, pp. 229–231, 2000.

[12] D. Bilu, D. J. Kouba, A. J. Mamelak, R. A. Kazin, and C. H. Nousari, "Neutrophilic dermatosis of the dorsal hand," *The Journal of Dermatology*, vol. 31, no. 6, pp. 464–468, 2004.

[13] C. Laguna, J. Vilata, and B. Martín, "Neutrophilic Dermatosis of the Dorsal Hands," *Actas Dermo-Sifiliográficas*, vol. 98, no. 2, pp. 102–104, 2007.

[14] J. W. Byun, W. K. Hong, H. J. Song et al., "A case of neutrophilic dermatosis of the dorsal hands with concomitant involvement of the lips," *Annals of Dermatology*, vol. 22, no. 1, pp. 106–109, 2010.

[15] M. Malik, W. Perkins, and I. Leach, "Anti-neutrophil cytoplasmic antibody-positive neutrophilic dermatosis of the dorsal hands," *Clinical and Experimental Dermatology*, vol. 37, no. 8, pp. 869-870, 2012.

[16] E. Behrangi, A. Rasi, B. Attar, and Z. Azizian, "Neutrophilic dermatosis of dorsal hands and legs," *Archives of Iranian Medicine*, vol. 19, no. 12, pp. 879–881, 2016.

[17] R. H. Weenig, A. J. Bruce, M. T. McEvoy, L. E. Gibson, and M. D. P. Davis, "Neutrophilic dermatosis of the hands: Four new cases and review of the literature," *International Journal of Dermatology*, vol. 43, no. 2, pp. 95–102, 2004.

[18] I. Hirai, T. Sakiyama, A. Konohana, Y. Takae, and S. Matsuura, "A case of neutrophilic dermatosis of the dorsal hand in acute leukemia - a distributional variant of Sweet's syndrome," *JDDG: Journal der Deutschen Dermatologischen Gesellschaft*, vol. 13, no. 10, pp. 1033-1034, 2015.

[19] F. J. Fernández-Fernández, J. C. Álvarez – Fernández, E. Romero – Picos, J. A. Garrido, and P. Sesma, "Neutrophilic Dermatosis of the Dorsal Hands Associated with a "Myeloproliferative Neoplasm, Unclassifiable" and a Simultaneous Cancer of Colon," *Acta Medica (Hradec Kralove)*, vol. 53, no. 3, pp. 153–156, 2010.

[20] A. Gonzalez, S. Vaziri, J. C. Brandt, W. Steffes, and Y. Perbtani, "Neutrophilic dermatosis of the dorsal hands in an elderly man," *Dermatology Online Journal*, vol. 17, no. 22, p. 2, 2016.

[21] M. Cravo, J. C. Cardoso, O. Tellechea, M. R. Cordeiro, J. P. Reis, and A. Figueiredo, "Neutrophilic dermatosis of the dorsal hands associated with hypopharyngeal carcinoma," *Dermatology Online Journal*, vol. 14, no. 7, p. 5, 2008.

[22] T. Leecy, A. Anderson, J. Von Nida, N. Harvey, and B. Wood, "Neutrophilic dermatosis of the dorsal hands: An often under recognised and mistreated entity," *Pathology*, vol. 45, no. 2, pp. 198–200, 2013.

[23] D. Brajon, J.-F. Cuny, A. Barbaud, and J.-L. Schmutz, "Neutrophilic dermatosis of the hands," *Annales de Dermatologie et de Venereologie*, vol. 138, no. 10, pp. 673–676, 2011.

[24] J. Benzimra, J. Low-Beer, and J. Twomey, "A case of peripheral ulcerative keratitis associated with neutrophilic dermatosis of the dorsal hand," *International Ophthalmology*, vol. 31, no. 2, pp. 149–151, 2011.

[25] S. Kaur, D. Gupta, B. Garg, and N. Sood, "Neutrophilic dermatosis of dorsal hands," *Indian Dermatology Online Journal (IDOJ)*, vol. 6, no. 1, pp. 42–45, 2015.

[26] K. Baz, A. C. Yazici, T. I. Kaya et al., "Neutrophilic dermatosis of the hands (localized Sweet's syndrome) in association with chronic hepatitis C and sarcoidosis," *Clinical and Experimental Dermatology*, vol. 28, no. 4, pp. 377–379, 2003.

[27] F. Aydin, N. Senturk, L. Yildiz, M. T. Canturk, and A. Y. Turanli, "Neutrophilic dermatosis of the dorsal hands in a farmer," *Journal of the European Academy of Dermatology and Venereology*, vol. 18, no. 6, pp. 716-717, 2004.

[28] S. Thatte and A. Aggarwal, "Neutrophilic dermatosis of the dorsal hands: A rare unilateral presentation," *Indian Dermatology Online Journal (IDOJ)*, vol. 6, no. 5, pp. 361-362, 2015.

[29] S. Mathieu, M. Soubrier, A. Tournadre, and J.-J. Dubost, "Neutrophilic dermatosis of the dorsal hands during thalidomide treatment," *International Journal of Dermatology*, vol. 53, no. 9, pp. 1133–1135, 2014.

[30] A. R. Hoverson, M. D. P. Davis, R. H. Weenig, and A. P. Wolanskyj, "Neutrophilic dermatosis (sweet syndrome) of the hands associated with lenalidomide," *Archives of Dermatology*, vol. 142, no. 8, pp. 1070-1071, 2006.

[31] K. M. Rockers and L. M. Fielder, "Neutrophilic dermatosis of the dorsal hands in a patient treated with chemotherapy for acute myelogenous leukemia," *Cutis*, vol. 83, pp. 37–39, 2009.

[32] E. Cook, R. Epstein, and R. Miller, "A rare case of idiopathic neutrophilic dermatosis of the hands," *Dermatology Online Journal*, vol. 15, 11, no. 17, p. 11, 2011.

Site Injection Reaction, Maculopapular Rash and Rosacea Exacerbation after COVID-19 Vaccination

Younes Benyamna,[1,2] Farah Marraha,[1,2] Ibtissam Al Faker,[1,2] Hanane Chahoub,[1,2] Najlae Rahmani,[1,2] Yasmine Rkiek,[1,2] Soukayna Kabbou,[1,2] Driss Soussi Tanani,[2,3] and Salim Gallouj[1,2]

[1]*Department of Dermatology, University Hospital Center of Tangier, Tetouan, Al Hoceima, Morocco*
[2]*Faculty of Medicine and Pharmacy Tangier, Abdelmalek Essaadi University, Tangier, Morocco*
[3]*Department of Pharmacology and Pharmacovigilance, University Hospital Center of Tangier, Tetouan, Al Hoceima, Morocco*

Correspondence should be addressed to Younes Benyamna; dr.benyamna@gmail.com

Academic Editor: Sergio A. Cuevas Covarrubias

To date, the occurrence of adverse events following immunization after COVID-19 vaccine is rare, and their report is still very poor; however, causality assessment is conducted to identify the associated cause, if they occur. In this case report, we present a case of an association of three cutaneous manifestations (maculopapular exanthem with enanthem, site injection reaction, and rosacea exacerbation) occurring three days after taking the first dose of AstraZeneca AZD1222 vaccine.

1. Introduction

In November 2019, the first cases of novel beta-corona virus SARS-CoV-2 were detected [1].

The virus has since spread globally at an alarming rate, and a SARS-CoV-2 global pandemic was declared by the World Health Organization (WHO) in March 2020 [2].

Beside its high spread rate, SARS-CoV-2 was shown to be responsible of severe acute respiratory distress syndrome and death. Thus, there was a race against time to find a solution that may slow down the coronavirus disease 2019 (COVID-19). Many pharmaceutic and nonpharmaceutic options were used [3], but only a vaccine seems efficient to stop or, at least, slow down the spreading of the virus by promoting herd immunity through massive vaccination campaigns.

Traditionally, vaccine development takes more than 10 years, but the COVID-19 pandemic has demonstrated the urgency for an unprecedented quick vaccine development. A safe and efficacious vaccine had to be developed in less than 6–18 months.

According to the WHO, the production of a vaccine passes conventionally through different stages. First, screenings and evaluations are necessary to determine which antigen should be used. The retained vaccine is then tested in animals. This is called the preclinical stage. If the vaccine triggers an immune response, it is then tested in human clinical trials in three phases. Safety of the vaccine is generally assessed in the clinical trials. Once the clinical trials are achieved, only approval is left. An authorized vaccine is now ready to be introduced, but a further monitoring is necessary; pharmacovigilance takes place [4].

Pharmacovigilance has been defined by the WHO as the "science and activities relating to the detection, assessment, understanding and prevention of adverse effects or any other possible drug-related problems" [5].

In Morocco, the vaccination is provided using either the inactivated vaccine Sinopharm BBIBP-CorV or the

AstraZeneca AZD1222 vaccine using adenoviral vectors. The two vaccines present overall a good safety [6, 7].

Since the first administrated doses, the clinicians focus was on the surveillance of possible adverse events due to vaccine.

In this article, we report a rare case of an association of three cutaneous reactions after a vaccination with the AZD1222 vaccine.

2. Case Presentation

A 21-year-old female patient with a medical history of iron deficiency anemia on oral iron supplementation consulted for generalized maculopapular exanthem with enanthem.

A careful history taking was established. In fact, the patient has beneficiated from COVID-19 vaccination, 5 days before consultation. The onset was marked 3 days after vaccination by redness with itching in the site of injection (left arm). The erythema quickly became generalized on the 3rd day, producing a maculopapular exanthem. Furthermore, our patient did not show any general signs or pruritus (except of the site of the injection). Of note, the patient does not report any allergic history.

On the clinical examination, 5 days after vaccination, there was a generalized skin eruption consisting of macules and papules which do not form a scale (maculopapular exanthem), involving the trunk and limbs and sparing the palmoplantar regions (Figure 1). On the face, the patient also presented erythema which was in favor of a rosacea (after clinical and dermoscopic examination) (Figure 2). At the injection site, the patient presented an erythematous patch (8 × 5 cm of diameter). In addition to that, enanthem was found at the mucosal examination (Figure 1).

There was no associated lymphadenopathy, and other systemic examinations were normal. Laboratory investigations revealed normal leucocyte count ($5.76 \times 103/\mu L$) with a slightly elevated granulocytes percentage (72.6%) and normal lymphocytes and eosinophils percentage (respectively, 22% and 0.2%). C-reactive protein, liver function tests, and renal profile were normal (CRP = 2.4 mg/l, ALT = 10.4 U/l, AST 15 U/l, urea = 0.14 g/l, and creatinine = 5.1 mg/l).

As it is invasive, skin biopsy has not been done.

The patient was started on H1 antihistamine pills and topical corticosteroids with emollients. For her rosacea, the patient was put under topic metronidazole. The MPE lesions and site injection erythema improved remarkably after 5 days of treatment, but the enanthem persisted and further follow-up was scheduled to monitor her rosacea.

3. Discussion

Just like any approved medicine, any approved vaccine carries some risk of side effects.

The cutaneous adverse effects of vaccines include local and generalized reactions. Some mechanisms of action are known, and others are not well elucidated yet. The main cause of those reactions is allergic or pseudoallergic. The hypersensitivity can be immediate-type or delayed-type, and it is due to the vaccine or one of its components [8].

As the size of the populations studied in the premarketing phase is limited and the period of observation is short (especially with the COVID-19 vaccine, which was produced in less than one year), safety data are usually very limited; then, the side effects reported to each vaccine are very limited. Some rare or severe reactions may be reported only after commercialization of the vaccine. Generally, postmarketing surveillance of vaccines relies mainly on the spontaneous reporting system (SRS) (which is the case for our patient). This method is crucial to generate alerts, but pharmacoepidemiology studies are necessary to confirm the alerts identified by spontaneous reporting. This is the huge importance of vaccines pharmacovigilance [9].

In our case, while the imputability of the skin manifestations observed to the administered vaccine is high (considering the onset and the evolution), scientific proof of a cause and effect relationship is very difficult to obtain.

Our patient presented three different adverse effects in which the severity risk was qualified as mild: injection site reaction, maculopapular exanthem (MPE) with enanthem, and rosacea exacerbation.

According to literature, injection-site reactions are the most common form of reaction that follows an injectable vaccine administration [10].

Clinical presentation includes erythema and/or swelling and/or tenderness. Generally, this reaction resolves spontaneously within a few days to weeks. However, local care can be taken to reduce the symptoms and accelerate healing. Of note, site injection reactions may occur with any vaccine and are not specifically related to any of the vaccine components [8].

What about the maculopapular exanthem? To answer this question, it would be interesting to take a look at the composition of the vaccine taken by our patient. In fact, AZD1222 vaccine consists of a replication-deficient chimpanzee adenoviral vector ChAdOx1, containing the SARS-COVID-19 structural surface glycoprotein antigen (spike protein; COVID-19) gene [6].

In addition to the principal fraction of this vaccine, AZD1222 contains some excipients: L-histidine, L-histidine hydrochloride monohydrate, magnesium chloride hexahydrate, polysorbate 80, ethanol, sucrose, sodium chloride, disodium edetate dihydrate, and water for injection [11]. Among all these excipients, the most interesting component to highlight is polysorbate 80. It is used as a synthetic nonionic surfactant commonly used in vaccines and drugs as a solubilizer, stabilizer, or emulsifier and also used to prevent protein adsorption and/or aggregation. In fact, it has been noted that polysorbate 80 is a biologically and possibly pharmacologically active compound and consequently may alter the pharmacologic properties of the drug it is formulated with or may itself directly mediate adverse events. Consequently, polysorbate 80 has been implicated in some of the adverse reactions associated with drugs formulated with this vehicle [12].

Its properties reside on its capacity of activating the complement system and then may lead to phagocytosis, stimulation, and recruitment of white blood cells or perforation of cell membranes. We believe that polysorbate 80

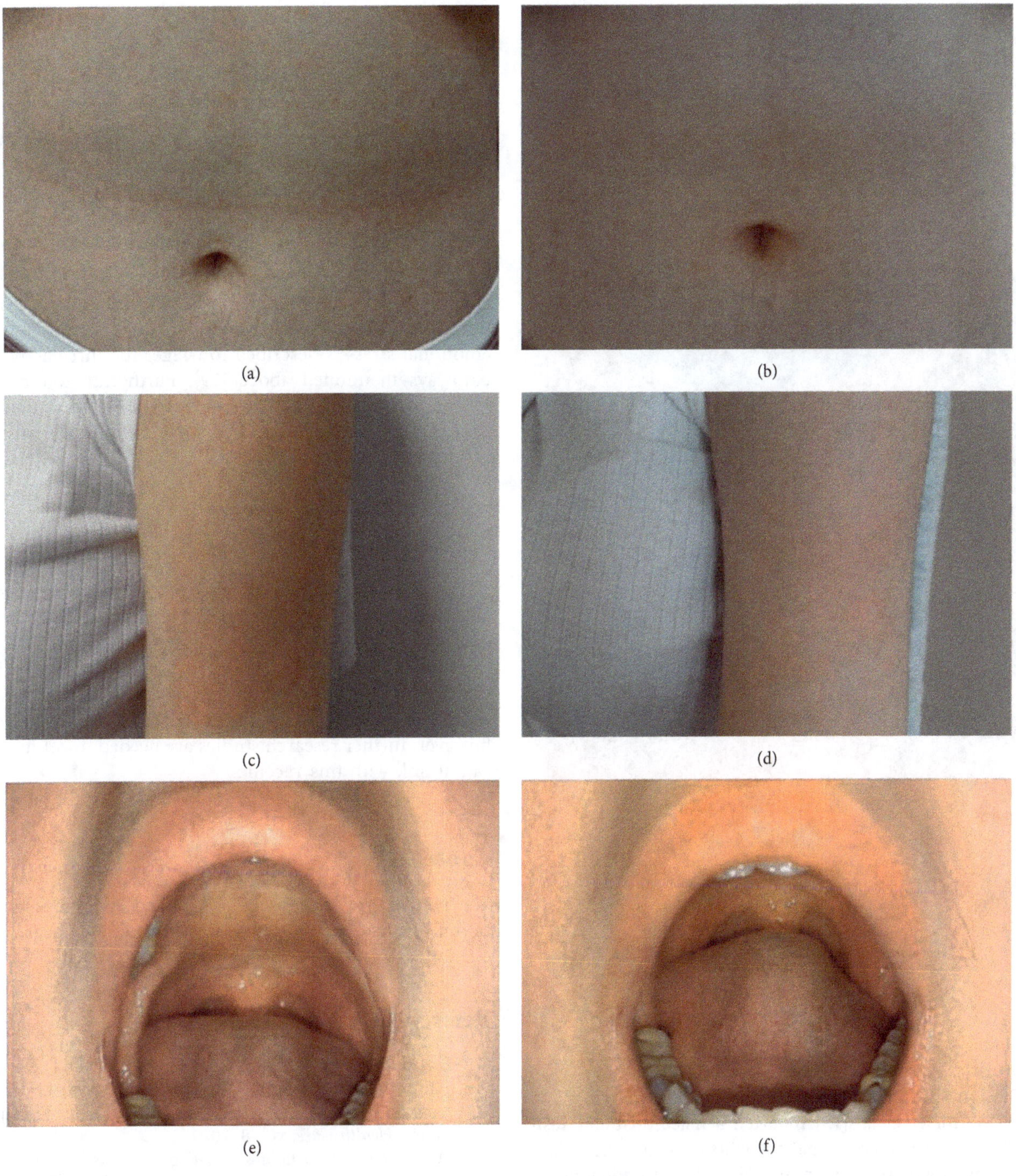

FIGURE 1: Clinical presentation. (a) The maculopapular exanthem at admission. (b) Regression of the maculopapular exanthem after a week. (c) Erythema of the injection site at admission. (d) Injection site after a week. (e) The enanthem at admission. (f) Persistence of enanthem after a week.

leads to immunologic side effects such as acute hypersensitivity and systemic immune reactions [13]. This explanation seems recomforting. Yet, in our case, the rash occurred 3 days after vaccination, which cannot be taken as an immediate hypersensitivity reaction.

Maculopapular rashes are described as a rare adverse event that may occur after immunization. It is also described as a delayed-type hypersensitivity reaction. In fact, the pathogenesis of this reaction is not fully understood. However, basophils activation and a reaction to circulating immune complexes take a major role in the pathogenesis [14].

Furthermore, giving that the commonest etiologies of a MPE are drugs and viral infections and that the vaccine taken by the patient is an adenovirus-vectored virus, we cannot discard a possible infection to adenovirus. Indeed, as described in literature, exposure to viruses may occur at mucosal surfaces or abraded skin sites and may or may not

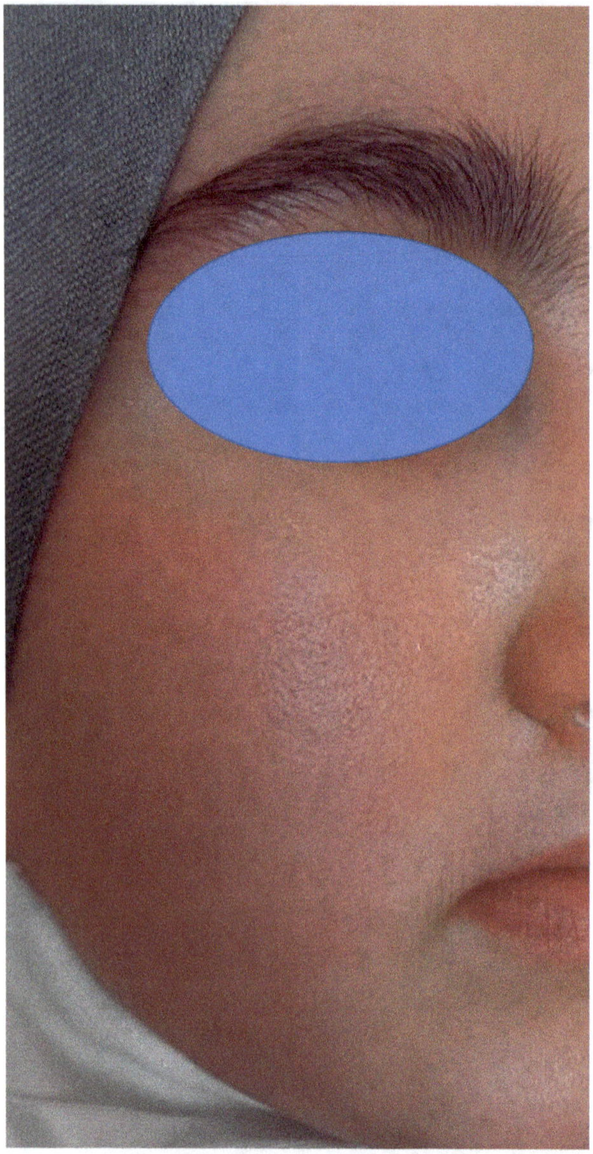

FIGURE 2: Face erythema.

be pruritic. Apropos, this rash is not directly due to viral replication, but a hypersensitivity reaction to the virus.

Niedermeier et al. [15] reported a maculopapular rash presented in a 6-year-old patient who presented, few days before, an upper respiratory tract infection to adenovirus. This eruption resolved spontaneously within 4 weeks.

In addition to the two previous presentations, our patient presented a facial erythema. After the clinical and dermoscopic examination, we retained rosacea as diagnosis.

Rosacea is a chronic inflammatory dermatological condition that concern the central facial skin [16].

It has rarely been described as an adverse effect of treatment or vaccination. However, some cases of rosacea associated with nicotinic acid (niacin, vitamin B3), high doses of vitamin B6 and B12, or etanercept have been reported in literature [16, 17]. On the other hand, several factors are well known to initiate or aggravate rosacea. These factors may be endogenous or exogenous, and they include ultraviolet (UV) radiation, heat, cold, stress, spicy food, and microbes [18].

The mechanisms in which those factors work are not well known. Yet, the role of immunity has been described.

Adaptive and innate immune systems might take a major role in the rosacea pathophysiology. Furthermore, several activation pathways have also been described, such as inflammasome (NALP3), TLR2, and TRPV1. These pathways are triggered in response to several factors previously mentioned.

For our patient, there is no clear cause and effect relationship between vaccination and rosacea. In contrast, emotional stress is described to trigger the three activation pathways mentioned above [19]. Furthermore, the body response to vaccine confers an adequate environment to rosacea, as both innate and adaptive immune systems are activated.

4. Conclusion

The postmarketing phase is crucial for monitoring possible adverse effects that may be related to new vaccines. In this case, we report three cutaneous adverse effects (site injection reaction, maculopapular rash, and rosacea exacerbation) observed in the same patient after taking her first dose of AstraZeneca AZD1222 vaccine. The imputability is high; however, further research studies are needed to confirm the causal link with this vaccine.

Consent

The patient provided written informed consent to publication of this case report and accompanying images.

References

[1] E. Amodio, F. Vitale, L. Cimino, A. Casuccio, and F. Tramuto, "Outbreak of novel coronavirus (SARS-Cov-2): first evidences from international scientific literature and pending questions," *Health Care*, vol. 8, 2020.

[2] WHO, *Director-General's Opening Remarks At The Media Briefing On COVID-19 - 11 March 2020*, WHO, Geneva, Switzerland, 2020.

[3] S. Felsenstein, J. A. Herbert, P. S. McNamara, and C. M. Hedrich, "COVID-19: immunology and treatment options," *Clinical Immunology*, vol. 215, Article ID 108448, 2020.

[4] WHO, *How Are Vaccines Developed?* WHO, Geneva, Switzerland, 2020.

[5] WHO, *Pharmacovigilance: Ensuring the Safe Use of Medicines*, WHO, Geneva, Switzerland, 2004.

[6] M. Voysey, S. A. C. Clemens, S. A. Madhi et al., "Safety and efficacy of the ChAdOx1 nCoV-19 vaccine (AZD1222) against SARS-CoV-2: an interim analysis of four randomised controlled trials in Brazil, South Africa, and the UK," *The Lancet*, vol. 397, pp. 99–111, 2021.

[7] F.-C. Zhu, Y.-H. Li, X.-H. Guan et al., "Safety, tolerability, and immunogenicity of a recombinant adenovirus type-5 vectored COVID-19 vaccine: a dose-escalation, open-label, non-randomised, first-in-human trial," *The Lancet*, vol. 395, pp. 1845–1854, 2020.

[8] E. Rosenblatt Adena and L. Stein Sarah, "Cutaneous reactions to vaccinations," *Clinics in Dermatology*, vol. 33, 2014.

[9] T. T. Shimabukuro, M. Nguyen, D. Martin, and F. DeStefano, "Safety monitoring in the vaccine adverse event reporting system (VAERS)," *Vaccine*, vol. 33, no. 36, pp. 4398–4405, 2015.

[10] C. Ponvert, "Les réactions d'hypersensibilité allergique et non allergique aux vaccins contenant des anatoxines," *Archives de Pediatrie*, vol. 16, no. 4, pp. 391–395, 2009.

[11] P. J. Turner, I. J. Ansotegui, D. E. Campbell et al., "COVID-19 vaccine-associated anaphylaxis: a statement of the world allergy organization anaphylaxis committee," *World Allergy Organization Journal*, vol. 14, no. 2, Article ID 100517, 2021.

[12] E. A. Coors, H. Seybold, H. F. Merk, and V. Mahler, "Polysorbate 80 in medical products and nonimmunologic anaphylactoid reactions," *Annals of Allergy, Asthma, & Immunology*, vol. 95, no. 6, pp. 593–599, 2005.

[13] L. S. Schwartzberg and R. M. Navari, "Safety of polysorbate 80 in the oncology setting," *Advances in Therapy*, vol. 35, no. 6, pp. 754–767, 2018.

[14] L. Sarti, G. Lezmi, F. Mori, M. Giovannini, and J.-C. Caubet, "Diagnosis and management of hypersensitivity reactions to vaccines," *Expert Review of Clinical Immunology*, vol. 16, 2020.

[15] A. Niedermeier, W. Pfützner, T. Ruzicka, P. Thomas, and R. Happle, "Superimposed lateralized exanthem of childhood: report of a case related to adenovirus infection," *Clinical and Experimental Dermatology*, vol. 39, no. 3, pp. 351–353, 2014.

[16] A. Yazici, A. S. Akturk, A. Cefle, D. Bayramgurler, and K. D. Yildiz, "Rosacée survenue sous-traitement par etanercept," *Revue Du Rhumatisme*, vol. 81, no. 3, pp. 269-270, 2014.

[17] T. Jansen, R. Romiti, A. Kreuter, and P. Altmeyer, "Rosacea fulminans triggered by high-dose vitamins B6 and B12," *Journal of the European Academy of Dermatology and Venereology*, vol. 15, no. 5, pp. 484-485, 2001.

[18] P. A. Gerber, B. A. Buhren, M. Steinhoff, and B. Homey, "Rosacea: the cytokine and chemokine network," *Journal of Investigative Dermatology - Symposium Proceedings*, vol. 15, no. 1, pp. 40–47, 2011.

[19] J. Buddenkotte and S. Martin, "Recent advances in understanding and managing rosacea," *F1000Research 7*, vol. 7, 2018.

38

Exclusive Cutaneous and Subcutaneous Sarcoidal Granulomatous Inflammation due to Immune Checkpoint Inhibitors: Report of Two Cases with Unusual Manifestations and Review of the Literature

Narciss Mobini,[1,2] Rummit Dhillon,[3] Jason Dickey,[3] Jordan Spoon,[4] and Kaviyon Sadrolashrafi[5]

[1] *University of Nevada, School of Medicine, Reno and Las Vegas, Nevada, USA*
[2] *Associated Pathologists Chartered, Las Vegas, Nevada, USA*
[3] *College of Osteopathic Medicine, Touro University, Henderson, Nevada, USA*
[4] *Thomas Dermatology, Las Vegas, Nevada, USA*
[5] *University of California, Los Angeles (UCLA), California, USA*

Correspondence should be addressed to Narciss Mobini; mscons@aol.com

Academic Editor: Soner Uzun

Recent emergence of immune checkpoint inhibitors (ICIs) has revolutionized the treatment of cancers and produced prolonged response by boosting the immune system against tumor cells. The primary target antigens are cytotoxic T-lymphocyte-associated antigen-4 (CTLA-4), a downregulator of T-cell activation, and programmed cell death-1 receptor (PD-1), a regulator of T-cell proliferation. This enhanced immune response can induce autoimmune adverse effects in many organs. Although skin toxicities are the most common, sarcoidal inflammation with exclusive cutaneous involvement is a rare occurrence with only 6 cases reported to date. We report 2 cases with unusual features. One patient is a female who was treated for metastatic renal cell carcinoma with combination of ipilimumab (anti-CTLA-4) and nivolumab (anti-PD-1). She developed deep nodules showing sarcoidal dermatitis and panniculitis on histopathologic exam. The second patient is a male with melanoma of eyelid conjunctiva who was treated prophylactically with ipilimumab. He presented with papules/plaques confined to black tattoos, where the biopsy revealed sarcoidal dermatitis. By a comprehensive literature review, we intend to raise awareness about this potential skin side effect in the growing number of patients receiving targeted immunotherapies. It is crucial to have a high index of suspicion and perform timely biopsies to implement appropriate management strategies.

1. Introduction

Despite their tremendous success in treatment of cancer, ICIs are capable of inducing a variety of immune-related adverse events in many organ systems. Skin is reported to be the most common organ affected among other organs such as gastrointestinal, hepatic, endocrine, and renal [1]. The incidence of dermatologic toxicities from ipilimumab (anti-CTLA-4) in metastatic melanoma patients ranges from 49% to 68%, compared to 24% risk of toxicity used for other cancers such as urothelial carcinoma, pancreatic adenocarcinoma, renal cell carcinoma, and non-small cell lung carcinoma [2]. The most common cutaneous side effects related to ipilimumab are pruritus, morbilliform rash, maculopapular eruptions resembling a dermal hypersensitivity reaction, vitiligo, and lichenoid reactions [3]. With anti-PD-1 drugs there may be a 34-39% chance of such adverse cutaneous reactions [1, 4]. Other less common cutaneous toxicities collectively include lichenoid mucositis (tongue, buccal, gingiva, and lips), exacerbation of psoriasis, immunobullous lesions, erythema multiforme, exfoliative dermatitis, prurigo nodularis,

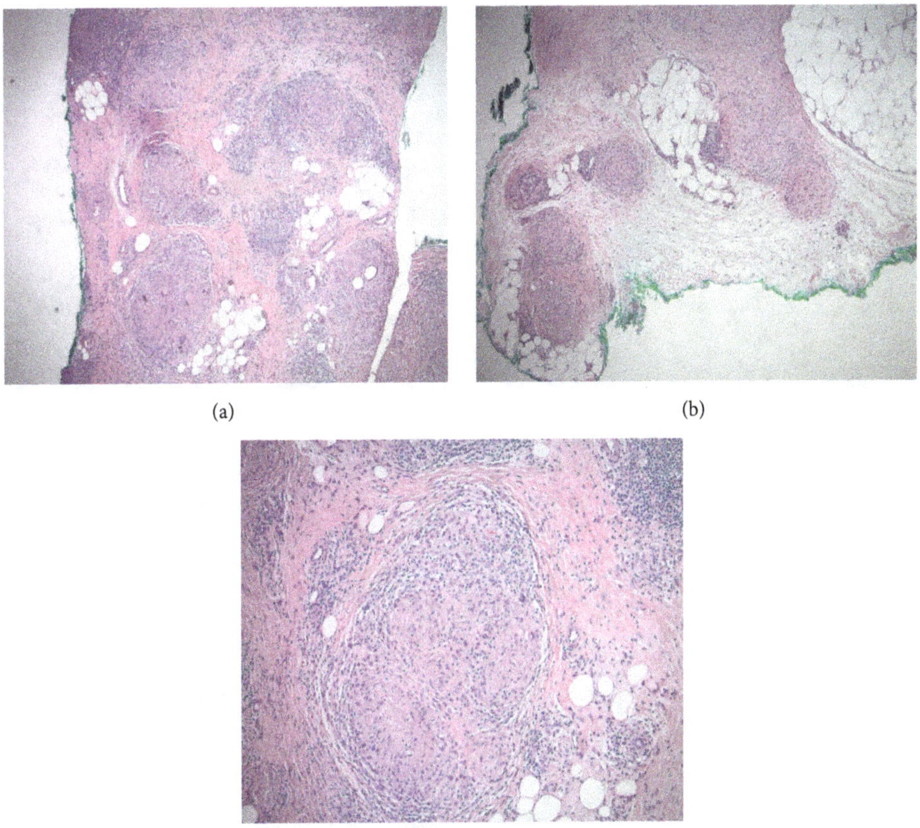

(a) (b) (c)

FIGURE 1: (a), (b), (c). Deep dermal and mainly subcutaneous sarcoidal granulomata characterized by multinodular infiltrate of mono- and multinucleated epithelioid histiocytes with some lymphocytes (hematoxylin-eosin stain, magnifications 10 X, 10X, 20X, respectively).

pyoderma gangrenosum-like ulceration, Sweet syndrome, DRESS syndrome, and toxic epidermal necrolysis [5–7]. Sarcoidal-type granulomatous dermatitis, a rare occurrence, was first introduced by Eckert et al. in 2009 as an adverse side effect of ipilimumab for metastatic melanoma [8]. In addition to ICI, it is noteworthy that sarcoidal lesions can also appear during treatments with kinase inhibitors such as BRAF/MEK inhibitors [6]. ICI-induced cutaneous sarcoidal reactions have been reported in only six patients in the literature to date [2, 9–12]. We present two new cases of such reactions with unique and exclusively skin manifestations following immune checkpoint inhibitors.

2. Case Reports

2.1. Case # 1. A 49-year-old female was referred by her oncologist for evaluation of deep nodules on the left elbow and left forearm for 2 months. She had a history of renal cell carcinoma, clear cell type, and was treated by radical nephrectomy one year prior to her visit. The tumor was reported to be limited to the kidney cortex with no lymphovascular invasion or regional lymph node metastasis (TNM:T2b, NX). Seven months later, the patient developed metastatic lung lesions. She was then treated with nivolumab (opdivo) and ipilimumab (yervoy). The patient started to develop slowly enlarging subcutaneous lesions on her left forearm and elbow one month after the first round of therapy. The patient has a family history of Fragile X syndrome in two of her three sisters and in two brothers, one of whom is also blind. Her parents and children are healthy. On physical examination, there were large nontender firm subcutaneous nodules and plaques on her left forearm and elbow, which were more palpable than visible. A skin biopsy was performed that revealed sarcoidal-type granulomatous inflammation in the dermis and subcutaneous tissue (Figures 1(a), 1(b), and 1(c)). Examination with polarized light failed to reveal foreign material. Special stains for fungi (PAS/periodic acid-Schiff) and atypical mycobacteria (AFB and Fite) were negative. In addition, due to the patient's immunocompromised state, appropriate cultures from the affected skin were also obtained that yielded negative results. The sarcoidal dermatitis and panniculitis was therefore believed to be secondary to combination therapy with opdivo and yervoy. Upon consultation with the treating oncologist, the checkpoint inhibitor therapy was decided to be discontinued after the third round. Systemic workup failed to reveal sarcoidal lesions elsewhere in her body. On the subsequent follow-up visit in three weeks, the patient reported that the lesions were decreasing in size and firmness. She started a new regimen at this time.

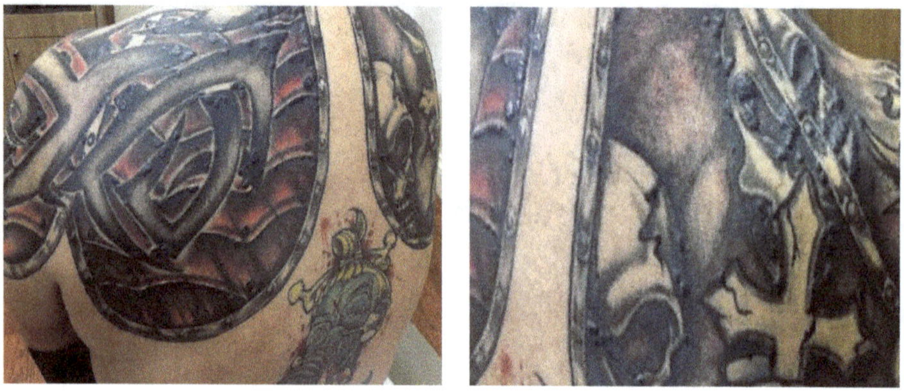

(a) (b)

FIGURE 2: (a), (b). Papulonodular lesions within the black tattoos in patient 2.

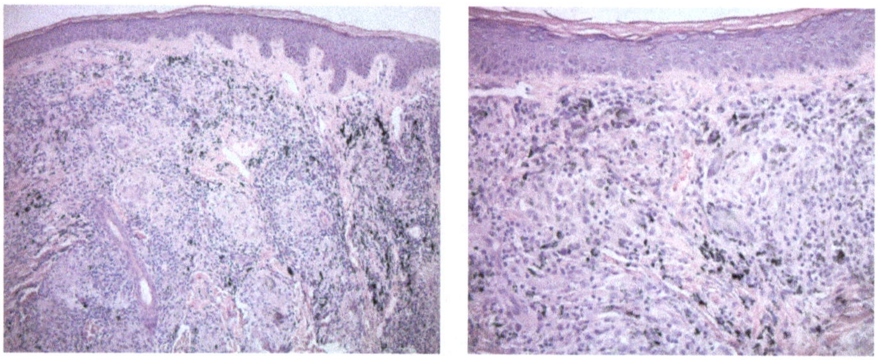

(a) (b)

FIGURE 3: (a), (b). Sarcoidal-type granulomatous inflammation confined to the areas harboring black tattoo pigment (hematoxylin-eosin stain, magnifications 10 X, 20X, respectively).

2.2. Case # 2. A 58-year-old male presented with lesions occurring only within his black tattooed skin on the chest, shoulders, back, left forearm, and right thigh for the past 3 months. The lesions were tender (only upon pressure), with no itching or pain. All tattoos were present for more than 5 years. The patient has a medical history of hypertension and eczema, with a family history of colon cancer in both parents. He was diagnosed with malignant melanoma on the left eyelid conjunctiva 8 months earlier, measuring 1.8 mm with ulceration (TNM stage: pTN2b). Sentinel lymph node from the left preauricular region was negative. Melanoma was treated with Mohs surgery and wide local excision. Metastatic workup was negative. He was later started on four rounds of adjuvant ipilimumab prophylaxis. The rash appeared after the first month of treatment. On physical examination, there were erythematous, scaly tender papules, plaques, and nodules, only confined to the black tattooed areas on his chest, shoulders, upper back, left forearm, and right thigh. The red, yellow, and green tattoos were completely uninvolved (Figures 2(a) and 2(b)). With the clinical diagnosis of possible allergic reaction, he was initially treated with oral prednisone 10 mg/day and 0.1% triamcinolone cream for two weeks with some improvement; however, the rash was persistent. Treatment was switched to topical clobetasol cream and he was given an intralesional triamcinolone acetonide (kenalog) injection to an area on the right upper arm. In his 4-week follow-up visit, due to the lack of significant clinical improvement, a punch biopsy from the left upper arm was performed that revealed sarcoidal-type granulomatous inflammation, associated with only the black tattoo areas (Figures 3(a) and 3(b)). Since the tattoos were present for many years prior to this occurrence with no such reactions, we concluded that the sarcoid reaction was secondary to his ICI therapy. The results were communicated to his oncologist and the ICI treatment was decided to be stopped. A systemic workup failed to reveal lesions elsewhere in his body. In subsequent follow-up visits, the lesions started to improve without further treatment. He is currently being seen by his oncologist at regular intervals, who will continue to monitor the patient for internal disease.

3. Discussion

Immune-related adverse events are well-recognized consequences of immunotherapies. Sarcoidal lesions can appear during treatments with both kinase inhibitors such as BRAF/MEK inhibitors and immune checkpoint inhibitors [6, 12]. During ICI therapies, sarcoidal reactions most commonly involve hilar, mediastinal, or thoracic lymph nodes and also pulmonary parenchyma. It is not certain if the development of sarcoidal lesions carries a better prognosis in patients receiving ICI treatments. In 71% of patients with sarcoidal reactions due to ICIs, the malignancy showed either a partial clinical response, remained stable, or went into remission. In 29% of reports, the malignancy progressed. More than 90% of sarcoidal lesions resolved or improved, irrespective of the medical intervention [13]. In 38-49% of the patients, immunotherapy was discontinued, 44-57% of patients were given systemic steroids for their lesions, and local steroid treatment was used in 8 to 24% of reported cases [4, 13]. Both of our patients showed only cutaneous and/or subcutaneous involvement, with no systemic involvement and there was no prior history of sarcoidosis in either one. Of note, the therapies were given for metastatic renal cell carcinoma (Pt1) and as adjuvant therapy and prophylactically for a conjunctival melanoma (Pt2). Sarcoidal lesions are mostly reported in the setting of treatment for metastatic melanomas. To our knowledge, we report the first case of sarcoidal granulomatous inflammation following ICI therapy that has remained confined within the black tattoo on the skin. Only one case of tattoo sarcoid has been reported, but additional skin areas and the hilar lymph nodes were also involved [14]. One interesting note is that papulonodular reactions in black tattoos are strong markers of sarcoidosis. The "Rush phenomenon" begins with a recent tattoo triggering a local papulonodular reaction. It is characterized by a concomitant reaction in many other black tattoos on the individual and has proven to be a sarcoidal reaction in the majority of cases. Sarcoidosis is estimated to be increased 500-fold in papulonodular reactions compared to the prevalence in the general population [15]. In our patient, the tattoos were present for more than 5 years with no history of any reactions. Therefore, we deduce that the ICI therapy must be the main culprit in producing this manifestation.

Table 1 summarizes all the previously reported cases of sarcoid/sarcoid-like reactions from ICI therapy so far that clinically involved the skin, with or without other organ involvement [13, 14, 16–32].

In summary, of 36 total cases (including our current two cases) reported to date, 24/36 or 67% were female and 12/36 or 33% were male. Exclusive cutaneous/subcutaneous involvement was reported in 8/36 or 22%, including our present cases. The most common site of skin involvement was upper and lower extremities. Other locations included face, scalp, chest, and trunk. Two cases showed tattoo involvement where in one, the sarcoid reaction was only confined to black tattoo (current report). In addition, localization to dermal scars was seen in two patients. Lymph nodes were the most common extracutaneous organ involved in 15/36 or 45% of cases, followed by pulmonary parenchyma in 11/36 or 30%. Ipilimumab was the culprit in 11/36 or 31%, nivolumab and pembrolizumab, each in 8/36 or 22%, and combination therapy was reported in 9/36 or 25%. The most common type of underlying cancer was melanoma in 30/36 or 83%, which is consistent with the previously published research on ICI-induced sarcoidal reactions reported to occur in more than %75 of the patients under melanoma treatment [13]. Melanomas are highly immunogenic and the neoantigen environment in these cells has a tremendous impact on antitumor activity of cytotoxic T cells and response to ICI. Enhanced destroying of melanoma cells induced by ICI therapy exposes additional neoantigens presenting by antigen presenting cells that promote Th1 response and release of cytokines that promote the development of granulomatous/sarcoidal lesions in ICI therapy. The pathogenesis of sarcoidal granulomas is complex and involves the interaction of mononocytes/macrophages and CD4 + Th1 cells. In response to antigens and possibly neoantigens secondary to destruction of melanoma in ICI therapy, macrophages produce TNF-alpha and interleukins that recruit CD4+ Th cells [33]. Cytokines that enhance Th1 differentiation are found to be upregulated in sarcoidosis where they secret IFN-gamma and IL-17 and organize granulomatous structure by promoting the maturation of epithelioid histiocytes and multinucleated giant cells. Sarcoidosis seen during ICI therapy supports a hyperactive immune response. Recent reports also highlight the possible role of Th17 cells in the pathogenesis of sarcoid, specifically a subset of CD4+T cells that produce IFN-gamma and IL-17 [34, 35]. Although the development of sarcoidal lesions in immunotherapies may represent a favorable sign of potential therapeutic response, it is not yet completely elucidated and requires further studies in larger scales for clearer guidelines in the clinical management of these patients.

4. Conclusion

Immune checkpoint targeted agents can induce nonspecific enhanced immune response and overstimulation of inflammatory pathways, leading to a spectrum of autoimmune side effects. Among these, sarcoidosis or sarcoid-like lesions are reported with the majority of cases, presenting with lymph node and pulmonary involvement, and less frequently skin and other organs. By reporting two new cases of exclusively cutaneous/subcutaneous sarcoid secondary to ipilimumab and nivolumab immunotherapies (so far there are a total of 8 cases in the literature) and a thorough review of existing published data, we intend to raise awareness of this potential adverse effect. To our knowledge, we report the first case of sarcoidal granulomatous dermatitis confined solely to black tattoo areas with no systemic involvement. In light of increased utilization of successful ICI therapies today, clinicians should have a high index of suspicion and perform timely biopsies of any newly developing, unusual, or persistent cutaneous lesions in the course of the treatment to avoid misinterpreting sarcoid reactions as progressive or recurrent disease and implement proper management strategies.

Table 1: Sarcoidal-type granulomatous reaction due to immune checkpoint inhibitors (anti-CTLA-4 and anti PD-1 antibodies), affecting skin, with and without other organ systems.

	Case	Age	Sex	Primary disease	Clinical manifestation	ICI therapy
1	Suozzi, 2016 [9]	60	F	Lung Adenocarcinoma	Cutaneous only	Ipilimumab & Nivolumab
2	Ogawa, 2018 [10]	63	F	Lung Adenocarcinoma	Cutaneous only	Nivolumab
3	Birnbaum, 2017 [11]	56	F	Melanoma	Cutaneous only	Nivolumab
4	Dimitriou, 2018 [12]	72	M	Melanoma	Cutaneous only	Pembrolizumab
5	Tetzlaff, 2017 [2]	57	F	Ovarian Cancer	Subcutaneous only (bilateral lower extremities, forearms)	Ipilimumab & Nivolumab
6	Tetzlaff, 2017 [2]	39	F	Melanoma	Subcutaneous only (bilateral lower extremities & buttocks)	Ipilimumab & Nivolumab
7	Current Report, 2019	49	F	Renal Cell Carcinoma	Cutaneous only (left forearm and elbow)	Ipilimumab & Nivolumab
8	Current Report, 2019	58	M	Melanoma	Cutaneous only (black tattoo on chest, shoulders, back, forearm, thigh)	Ipilimumab
9	Kim, 2016 [14]	52	M	Urothelial Carcinoma	Cutaneous (tattoo & face), Hilar Lymph Nodes (LN)	Ipilimumab & Nivolumab
10	Cotliar, 2016 [16]	72	F	Hodgkin Lymphoma	Subcutaneous (bilateral arms), Pulmonary, Hilar LN, Bone	Pembrolizumab
11	Tetzlaff, 2018 [13]	44	F	Melanoma	Subcutaneous (peripatellar), Hilar LN	Ipilimumab
12	Tetzlaff, 2018 [13]	79	M	Melanoma	Cutaneous (bilateral forearms, elbows, hands), Hilar LN	Pembrolizumab & Nivolumab
13	Le Burel, 2017 [17]	71	F	Melanoma	Cutaneous, Pulmonary Parenchyma	Nivolumab
14	Lomax, 2017 [18]	75	F	Melanoma	Cutaneous, Pulmonary	Nivolumab
15	Oommen, 2017 [19]	54	M	Melanoma	Cutaneous, Pulmonary	Ipilimumab
16	Reddy, 2017 [20]	57	F	Melanoma	Cutaneous, Pulmonary	Ipilimumab
17	Reddy, 2017 [20]	55	F	Melanoma	Cutaneous, Pulmonary	Ipilimumab & Nivolumab
18	Toumeh, 2016 [21]	26	F	Melanoma	Cutaneous, Pulmonary	Ipilimumab
19	Yatim, 2018 [22]	72	F	Melanoma	Subcutaneous (left flank, right leg, scar), Pulmonary, hilar LN, Eye	Pembrolizumab
20	Firwana, 2017 [23]	37	F	Melanoma	Cutaneous (right forearm, bilateral shins), Hilar LN & other LN	Ipilimumab & Pembrolizumab
21	Firwana, 2017 [23]	57	F	Melanoma	Cutaneous (bilateral lower extremities), Hilar LN	Ipilimumab
22	Danlos, 2016 [24]	57	M	Melanoma	Cutaneous (lip, scar), Hilar and Mediastinal LN	Nivolumab
23	Martinez, 2016 [25]	46	F	Melanoma	Cutaneous, Pulmonary	Ipilimumab
24	Tissot, 2013 [26]	57	M	Melanoma	Cutaneous (elbow, arm), Pulmonary, Hilar LN	Ipilimumab
25	Eckert, 2009 [8]	67	F	Melanoma	Cutaneous, Pulmonary	Ipilimumab
26	Reule, 2013 [27]	55	M	Melanoma	Cutaneous (finger, forearm, knee), Pulmonary, Hilar LN	Ipilimumab
27	Lomax, 2017 [18]	57	F	Melanoma	Subcutaneous & Cutaneous (elbows, wrists, thighs), Pulmonary, Hilar LN	Pembrolizumab
28	McKenna, 2018 [28]	69	F	Melanoma	Cutaneous, Pulmonary	Nivolumab
29	Jespersen, 2018 [29]	57	F	Melanoma	Cutaneous, Pulmonary, Bone	Pembrolizumab
30	Dimitriou, 2018 [12]	65	M	Melanoma	Cutaneous (elbow), Hilar LN	Pembrolizumab

TABLE 1: Continued.

	Case	Age	Sex	Primary disease	Clinical manifestation	ICI therapy
31	Dimitriou, 2018 [12]	57	M	Melanoma	Cutaneous (scar), Hilar LN, Thyroid	Ipilimumab & Nivolumab
32	Burillo-Martinez, 2017 [30]	69	F	Melanoma	Subcutaneous (forearms, legs, blue nevus), Hilar LN	Pembrolizumab
33	Paolini, 2018 [31]	56	F	Non-small Cell Lung Cancer	Cutaneous, Pulmonary	Nivolumab
34	Wilgenhof, 2012 [32]	37	M	Melanoma	Cutaneous, Pulmonary, Lymph Nodes, Spleen	Ipilimumab
35	Lomax, 2017 [18]	44	M	Melanoma	Cutaneous (elbow and occipital region), Pulmonary, Hilar and Mediastinal LN, Colitis	Nivolumab
36	Lomax, 2017 [18]	65	F	Melanoma	Cutaneous (face, knees), Thyroiditis, Pulmonary, Hilar LN	Pembrolizumab

References

[1] L. Hoffman, A. Forschner, C. Loquai et al., "Cutaneous, gastrointestinal, hepatic,endocrine, and renal side-effects of anti-PD-1 therapy," *European Journal of Cancer*, vol. 60, pp. 190–209, 2016.

[2] M. T. Tetzlaff, A. A. Jazaeri, C. A. Torres-Cabala et al., "Erythema nodosum-like panniculitis mimicking disease recurrence: A novel toxicity from immune checkpoint blockade therapy. Report of two patients," *Journal of Cutaneous Pathology*, vol. 44, no. 12, pp. 1080–1086, 2017.

[3] J. L. Curry, M. T. Tetzlaff, P. Nagarajan et al., "Diverse types of dermatologic toxicities from immune checkpoint blockade therapy," *Journal of Cutaneous Pathology*, vol. 44, no. 2, pp. 158–176, 2017.

[4] C. M. Cornejo, P. Haun, J. English, and M. Rosenbach, "Immune checkpoint inhibitors and the development of granulomatous reactions," *Journal of the American Academy of Dermatology*, 2018.

[5] L. K. Collins, M. S. Chapman, J. B. Carter, and F. H. Samie, "Cutaneous adverse effects of the immune checkpoint inhibitors," *Current Problems in Cancer*, vol. 41, no. 2, pp. 125–128, 2017.

[6] L. Zimmer, J. Vaubel, E. Livingstone, and D. Schadendorf, "Side effects of systemic oncological therapies in dermatology," *Journal der Deutschen Dermatologischen Gesellschaft*, vol. 10, no. 7, pp. 475–486, 2012.

[7] C. J. Voskens, S. M. Goldinger, C. Loquai et al., "The price of tumor control: an analysis of rare side effects of anti-CTLA-4therapy in metastatic melanoma from ipilimumab network," *PLoS One*, vol. 8, Article ID e57345, 2013.

[8] A. Eckert, A. Schoeffler, S. Dalle, A. Phan, L. Kiakouama, and L. Thomas, "Anti-CTLA4 monoclonal antibody induced sarcoidosis in a metastatic melanoma patient," *Dermatology*, vol. 218, no. 1, pp. 69-70, 2009.

[9] K. C. Suozzi, M. Stahl, C. J. Ko et al., "Immune-related sarcoidosis observed in combination ipilimumab and nivolumab therapy," *JAAD Case Reports*, vol. 2, no. 3, pp. 264–268, 2016.

[10] T. Ogawa, Y. Ishitsuka, K. Iwamoto et al., "Programmed cell death 1 blockade-induced cutaneous sarcoid-like epithelioid granulomas in advanced melanoma: a case report," *Journal of the European Academy of Dermatology and Venereology*, vol. 32, no. 7, pp. e260–e261, 2018.

[11] M. R. Birnbaum, M. W. Ma, S. Fleisig et al., "Nivolumab-related cutaneous sarcoidosis in a patient with lung adenocarcinoma," *JAAD Case Reports*, vol. 3, no. 3, pp. 208–211, 2017.

[12] F. Dimitriou, A. L. Frauchiger, M. Urosevic-Maiwald et al., "Sarcoid-like reactions in patients receiving modern melanoma treatment," *Melanoma Research*, vol. 28, no. 3, pp. 230–236, 2018.

[13] M. T. Tetzlaff, K. C. Nelson, A. Diab et al., "Granulomatous/sarcoid-like lesions associated with checkpoint inhibitors: a marker of therapy response in a subset of melanoma patients," *Journal for ImmunoTherapy of Cancer*, vol. 6, no. 1, p. 14, 2018.

[14] C. Kim, J. Gao, V. R. Shannon, and A. Siefker-Radtke, "Systemic sarcoidosis first manifesting in a tattoo in the setting of immune checkpoint inhibition," *BMJ Case Reports*, vol. 2016, 2016.

[15] M. Sepehri, K. Hutton Carlsen, and J. Serup, "Papulo-nodular reactions in black tattoos as markers of sarcoidosis: study of 92 tattoo reactions from a hospital material," *Dermatology*, vol. 232, no. 6, pp. 679–686, 2017.

[16] J. Cotliar, C. Querfeld, W. J. Boswell, N. Raja, D. Raz, and R. Chen, "Pembrolizumab-associated sarcoidosis," *JAAD Case Reports*, vol. 2, no. 4, pp. 290–293, 2016.

[17] S. Le Burel, S. Champiat, C. Mateus et al., "Prevalence of immune-related systemic adverse events in patients treated with anti-Programmed cell Death 1/anti-Programmed cell Death-Ligand 1 agents: a single-centre pharmacovigilance database analysis," *European Journal of Cancer*, vol. 82, pp. 34–44, 2017.

[18] A. J. Lomax, H. M. McGuire, C. McNeil et al., "Immunotherapy-induced sarcoidosis in patients with melanoma treated with PD-1 checkpoint inhibitors: Case series and immunophenotypic analysis," *International Journal of Rheumatic Diseases*, vol. 20, no. 9, pp. 1277–1285, 2017.

[19] E. Oommen and J. Allam, "Ipilimumab lung toxicity," *CHEST*, vol. 152, no. 4, Article ID A724, 2017.

[20] S. B. Reddy, J. D. Possick, H. M. Kluger, A. Galan, and D. Han, "Sarcoidosis following anti-PD-1 and anti-CTLA-4 therapy for metastatic melanoma," *Journal of Immunotherapy*, vol. 40, no. 8, pp. 307–311, 2017.

[21] A. Toumeh, R. Sakhi, S. Shah, S. K. Arudra, L. E. De Las Casas, and R. T. Skeel, "Ipilimumab-induced granulomatous disease occurring simultaneously with disease progression in a patient with metastatic melanoma," *American Journal of Therapeutics*, vol. 23, no. 4, pp. e1068–e1071, 2016.

[22] N. Yatim, C. Mateus, and P. Charles, "Sarcoidosis post-anti-PD-1 therapy, mimicking relapse of metastatic melanoma in a patient undergoing complete remission," *La Revue de Médecine Interne*, vol. 39, no. 2, pp. 130–133, 2018.

[23] B. Firwana, R. Ravilla, M. Raval, L. Hutchins, and F. Mahmoud, "Sarcoidosis-like syndrome and lymphadenopathy due to checkpoint inhibitors," *Journal of Oncology Pharmacy Practice*, vol. 23, no. 8, pp. 620–624, 2017.

[24] F.-X. Danlos, C. Pagès, B. Baroudjian et al., "Nivolumab-induced sarcoid-like granulomatous reaction in a patient with advanced melanoma," *Chest*, vol. 149, no. 5, pp. e133–e136, 2016.

[25] L. Martínez Leboráns, A. Esteve Martínez, A. M. Victoria Martínez, V. Alegre de Miquel, and A. Berrocal Jaime, "Cutaneous sarcoidosis in a melanoma patient under Ipilimumab therapy," *Dermatologic Therapy*, vol. 29, no. 5, pp. 306–308, 2016.

[26] C. Tissot, A. Carsin, N. Freymond, Y. Pacheco, and G. Devouassoux, "Sarcoidosis complicating anti-cytotoxic T-lymphocyte-associated antigen-4 monoclonal antibody biotherapy," *European Respiratory Journal*, vol. 41, no. 1, pp. 246-247, 2012.

[27] R. B. Reule and J. P. North, "Cutaneous and pulmonary sarcoidosis-like reaction associated with ipilimumab," *Journal of the American Academy of Dermatology*, vol. 69, no. 5, pp. e272–e273, 2013.

[28] M. C. McKenna, K. Molloy, S. Crowther et al., "Pembrolizumab-related sarcoid-like reaction presenting as reactivation of quiescent scars," *Journal of Oncology Practice*, vol. 14, no. 3, pp. 200-201, 2018.

[29] H. Jespersen, S. Bjursten, L. Ny, and M. Levin, "Checkpoint inhibitor-induced sarcoid reaction mimicking bone metastases," *The Lancet Oncology*, vol. 19, no. 6, Article ID e327, 2018.

[30] S. Burillo-Martinez, C. Morales-Raya, M. Prieto-Barrios, J. Rodriguez-Peralto, and P. Ortiz-Romero, "Pembrolizumab-induced extensive panniculitis and nevus regression: two novel cutaneous manifestations of the post-immunotherapy granulomatous reactions spectrum," *JAMA Dermatology*, vol. 153, no. 7, pp. 721-722, 2017.

[31] L. Paolini, C. Poli, S. Blanchard et al., "Thoracic and cutaneous sarcoid-like reaction associated with anti-PD-1 therapy: longitudinal monitoring of PD-1 and PD-L1 expression after stopping treatment," *Journal for ImmunoTherapy of Cancer*, vol. 6, no. 1, p. 52, 2018.

[32] S. Wilgenhof, V. Morlion, A. C. Seghers et al., "Sarcoidosis in a patient with metastatic melanoma sequentially treated with anti-CTLA-4 monoclonal antibody and selective BRAF inhibitor," *Anticancer Reseach*, vol. 32, no. 4, pp. 1355–1359, 2012.

[33] W. M. Timmermans, J. A. van Laar, P. M. van Hagen, and M. C. van Zelm, "Immunopathogenesis of granulomas in chronic autoinflammatory diseases," *Clinical & Translational Immunology*, vol. 5, no. 12, Article ID e118, 2016.

[34] S. N. Georas, T. J. Chapman, and E. D. Crouser, "Sarcoidosis and T-helper cells. Th1, Th17, or Th17.1?" *American Journal of Respiratory and Critical Care Medicine*, vol. 193, no. 11, pp. 1198–1200, 2016.

[35] J. Ramstein, C. E. Broos, L. J. Simpson et al., "IFN-gamma-producing T-helpr 17.1 cells are increased in sarcoidosis andare moreprevalent than T-helper type 1 cells," *American Journal of Respiratory and Critical Care Medicine*, vol. 193, pp. 1281–1291, 2016.

39

Metastatic Multiple Myeloma to the Skin

Alex C. Holliday,[1] Mohammed I. Khan,[1] Sean E. Mazloom,[1] Rahul N. Chavan,[2] and Douglas J. Grider[1,3]

[1]*Carilion Clinic and Virginia Tech Carilion School of Medicine, Department of Internal Medicine, Section of Dermatology, Roanoke, VA, USA*
[2]*Alabama College of Osteopathic Medicine, Dothan, AL, USA*
[3]*Virginia Tech Carilion School of Medicine, Department of Basic Science Education, Roanoke, VA, USA*

Correspondence should be addressed to Douglas J. Grider; djgrider@carilionclinic.org

Academic Editor: Jaime A. Tschen

Cutaneous involvement of multiple myeloma (MM) is uncommon, typically occurs in late stage disease, and is a poor prognostic indicator with an approximate eight month median survival. We present a 51-year-old man with relapsed lambda light chain MM who developed abrupt asymptomatic skin metastases. Biopsy revealed a dermis replete of atypical plasma cells, positive for CD138 and CD45. In situ hybridization confirmed lambda light chain restriction. Despite rescue antimyeloma therapy with the anti-CD38 drug daratumumab, he rapidly declined clinically and succumbed to the disease four weeks after presentation. A standard treatment approach for cutaneous MM does not currently exist; however, various techniques to detect cytogenetic abnormalities are emerging and will provide additional prognostic value and direct individualized therapy.

1. Case Presentation

A 51-year-old man with relapsed lambda light chain multiple myeloma (MM) was hospitalized due to uremic encephalopathy. Three years prior he experienced remission from MM after treatment with lenalidomide, bortezomib, and dexamethasone (RVD). At that time, he declined maintenance therapy and autologous stem cell transplant. After a relapse involving his cervical spine, he underwent de-compressive surgery, radiation, and restarted RVD. Subsequent bone marrow biopsy revealed disease progression. Dermatology was consulted regarding asymptomatic erythematous papules, plaques, and nodules involving his upper trunk, face, and scalp that had abruptly appeared over the prior three weeks (Figure 1). Punch biopsies from the chin nodule and a scalp plaque were obtained (Figure 2(a)). The papillary and reticular dermis were replete with atypical plasma cells, focally resembling plasmablasts, positive for CD138 (Figure 2(b)) and CD45 (Figure 2(c)) by immunohistochemistry. A Grenz zone underlined the epidermis and foci of malignant cells involving adnexal structures including pilosebaceous units were apparent. Dutcher bodies were rare; no Russell bodies were appreciated. In situ hybridization (ISH) confirmed lambda light chain restriction (Figures 2(d) and 2(e)).

The patient's renal failure was attributed to myeloma kidney; and hemodialysis, apheresis, and daratumumab were initiated. While his encephalopathy initially improved, the patient declined clinically and he was transitioned to comfort care three weeks after the biopsy, dying 5 days later.

2. Discussion

Multiple myeloma results from the accumulation of monoclonal protein producing plasma cells and principally affects the bone marrow. Common clinical manifestations are represented by the acronym CRAB: hyper*C*alcaemia, *R*enal insufficiency, *A*nemia, and *B*one lesions [1]. As of 2014, guideline revisions allow patients with a positive bone marrow biopsy and one CRAB feature or patients with smoldering myeloma and positive biomarkers predicting progression be offered treatment [1].

Cutaneous involvement of MM is uncommon. It usually occurs in late stage disease and reflects a high tumor

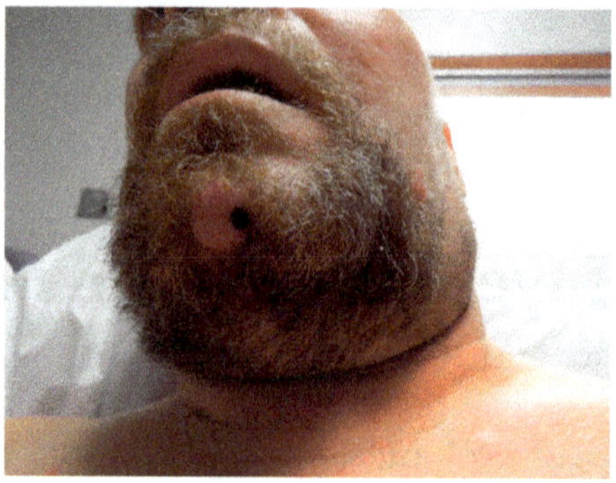

Figure 1: Physical examination revealed a pink nodule (with a 4 mm punch biopsy defect) on his chin and a pink plaque on his left cheek. Similar plaques and papules were evident on his upper trunk and scalp.

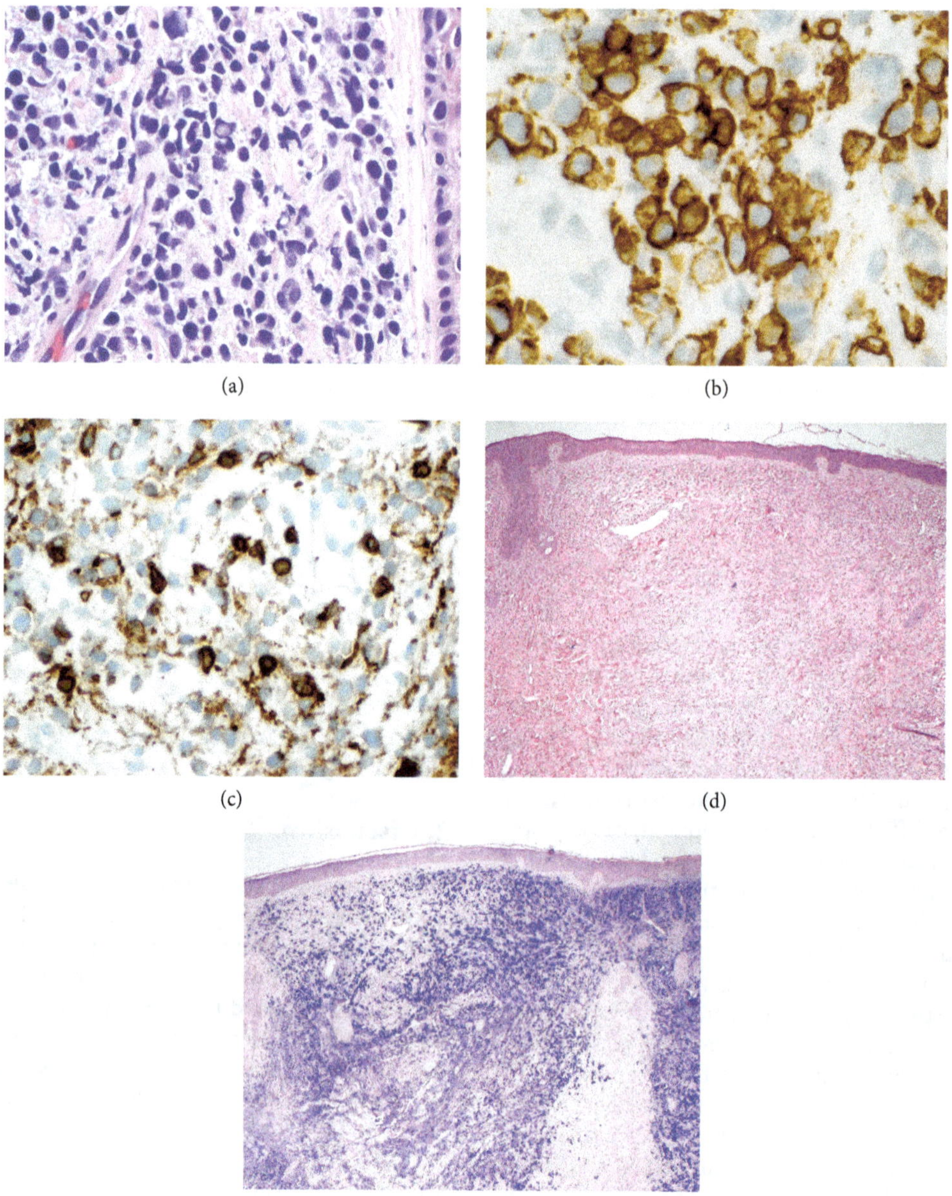

(a) (b) (c) (d) (e)

Figure 2: (a) Haematoxylin and Eosin stained tissue section from the chin punch biopsy. Atypical plasma cells with a Dutcher body apparent in the middle left (400 magnification; 40x). (b) CD138 positive (400 magnification, 40x). (c) CD45 positive (400 magnification, 40x). (d) Kappa light chain negative (40 magnification, 4x). (e) Lambda light chain positive (40 magnification, 4x).

burden. The median time from diagnosis to skin involvement is 2.2 years, but cutaneous MM may present at any time or in any stage of the disease [2]. There is an approximate eight month median survival after the appearance of cutaneous metastases [2, 3].

When skin lesions manifest in a MM patient, biopsy provides rapid assessment of disease severity. Histology is useful to differentiate direct tumor involvement from paraneoplastic processes like Sweet syndrome and complications from manufactured proteins such as those seen in amyloidosis [4].

Histopathologically, nodular and diffuse interstitial patterns exist. The neoplastic plasma cells typically stain strongly with CD79a, CD138, and epithelial membrane antigen; and variably with VS38c and CD43 [5]. Staining with CD138 (collagen-1 binding proteoglycan, syndecan) is particularly helpful as it is a specific marker for bone marrow derived plasma cells, both benign and malignant [5]. CD45 (leukocyte common antigen) immunohistochemical positivity is seen in relapsed MM [6]. Plasmablastic morphology can be misleading as it can mimic other blastic proliferations or be misinterpreted as a pseudolymphoma. A benign, dermal plasma cell rich proliferation can also be present at cutaneous-mucosal junctions or in special site areas like the scalp or the genitals. Thus, studies proving clonality, such as in situ hybridization for kappa and lambda light chains are important [2]. Light chain restriction does not occur in reactive plasma cell-rich infiltrates [3].

Acute renal insufficiency is a myeloma emergency, a poor prognostic indicator, and is attributed to the toxic effects of monoclonal light chains on the kidney [7]. Antimyeloma therapy coupled with aggressive hydration and avoidance of nephrotoxic agents is standard for acute renal insufficiency in MM patients [7].

Treatment and maintenance regimens include numerous combinations of traditional chemotherapy drugs, corticosteroids, proteasome inhibitors, immunomodulating agents, histone deacetylase inhibitors, interferon, monoclonal antibodies, and stem cell transplants. Although unsuccessful in our patient, the monoclonal antibody daratumumab targeting CD38 (a molecule overexpressed by MM cells) has been effective monotherapy in resistant and refractory disease [8].

3. Conclusion

With a dismal median survival, cutaneous MM confers a poor prognosis and treatment challenge for physicians. Research into cytogenetic abnormalities detected by fluorescent in situ hybridization is providing additional prognostic value and therapeutic application [9].

Disclosure

This case was originally presented in 2015 as a poster at the 53rd Annual Meeting of the American Society of Dermatopathology.

References

[1] S. V. Rajkumar, M. A. Dimopoulos, A. Palumbo et al., "International myeloma working group updated criteria for the diagnosis of multiple myeloma myeloma," *The Lancet Oncology*, vol. 15, no. 12, pp. e538–e548, 2014.

[2] A. Jurczyszyn, M. Olszewska-Szopa, V. Hungria et al., "Cutaneous involvement in multiple myeloma: a multi-institutional retrospective study of 53 patients," *Leukemia & Lymphoma*, vol. 57, no. 9, pp. 2071–2076, 2016.

[3] J. Malysz, G. Talamo, J. Zhu et al., "Cutaneous involvement in multiple myeloma (MM): a case series with clinicopathologic correlation," *Journal of the American Academy of Dermatology*, vol. 74, no. 5, pp. 878–884, 2016.

[4] I. B. Bayer-Garner and B. R. Smoller, "The spectrum of cutaneous disease in multiple myeloma," *Journal of the American Academy of Dermatology*, vol. 48, no. 4, pp. 497–507, 2003.

[5] L. Requena, H. Kutzner, G. Palmedo et al., "Cutaneous involvement in multiple myeloma: a clinicopathologic, immunohistochemical, and cytogenetic study of 8 cases," *Archives of Dermatology*, vol. 139, no. 4, , 2003.

[6] S. Kumar, R. Kimlinger, and W. Morice, "Immunophenotyping in multiple myeloma and related plasma cell disorders," *Best Practice & Research Clinical Haematology*, vol. 23, no. 3, pp. 433–451, 2010.

[7] M. A. Dimopoulos, P. Sonneveld, N. Leung et al., "International myeloma working group recommendations for the diagnosis and management of myeloma-related renal impairment," *Journal of Clinical Oncology*, vol. 34, no. 13, pp. 1544–1557, 2016.

[8] H. M. Lokhorst, T. Plesner, J. P. Laubach et al., "Targeting CD38 with daratumumab monotherapy in multiple myeloma," *New England Journal of Medicine*, vol. 373, no. 13, pp. 1207–1219, 2015.

[9] P. Sonneveld, H. Avet-Loiseau, S. Lonial et al., "Treatment of multiple myeloma with high-risk cytogenetics: a consensus of the international myeloma working group," *Blood*, vol. 127, no. 24, pp. 2955–2962, 2016.

A Guttate Psoriasis that Tends to Spare Three Tattoos: A Macrophage Liaison

Panagiota Spyridonos,[1] Vasiliki Zampeli,[2] Sophia-Nefeli Rapti,[3] and Ioannis D. Bassukas[2,3]

[1]*Department of Medical Physics/Informatics, Faculty of Medicine, School of Health Sciences, University of Ioannina, Ioannina, Greece*
[2]*Department of Skin and Venereal Diseases, Faculty of Medicine, School of Health Sciences, University of Ioannina, Ioannina, Greece*
[3]*Department of Dermatology, University Hospital of Ioannina, Ioannina, Greece*

Correspondence should be addressed to Ioannis D. Bassukas; ibassuka@uoi.gr

Academic Editor: Alireza Firooz

Induction of new psoriasis sites was reported in only a small amount of psoriasis patients undergoing tattooing, despite the intuitive belief that tattoo trauma might awaken the disease due to the isomorphic phenomenon of Koebner. In this case report, we discuss a patient who presented with a remarkable sparing of his three tattoo sites during a guttate psoriasis flare-up that was unrelated to tattooing. The spatial concordance of tattoo and psoriasis lesions was analyzed on clinical pictures of tattoo sites taken during the psoriasis episode. For the quantification of the spatial distribution of the psoriasis lesions, Voronoi diagrams were generated, and coefficients of variation and the two-sample *t*-test were employed to compare the distributions of Voronoi patch sizes in different settings. Compared to skin areas without tattoos, a tattoo introduced a higher variation in the sizes of the Voronoi patches centered around psoriasis lesions. Based on our findings, we would like to discuss the possible role of macrophages as the key cellular link in the complex pathophysiologic relationship between tattooing/tattoo and psoriasis. Taking into account the relationship of autophagy and psoriasis lesions, we propose the hypothesis that tattoos represent a "psoriasis-hostile" tissue environment pertained by a population of LAP active M2-polarized macrophages. Further clinical studies of the relationship of psoriasis lesions to the tattooed skin are needed and may provide important insights into the role of macrophages in the pathogenesis of psoriasis.

1. Introduction

The nosologic relationship of psoriasis and tattoo remains a matter of debate. Despite the intuitive concern that tattoo trauma might induce the disease (Koebner phenomenon, KP), a KP was reported in only 3.2% of psoriasis patients undergoing tattooing [1], an overall rather moderate rate [2]. Moreover, Grodner and colleagues [3] observed that much more patients with psoriasis did not recall lesions that had affected their tattoo sites during episodes of disease flare-ups (47.6%) than recalling them (19.8%). Herein, on the occasion of a patient who presented with a distinct sparing of three tattoo sites during a guttate psoriasis episode that was unrelated to tattooing, we would like to comment on the putative role of macrophages as the key cellular link in the complex pathophysiologic relationship between tattooing/tattoo and psoriasis.

2. Case Presentation

An afebrile, 27-year-old male patient, in otherwise good general condition, presented with a rash of scattered, up to 1.0 cm large psoriasiform lesions that progressively affected his torso (shown in Figure 1) and the extremities during the past two weeks. The rash was accompanied by moderate itching and an apparent tendency to coalesce in typical for

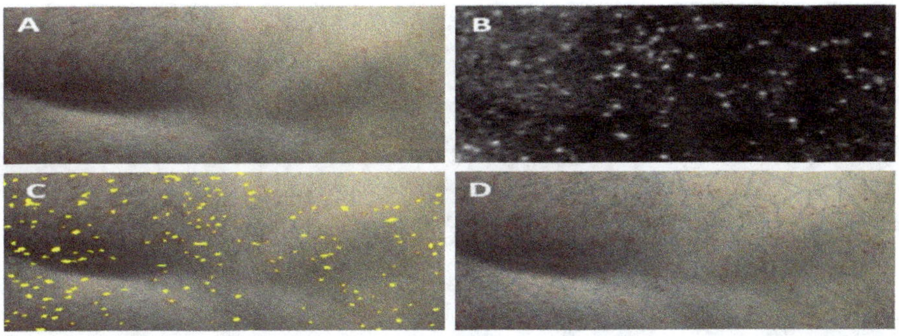

Figure 1: (a) Skin area affected with psoriasis. (b) Enhanced lesion representation by a* color channel of lab space. (c) Segmented lesions (yellow spots) superimposed on the initial image to visualize the result of morphological processing. (d) Lesions' centroids generating Voronoi tessellation.

plaque psoriasis skin localizations, i.e., the knees. The patient was diagnosed with plaque psoriasis at the age of 15 years, which was treated successfully with topical regimens. The laboratory evaluation including chest X-ray, ASO, syphilis, and hepatitis A, B, and C serology returned no pathologic findings. Based on patient's history, the macromorphology of the rash, and a lesional skin biopsy, guttate psoriasis was diagnosed. Except for psychosocial stress, no other triggering events of the dermatosis could be elucidated. Remarkably, the rash spared almost completely the sites of his three tattoos (lower leg, forearm, and shoulder; larger diameters 15–25 cm, shown in Figures 2 and 3). The tattoos (two of them monochrome black and the third black contours on whitish background; Figures 2 and 3) were performed on different occasions over the last 3 years (the last one about 9 months before the flare-up) in the same tattoo studio. The patient reported no KP on previous tattooing with either local or generalized exacerbations of his psoriasis.

The spatial concordance of tattoo and psoriasis lesions was analyzed on clinical pictures of tattoo sites taken during the flare-up. For the detection of psoriasis lesions, RGB clinical images (shown in Figure 1(a)) were converted into the L*a*b* color space. The high-peak intensity areas ("spots") in the a*color channel (shown in Figure 1(b)), which correspond to psoriasis lesions, were extracted by serially applying the h-maxima transform and the regional maxima morphological operations [4] (shown in Figure 1(c)). To quantify the spatial distribution of the psoriasis lesions, Voronoi diagrams [5] were generated with generator points the centroids of above intensity spots (shown in Figure 1(d)). Figure 2 exemplifies this procedure in the case of a tattoo (arbitrary designated tattoo #1). Coefficients of variation (CV) and two-sample t-test were employed to compare the distributions of Voronoi patch sizes in different settings. Skin areas without a tattoo, like the front of the torso (Figure 1), are characterized by a rather homogeneous, unimodal size distribution of the Voronoi patches centered on psoriasis lesions (CV = 0.46, Table 1). However, the presence of a tattoo introduces a higher variation in the size distributions of the corresponding Voronoi patches in its neighborhood (CV = 0.60–1.23; shown in Figures 2 and 3; Table 1). Moreover, it seems that the presence of a tattoo induces a bimodal size distribution of the Voronoi polygons, with the patches that intersect tattoo lines, i.e., those patches that are localized within the tattooed skin area or are located in the vicinity of the tattoo contours, being significantly larger compared to the rest, more remote polygons ($p < 0.001$; Table 1).

3. Discussion/Conclusion

Sparing of skin lesions by an evolving psoriasis has been observed, so psoriasis spared a polio-affected limb [6–8] or a guttate psoriasis spared Becker's melanosis [9]. Also, a purpuric rash and a leukocytoclastic vasculitis that spared tattoos have been described [10, 11]. However, to the best of authors' knowledge, this is the first report of guttate psoriasis sparing tattoos. Remarkable is also the case of a patient with a reverse Koebner phenomenon, i.e., clearing of psoriasis lesions after tattooing [12]. All these observations, together with evidence for lower than anticipated KP risk in association with tattooing, indicate to a distinct pathophysiologic interaction of tattoo and psoriasis. We suggest that the macrophage, the key cell species involved in tattoo pathophysiology, is the cellular link of tattoo and the psoriasis sparing in this patient.

Dermal macrophages, both resident and blood-borne monocyte-derived, comprise a slowly renewing and in loco relatively long-lived cell species [13]. Macrophages are the key effector cells in the pathophysiology of tattoos, as they phagocytose and carry locally most of the tattoo pigment [14]. Moreover, they enable the stability of the tattoo via a process of capture-release-recapture of the pigment in situ during successive cell death and renewal cycles [15]. Zaba et al. [16] have previously shown that macrophages in normal skin that have ingested tattoo pigment was not able to stimulate T cell activation. This is probably the result of a LC3-associated phagocytosis (LAP) process [17], which ensures the shift of the local immune state towards sustained anti-inflammation by dampening of proinflammatory signals and preventing the presentation of autoantigens to other immune cells [18, 19]. Accordingly, a tattoo site can be conceptualized as a noninflammatory skin area with pigment-laden macrophages in a predominantly "deactivated," immunologically inert, or "anti-inflammatory," M2-polarized state [20], resembling a tissue milieu that corresponds to a sustained resolution phase of an inflammatory process.

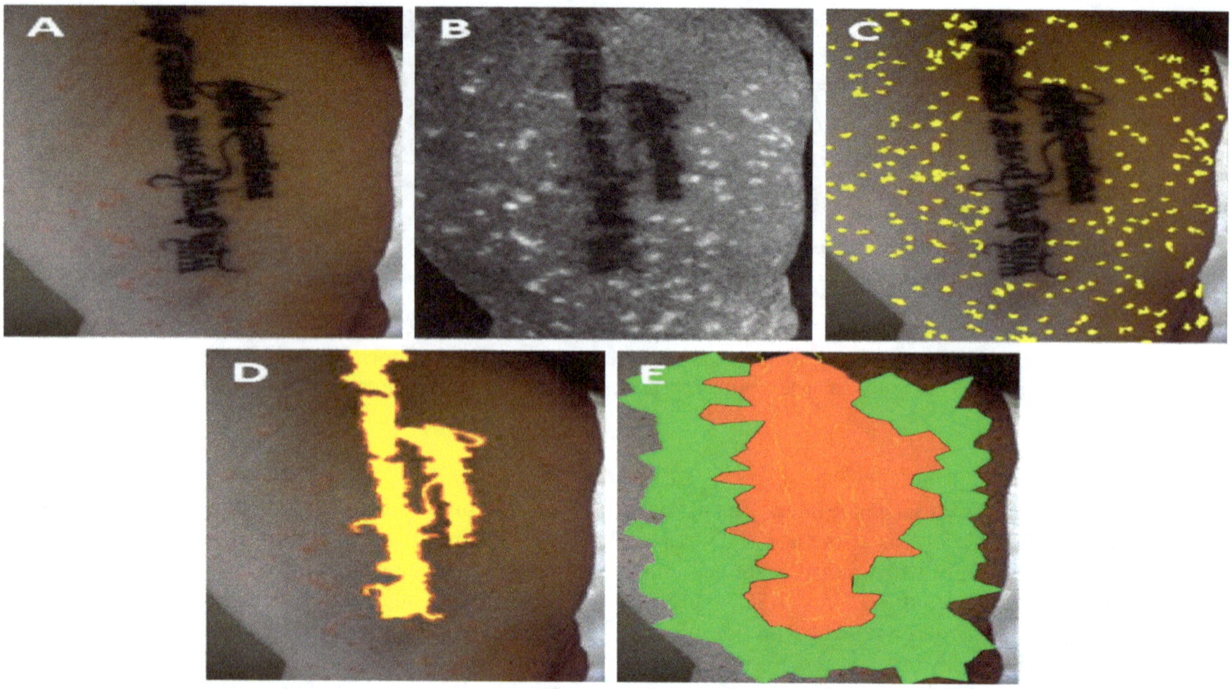

FIGURE 2: Psoriasis and tattoo #1. (a) Clinical picture. (b) Retained a* color channel of L*a*b* color space: high-peak intensity areas mark psoriasis lesions and low-level intensity areas correspond to tattooed skin segments. (c) Applying h-maxima transform followed by regional maxima, the lesional skin spots (patches) were extracted and are displayed in yellow pseudocolor. (d) Equivalently, the tattoo area was extracted by applying h-minima transform, followed by regional minima and is shown in yellow pseudocolor to enhance visualization. (e) The extracted psoriasis skin lesions' centroids (panel (C) applied to generate Voronoi diagrams (tessellation) of the tattoo area. Voronoi polygons with and without overlapping with the tattoo area (yellow border) are displayed in red and green pseudocolors, respectively.

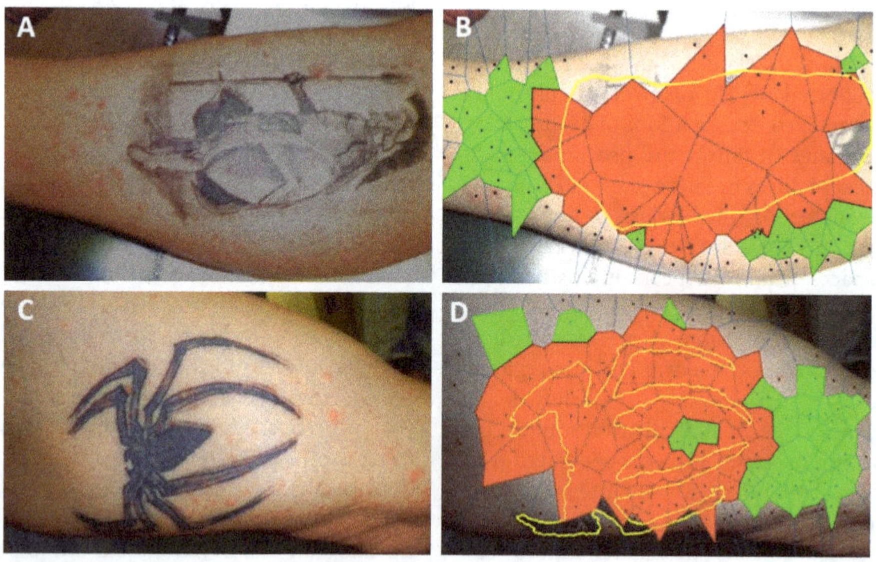

FIGURE 3: Tattoo #2 (panels (a) and (b)) and tattoo #3 (panels (c) and (d)). (a)–(c) Clinical pictures. (b)–(d) Voronoi patches intersecting (red) or not intersecting (green) tattooed skin areas (yellow contoured).

On the other hand, macrophages emerge also as a key cell species in the pathophysiology of psoriasis. In human psoriasis, a subpopulation of classically activated proinflammatory macrophages plays a crucial role in the pathogenesis of skin lesions, and a preponderance of M1 macrophage activation state is also associated with increased PASI scores [21]. In accordance with above, markers of M2 macrophage polarization are reduced in psoriasis [22], and the improvement of psoriasis with TNF-α inhibitors correlates with the inhibition of the M1 macrophage polarization pathway [23]. Stimulated macrophages are the main immune-effector cell species in animal psoriasis models, like the inducible human TNF transgenic mouse line [24]. Furthermore, in the K14-VEGF-A-Tg mice psoriasis model,

Table 1: Effect of tattoo on psoriasis lesions centered Voronoi patches.

Skin site	CV[1]	Mean size (SD)[2] V_{out}[4]	Mean size (SD)[2] V_{in}[5]	t-test P value[6]	Figure[3]
Tattoo-free	0.46	13416 (6244)	N/A[7]	N/A	1
Tattoo #1	0.60	12878 (4791)	28972 (12205)	<0.001	2
Tattoo #2	1.23	15504 (8658)	6680000 (58326)	<0.001	3
Tattoo #3	0.73	12173 (9700)	25902 (14564)	<0.001	3

[1]CV, coefficient of variation of the sizes of the Voronoi patches. [2]Mean size of Voronoi polygons (SD, standard deviation). [3]Figure number in text, where the corresponding skin site is displayed. [4]V_{out}, Voronoi patches not crossing tattoo contours. [5]V_{in}, Voronoi patches that intersect with tattoo. [6]P value for the comparison V_{out} vs. V_{in} (two-sample t-test). [7]N/A, not applicable.

IL-35 therapy was shown to alleviate the development of skin lesions through the reduction of macrophage infiltration and a shift from a M1- to M2-dominated tissue milieu [25]. Finally, in the imiquimod psoriasis model, the skin lesions are characterized by a distinct accumulation of macrophages and monocytes with the concomitant activation of the proinflammatory M1 over the anti-inflammatory M2 macrophage polarization [26]. Within the framework of this latter model, the induction of a M2-polarization predominated tissue milieu may attenuate the development of psoriasis lesions [27].

Based on above evidence and recent findings, considering the relationship of autophagy and psoriasis lesions [22], we propose the hypothesis that tattoos represent a "psoriasis-hostile" tissue environment pertained by a population of LAP active M2-polarized macrophages. Expanding our above observation of guttate psoriasis tending to spar tattoo areas, we assume that further study of the relationship of psoriasis lesions to tattooed skin may provide important insights into the role of macrophages in the pathogenesis of this disease. However, sparing or not of a tattoo site by evolving psoriasis can be conclusively decided only during a generalized disease flare-up, like a guttate one, with lesions not just confided on the typical for psoriasis skin localizations, which generally do not comprise popular sites for tattooing. In the framework of the current world-wide "tattooing epidemic," awareness is mandatory to document psoriasis cases in relation to tattooing and tattoos that may provide important insights into the role of the macrophage in the pathogenesis of psoriasis.

Authors' Contributions

P. S. contributed to the concept of the work, performed imaging and statistical analysis, interpreted, and contributed to the first draft of the manuscript. V. Z. contributed to the concept of the study, data interpretation, and drafting. S.-N. R. contributed to data acquisition, interpretation, and manuscript drafting. IDB was responsible for the concept and design of the work and contributed to the first draft. All authors contributed to the drafting and revision of the manuscript and read and approved the final submitted version.

References

[1] N. Kluger, E. Estève, S. Fouéré, F. Dupuis-Fourdan, M.-H. Jegou, and C. Lévy-Rameau, "Tattooing and psoriasis: a case series and review of the literature," *International Journal of Dermatology*, vol. 56, no. 8, pp. 822–827, 2017.

[2] A. S. Boyd and K. H. Neldner, "The isomorphic response of Koebner," *International Journal of Dermatology*, vol. 29, no. 6, pp. 401–410, 1990.

[3] C. Grodner, A. Beauchet, A. C. Fougerousse et al., "Tattoo complications in treated and non-treated psoriatic patients," *Journal of the European Academy of Dermatology and Venereology*, vol. 34, no. 4, pp. 888–896, 2020.

[4] P. Soille, *Morphological Image Analysis*, Springer, Berlin-Heidelberg, Germany, 2nd edition, 2004.

[5] N. Ahuja, "Dot pattern processing using Voronoi neighborhoods," *IEEE Transactions on Pattern Analysis and Machine Intelligence; PAMI-PAMI-4*, vol. 3, pp. 336–343, 1982.

[6] K. Krishna, "Koebner response in psoriasis," *Indian Journal of Dermatology Venereology and Leprology*, vol. 64, pp. 42-43, 1998.

[7] B. Ravikumar and A. Sinhasan, "Psoriasis sparing the polio-affected limb: is it merely the Koebner phenomenon?" *Indian Journal of Dermatology*, vol. 59, no. 5, pp. 505-506, 2014.

[8] T.-S. Wang and T.-F. Tsai, "Psoriasis sparing the lower limb with postpoliomyelitis residual paralysis," *British Journal of Dermatology*, vol. 171, no. 2, pp. 429–431, 2014.

[9] R. M. Weiss and E. J. Schulz, "Guttate psoriasis sparing becker's melanosis-a case report," *Dermatology*, vol. 180, no. 3, pp. 160–162, 1990.

[10] C. Chen, A. Mikailov, B. Faulkner-Jones, and P. A. Wu, "Leukocytoclastic vasculitis sparing a tattoo with halo effect," *JAAD Case Reports*, vol. 1, no. 5, pp. 269–271, 2015.

[11] I. Pinal-Fernandez and R. Solans-Laqué, "The "sparing phenomenon" of purpuric rash over tattooed skin," *Dermatology*, vol. 228, pp. 27–30, 2014.

[12] N. Kluger and M.-H. Jegou, "Psoriasis et phénomène de Koebner inversé après tatouage," *Annales de Dermatologie et de Vénéréologie*, vol. 145, no. 1, pp. 48-49, 2018.

[13] S. Epelman, K. J. Lavine, and G. J. Randolph, "Origin and functions of tissue macrophages," *Immunity*, vol. 41, no. 1, pp. 21–35, 2014.

[14] H. Strandt, O. Voluzan, T. Niedermair et al., "Macrophages and fibroblasts differentially contribute to tattoo stability," *Dermatology (Basel, Switzerland)*, vol. 237, no. 2, pp. 296–302, 2021.

[15] A. Baranska, A. Shawket, M. Jouve et al., "Unveiling skin macrophage dynamics explains both tattoo persistence and

strenuous removal," *Journal of Experimental Medicine*, vol. 215, no. 4, pp. 1115–1133, 2018.

[16] L. C. Zaba, J. Fuentes-Duculan, R. M. Steinman, J. G. Krueger, and M. A. Lowes, "Normal human dermis contains distinct populations of CD11c+BDCA-1+ dendritic cells and CD163+FXIIIA+ macrophages," *Journal of Clinical Investigation*, vol. 117, no. 9, pp. 2517–2525, 2007.

[17] B. L. Heckmann, E. Boada-Romero, L. D. Cunha, J. Magne, and D. R. Green, "LC3-associated phagocytosis and inflammation," *Journal of Molecular Biology*, vol. 429, no. 23, pp. 3561–3576, 2017.

[18] A. J. Clarke and A. K. Simon, "Autophagy in the renewal, differentiation and homeostasis of immune cells," *Nature Reviews Immunology*, vol. 19, no. 3, pp. 170–183, 2019.

[19] M.-Y. Wu and J.-H. Lu, "Autophagy and macrophage functions: inflammatory response and phagocytosis," *Cells*, vol. 9, no. 1, p. 70, 2019.

[20] T. Lawrence and G. Natoli, "Transcriptional regulation of macrophage polarization: enabling diversity with identity," *Nature Reviews Immunology*, vol. 11, no. 11, pp. 750–761, 2011.

[21] J. Fuentes-Duculan, M. Suárez-Fariñas, L. C. Zaba et al., "A subpopulation of CD163-positive macrophages is classically activated in psoriasis," *Journal of Investigative Dermatology*, vol. 130, no. 10, pp. 2412–2422, 2010.

[22] H. J. Kim, J. Jang, E.-H. Lee, S. Jung, J. Y. Roh, and Y. Jung, "Decreased expression of response gene to complement 32 in psoriasis and its association with reduced M2 macrophage polarization," *The Journal of Dermatology*, vol. 46, no. 2, pp. 166–168, 2019.

[23] S.-H. Lin, H.-Y. Chuang, J.-C. Ho, C.-H. Lee, and C.-C. Hsiao, "Treatment with TNF-α inhibitor rectifies M1 macrophage polarization from blood CD14+ monocytes in patients with psoriasis independent of STAT1 and IRF-1 activation," *Journal of Dermatological Science*, vol. 91, no. 3, pp. 276–284, 2018.

[24] R. Leite Dantas, D. Masemann, T. Schied et al., "Macrophage-mediated psoriasis can be suppressed by regulatory T lymphocytes," *The Journal of Pathology*, vol. 240, no. 3, pp. 366–377, 2016.

[25] J. Zhang, Y. Lin, C. Li et al., "IL-35 decelerates the inflammatory process by regulating inflammatory cytokine secretion and M1/M2 macrophage ratio in psoriasis," *The Journal of Immunology*, vol. 197, no. 6, pp. 2131–2144, 2016.

[26] C. H. Lu, C. Y. Lai, D. W. Yeh et al., "Involvement of M1 macrophage polarization in endosomal Toll-like receptors activated psoriatic inflammation," *Mediators of Inflammation*, vol. 2018, Article ID 3523642, 14 pages, 2018.

[27] S. Morimura, T. Oka, M. Sugaya, and S. Sato, "CX3CR1 deficiency attenuates imiquimod-induced psoriasis-like skin inflammation with decreased M1 macrophages," *Journal of Dermatological Science*, vol. 82, no. 3, pp. 175–188, 2016.

41

Generalized Acquired Cutis Laxa Associated with Monoclonal Gammopathy of Dermatological Significance

Sophia Z. Shalhout,[1] Myrna R. Nahas,[2] Reed E. Drews,[2] and David M. Miller[1]

[1]*Division of Hematology/Oncology and Department of Dermatology, Massachusetts General Hospital, Harvard Medical School, Boston, MA 02114, USA*
[2]*Division of Hematology/Oncology, Beth Israel Deaconess Medical Center, Harvard Medical School, Boston, MA 02215, USA*

Correspondence should be addressed to David M. Miller; dmiller4@mgh.harvard.edu

Academic Editor: Michihiro Hide

Background. Cutis laxa is a rare dermatosis that is inherited or acquired and clinically features loose, wrinkled, and redundant skin with decreased elasticity. This heterogeneous connective tissue disorder may be localized or generalized, with or without internal manifestations. Generalized cutis laxa often has a cephalocaudal progression and is attributed to inflammatory cutaneous eruptions, medications, and infections. Cutis laxa is also associated with several other conditions including rheumatoid arthritis, systemic lupus erythematosus, and plasma-cell dyscrasias. *Case Presentation.* We report an unusual case of a 35-year-old male with progression of generalized acquired cutis laxa and vasculitis that occurred over a period of one year. No cutaneous inflammatory eruption preceded or accompanied his decreased skin elasticity, and a biopsy of the skin showed elastolysis. His cutaneous manifestation led to systemic evaluation and an eventual diagnosis of smoldering multiple myeloma accompanied by aortitis and anemia. His myeloma and vasculitis were successfully treated with cyclophosphamide, bortezomib, and dexamethasone and high-dose prednisone, respectively, with no improvement to his cutis laxa. *Conclusions.* The presence of monoclonal gammopathy is strongly associated with several dermatological entities such as acquired cutis laxa. We propose a new term for the dermatological manifestations caused by paraproteinemia: monoclonal gammopathy of dermatological significance, or MGODS, and stress the evaluation of an underlying gammopathy in the setting of certain dermatologic conditions, including scleromyxedema and amyloidosis. We present a case of a newly acquired cutis laxa secondary to plasma-cell dyscrasias that exemplifies MGODS, alongside a brief literature review, and underscore the clinical relevance of monoclonal gammopathies of dermatological significance.

1. Background

Cutis laxa (CL), or elastolysis, is a rare heterogeneous dermatosis with several etiologies. CL is typically inherited as a dominant, recessive, or X-linked recessive condition. Clinically, CL is characterized by loosely hanging, pendulous skin folds, resulting in the appearance of premature aging. Histologically, degeneration of the dermal elastic fibers is observed. Internal organ involvement is often seen in patients with CL and can affect the pulmonary, gastrointestinal, urogenital, and cardiovascular systems. Prognosis of CL may vary and largely depends on the implicated gene mutation as well as the extent of systemic involvement. It may range from a fatal outcome in certain cases of inherited CL to a normal life expectancy in the less severe forms. CL is a progressive disorder with insidious onset that worsens with age. In rare cases, CL may be acquired *de novo* or associated with preceding cutaneous inflammatory eruptions with adult-onset of disease. CL is also associated with infections, drug hypersensitivity reactions, and plasma-cell dyscrasias. We report a rare case of generalized acquired CL and aortitis, without preceding inflammatory lesions or eruptions, most likely secondary to multiple myeloma. The presence of monoclonal gammopathy is strongly associated with several dermatological entities and cutaneous manifestations. We suggest these should be referred to as monoclonal gammopathy of dermatological significance, or MGODS, and stress the evaluation of an underlying gammopathy in the setting of several well-established dermatological features. We present a case of MGODS and provide a brief literature review of other cases of acquired cutis laxa associated with monoclonal gammopathy.

2. Case Presentation

A 35-year-old male noticed the progression of loosening and thinning of his skin over the period of one year. These areas had been asymptomatic with no preceding inflammatory dermatosis. The patient's past medical history included hypertension and long-standing anemia of uncertain etiology.

On physical exam, profound laxity of the periocular skin, neck, axillary, and back was appreciated (Figures 1 and 2). The clinical presentation was suggestive of an acquired cutis laxa. A biopsy of involved skin demonstrated sparse superficial perivascular lymphocytic inflammation with rare giant cells. An elastic stain showed a decrease in the elastic fibers in the reticular dermis compared to a biopsy of uninvolved skin; no significant changes in the dermal collagen were appreciated on Masson's Trichome staining. Findings consistent with granulomatous slack skin were absent. In aggregate, the clinical and pathological presentation were consistent with an acquired cutis laxa (ACL).

Serology work-up for autoimmune connective tissue disease was negative for rheumatoid factors, antineutrophil cytoplasm antibodies, and anti-nuclear antibodies. Chromosomal microarray analysis performed on DNA extracted from a peripheral blood specimen returned normal findings. Anemia work-up demonstrated normal iron stores, normal renal function, and decreased reticulocyte count. He was found to have an elevated C-reactive protein (CRP) and erythrocyte sedimentation rate (ESR), and an IgG-kappa paraprotein of 1.36 g/dL. The patient was initially diagnosed with monoclonal gammopathy of undetermined significance (MGUS) and anemia of inflammation. Due to suspicion of a connection between his MGUS and cutis laxa, further evaluation revealed an abnormal kappa/lambda free-light chain ratio of 5.86. A PET-CT (Positron emission tomography-computed tomography) did not reveal evidence of skeletal lytic lesions or extraosseous findings of plasmacytoma. However, mild fluorodeoxyglucose avidity of the vascular walls of the aorta and branching vessels was seen, and in the setting of elevated CRP and ESR, was consistent with aortitis and mild vasculitis (Figure 3). Subsequent bone marrow biopsy demonstrated 20% plasma cells in the bone marrow core and 13% of aspirate.

In the setting of end-organ dysfunction presumed to be secondary to a plasma-cell dyscrasia (cutis laxa and vasculitis), the patient was started on CyBorD (cyclophosphamide, bortezomib, dexamethasone). His second cycle was delayed due to a left inguinal herniorrhaphy with unremarkable wound healing. CyBorD was tolerated well by the patient. Upon completion of his sixth cycle of CyBorD, a PET-CT revealed continued aortitis, a hiatal hernia, umbilical hernia, and small bowel-containing right inguinal hernia. The level of monoclonal IgG-kappa protein continued to decline (280 mg/dL), but C-reactive protein levels remained elevated. He was given high-dose oral prednisone, 60 mg/d, to treat his vasculitis which resulted in near normal C-reactive protein levels. His cutis laxa did not improve in response to corticosteroids and immunosuppressive therapy. However, at one-year posttreatment, his cutis laxa did not clinically appear to have progressed.

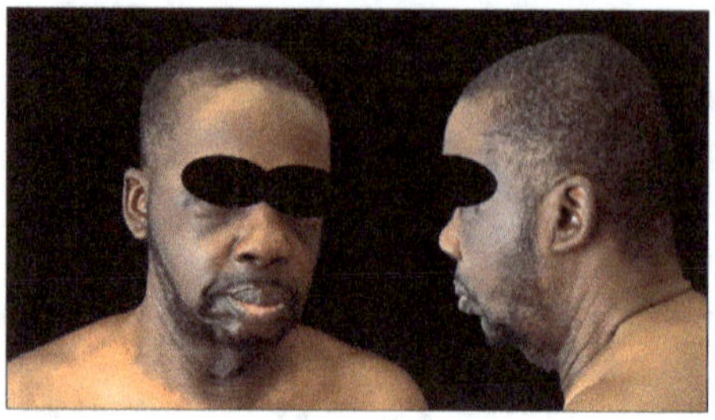

Figure 1: At the age of 35: appearance of premature aging; wrinkly face with profound laxity notable in the periocular skin and neck region.

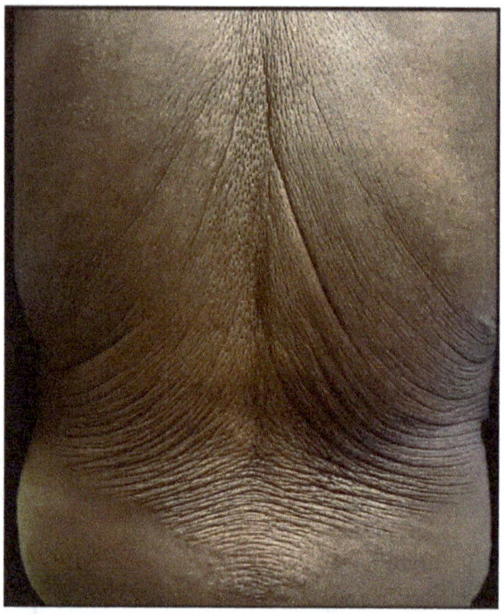

Figure 2: Back with evident loose, wrinkly, redundant skin folds.

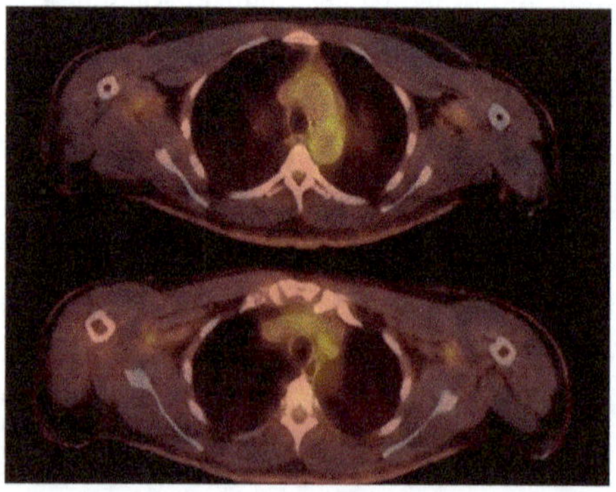

Figure 3: PET-CT shows FDG avidity of the vascular walls of the aorta.

Table 1: Summary of acquired cutis laxa associated with monoclonal gammopathies/plasma-cell dyscrasia.

Reference	Sex, age	Preceding cutaneous eruptions	Clinical features	Associated plasma-cell dyscrasia/ monoclonal gammopathy	Treatment	Outcome
Scott et al. [5]	F, 44	Edema of face and neck from hypersensitivity reaction to penicillin	Skin laxity to face and neck, followed by progression to extremities and torso; systemic involvement (gastrointestinal and urogenital)	Multiple myeloma	Surgical repair of hernias/ prolapses	Not reported
Ting et al. [6]	F, 45	Intermittent "puffiness" of eyelids	Progressive laxity of the skin starting from the eyelids and spreading gradually to the face, neck, trunk, lungs, rectum, bladder, and perineum	Multiple myeloma	Not reported	Not reported
Frémont et al. [7]	F, 59	None reported	Skin hyperlaxity present for several years	IgG lambda myeloma	Thalidomide	One year after treatment, skin laxity stabilized
Gupta and Helm [8]	F, 62	Denied any prior inflammatory skin disorder or exanthema	Progressive laxity to face, neck, chest, and back; no rectal or vaginal prolapse, emphysema, or cardiac problems detected	Multiple myeloma	Prior to CL onset, patient received vincristine, melphalan, doxorubicin, cyclophosphamide, and prednisone with improvement to hematological disease	Patient was on prednisone during onset of CL; thalidomide gradually increased; but no improvement to cutis laxa was observed
Turner et al. [9]	M, 29	2-year history of asymptomatic urticarial red papules and plaques on the neck, chest, and back lasting days at a time, urticarial vasculitis	Wrinkling and sagging skin on the face, neck, axillae, shoulders, and arms with transverse striae on abdomen, leukocytoclastic vasculitis, and immune complex-mediated glomerulonephritis	IgA myeloma involving kidneys	High-dose methyl prednisolone, and intravenous cyclophosphamide	Initially, all urticarial skin lesions resolved; eventually, renal function deteriorated, and the patient became dependent on dialysis; patient eventually succumbed to his disease
Kluger et al. [10]	M, 40	Chronic urticarial dermatosis of the extremities, mostly involving the hands, progressively worsened, with repeated swelling of the fingers	Acral localization of cutis laxa, joint hyperlaxity, and recurrent neutrophilic urticarial dermatosis	IgA multiple myeloma	Methotrexate, colchicine, hydroxychloroquine, intravenous gamma globulins, and dapsone, oral prednisone	Treatment with oral prednisone resulted in complete remission of the urticarial lesions, with steroid dependence; prevention of the progression in joint laxity or cutis laxa was not achieved

Table 1: Continued.

Reference	Sex, age	Preceding cutaneous eruptions	Clinical features	Associated plasma-cell dyscrasia/ monoclonal gammopathy	Treatment	Outcome
Lavorato et al. [11]	F, 57	Bilateral eyelid hyperchromia, and increase in palpebral volume	Cutaneous laxity in skin folds, bilateral palpebral ptosis, pain and paresthesia, histological and clinical features consistent with primary systemic amyloidosis, cutaneous mucinosis, and acquired cutis laxa	Multiple myeloma associated amyloidosis	Bortezomib and dexamethasone, followed by autologous bone marrow transplantation	"Clinically important dermatological improvement" was achieved
Yoneda et al. [12]	M, 62	None reported, but presented with lumbago and shoulder pain, with a history of severe fatigue and night sweats	Soft, redundant, cutaneous laxity to acral sites on fingertips and soles of feet, lumbago	Myeloma associated amyloidosis	Cyclophosphamide and prednisolone	Treatment decreased hematological disease but the cutis laxa of acral sites progressed; patient eventually succumbed to his disease
Yoneda et al. [12]	M, 71	None reported, but presented with lumbar and back pain, with a history of leg pain, weakness, and night sweats	Soft, loose skin changes to both thumbs	Myeloma associated amyloidosis	Cyclophosphamide	Chemotherapy resulted in a decrease of hematological disease, but cutaneous lesions did not regress; continued follow-up at time of report
Nikko et al. [3]	F, 40	Denied any prior inflammatory skin disorder	Progressive wrinkling, and laxity of the skin on back, chest, abdomen, upper arms, neck, thighs but face was spared	Plasma-cell dyscrasia	None reported	Careful follow-up in case of systemic complication at the time of report.
Lee et al. [13]	F, 54	One-year previous history of easy bruising	Hypopigmented patches with skin laxity, purpura on both flanks, periorbital purpura, lax skin of thumbs; histological, and clinical features consistent with acquired cutis laxa, and primary systemic amyloidosis	Multiple myeloma associated amyloidosis	Bortezomib, thalidomide, dexamethasone followed by autologous peripheral blood stem cell transplant	Slight clinical improvement of skin was noted
Dicker et al. [14]	F, 59	"Puffiness" in fingertips, tender with pressure, tense before resolving to lax skin	Persistent laxity of skin on finger pads, and tongue swelling	Plasma cell dyscrasia	Cyclophosphamide, vincristine, adriamycin, and methylprednisolone	Reduction in size of tongue and a decrease in laxity of skin lesions were achieved

TABLE 1: Continued.

Reference	Sex, age	Preceding cutaneous eruptions	Clinical features	Associated plasma-cell dyscrasia/ monoclonal gammopathy	Treatment	Outcome
Appiah et al. [15]	F, 64	History of multiple asymptomatic skin lesions in groin and axillae	Flesh-colored papules in axillae and groin, papules with purpura on eyelids, translucent papules and nodules on labia majora, wrinkled loose skin on fingertips	Myeloma associated amyloidosis	Not reported	Not reported
Ferrandiz-Pulido et al. [16]	M, 63	3-month history of asymptomatic skin lesions on ventral aspect of fingers	Soft redundant loose skin on all fingertips and hands	Multiple myeloma-associated amyloidosis	Not reported	Not reported
Silveira et al. [17]	M, 29	Diffuse erythematous plaques, mildly infiltrated papules, and plaques on his trunk	Multiple flaccid erythematous plaques on trunk, neck, and skinfolds with flaccidity of face, axillae, groin, neck, hiatal hernia, eventually developed nephrotic syndrome and acute renal failure	IgG lambda monoclonal gammopathy	Bortezomib, dexamethasone, and thalidomide	No improvement to dermatological lesions observed
New and Callen [4]	M, 48	No preceding cutaneous changes, but he developed erythematous plaques and granuloma annulare like features on his buttocks and lateral hips	4-year history of loose wrinkled skin of his face, chest, upper back, lateral hips, buttocks, and proximal upper extremities	Multiple myeloma	Lenalidomide, dexamethasone, oral pamidronate, and aspirin	With 5 months of therapy, patient had hematological and skeletal lesion stabilization, but his cutis laxa progressed during treatment.
Gonzalez-Ramos et al. [18]	M, 68	3-month history of stable asymptomatic multiple myeloma (progressed after 5 years with MGUS) and 2-month history of hemorrhagic bullae in oral buccal and labial mucosa before presentation	Numerous large hemorrhagic oral bullae, yellowish and purple purpura plaques on eyelids and macroglossia, cutis laxa of axilla and antecubital flexure; clinical and histological features consistent with primary systemic amyloidosis and acquire cutis laxa	Multiple myeloma associated amyloidosis	Intensive chemotherapy	No recurrence of skin lesions; at the time of the report, the patient was awaiting an autologous bone marrow transplant

Table 1: Continued.

Reference	Sex, age	Preceding cutaneous eruptions	Clinical features	Associated plasma-cell dyscrasia/ monoclonal gammopathy	Treatment	Outcome
Tan et al. [19]	M, 50	No preceding skin lesions, and his skin was otherwise asymptomatic, a history of heavy chain deposition disease without evidence of multiple myeloma preceding any cutaneous findings	Weight loss and significant lax skin of axillae, groin, neck, face with periocular involvement with upper lid ptosis and lower lid laxity; subsequent emphysema, leg weakness and peripheral polyneuropathy; no known herniations, diverticula, or aneurysms	Heavy chain deposition disease/ monoclonal gammopathy	Prednisone and cyclophosphamide but he presented to dermatological service with end-stage disease, medical therapy for the skin condition was not attempted	There was a transient improvement in renal function; the patient underwent functional blepharoplasty to relieve the ectropion/epiphora
O'Malley et al. [20]	F, 60–69	No preceding cutaneous eruptions; a history of nephrotic syndrome and renal insufficiency due to renal heavy chain deposition disease	Extensive emphysema, lower extremity edema with relapse of her heavy chain deposition disease, marked "hound-dog" facies with lax skin encompassing face, neck, and arms; onset correlating with the time renal involvement was first diagnosed	Heavy chain deposition disease/low-grade plasma-cell neoplasm (complement components on dermal elastic fibers also detected)	Bortezomib and pulse dexamethasone	The patient had subsequent improvement of her nephrotic syndrome and resolution of her acute kidney injury; cutaneous outcome not discussed.
Harrington et al. [21]	F, 38	A history of urticaria, renal insufficiency, heavy chain deposition in heart and kidneys, bilateral lower extremity edema	Excessive wrinkling of the skin that began in the axillae a few years before presentation and progressed to involve her face, extremities, and trunk	Heavy chain deposition disease/ monoclonal gammopathy	Lenalidomide with progression of renal failure, requiring temporary dialysis and the discontinuation of this medication; stabilized on bortezomib and dexamethasone	The cutaneous outcome was not described
de Larrea et al. [22]	M, 52	None reported	Cutis laxa of the face, neck, axillae, and groin in the setting of MGUS, renal failure	IgG lambda monoclonal gammopathy	Initially, he was treated with granulocyte CSF but developed alveolar hemorrhage and decreased renal function; he was later treated with bortezomib and oral dexamethasone	A complete hematological response without an increase in bone marrow plasma cells was achieved; he was still on chronic hemodialysis at time of report but his cutis laxa had not progressed, and the patient planned for surgical correction of redundant skin folds.

Table 1: Continued.

Reference	Sex, age	Preceding cutaneous eruptions	Clinical features	Associated plasma-cell dyscrasia/ monoclonal gammopathy	Treatment	Outcome
Majithia et al. [23]	M, 40	None reported; but gave a history of fatigue, shortness of breath, and edema	Loose hanging ear lobes, blepharochalasis, lax nasolabial folds, and increased folds over the neck, axilla, and trunk progressing over two years.	Light and heavy chain deposition disease (LHCDD)	Dexamethasone, cyclophosphamide, and bortezomib	Patient had significant improvement clinically and with hematological disease but was lost to follow-up.
Kim and Klein [24]		She had no history of an inflammatory preceding cutaneous process.	Patient presented with a 10-year history of lax skin with progression in recent years to face, neck, and legs; she was diagnosed with MGUS and eventually light chain multiple myeloma, anemia, and immune-mediated glomerular nephritis; in aggregate, findings were consistent with acquired cutis laxa and systemic lupus erythematosus associated with multiple myeloma	Multiple myeloma and systemic lupus erythematosus	Lenalidomide and low-dose dexamethasone for multiple myeloma. Later, she was treated with bortezomib and dexamethasone, followed by IVIG and danazol	She had a good response to lenalidomide and dexamethasone in terms of reduction of light chain disease, but therapy was discontinued due to cytopenia; excellent response to bortezomib and dexamethasone but discontinued therapy due to cytopenia; IVIG and danazol stabilized her blood counts.
Current case	M, 35	None reported	Profound laxity of the periocular skin, neck, axillary and back which progressed over the period of one year; aortitis, several hernias and diverticula.	Multiple myeloma	Cyclophosphamide, bortezomib, dexamethasone, (CyBorD) herniorrhaphy, and high-dose prednisone	His hematological disease stabilized on CyBorD, and high-dose prednisone improved vasculitis; his cutis laxa has not progressed one-year posttreatment.

Table 2: Summary of monoclonal gammopathies of dermatological significance.

Disease/Condition	Dermatological presentation	Monoclonal gammopathy
Acquired cutis laxa	Lax, wrinkled, sagging, redundant, inelastic skin	IgG, IgA, light and/or heavy chain deposition disease
Scleromyxedema	Mucinosis, papular and sclerodermoid eruption	IgG (lambda) [30]
Light chain amyloidosis	Purpura, hemorrhagic bullous lesions	IgG (lambda) [31]
Nodular amyloidosis	Papulonodules	IgG, IgA [32]
Waldenstrom macroglobulinemia	Nonspecific ulcers, purpura, and urticarial lesions	IgM [33]
Cryoglobulin vasculitis	Palpable purpura	Type I (IgM) and mixed (IgM and IgG, few polyclonal) [34]
Schnitzler's syndrome	Rose or red macules, urticarial plaques	IgM (few have IgG component) [35]
Necrobiotic xanthogranuloma	Waxy, yellow, plaques, nodules	IgG (kappa) [36]
POEMS syndrome	Hyperpigmentation, glomeruloid hemangioma	IgA or IgG (lambda) [37]
Pyoderma gangrenosum	Pustules, ulcerated plaques	IgA [38]
Cold agglutinin disease	Livido reticularis, raynaud phenomenon, acrocyanosis, ulceration	IgM (kappa) (few have IgA, few polyclonal) [39]
Papular mucinosis	Small, generally localized, lichenoid papular lesions	IgG (lambda) [30]
Subcorneal pustular dermatosis	Vesiculopustular eruptions	IgA [40]
Erythema elevatum diutinum	Plaques, nodules often localized to extensor surfaces	IgA [41]
Scleredema	Thickened, indurated plaques, most often affecting trunk	IgG and IgA [42]

3. Discussion and Conclusions

ACL is extremely rare and can be generalized or localized. Several conditions warrant discussion in the differential diagnosis of the skin manifestations in this patient, including anetoderma, and mid-dermal elastolysis. Anetoderma usually involves the trunk and extremities and consists of well-circumscribed atrophic or depressed patches or saccular outpouchings of wrinkled skin. The histological finding of anetoderma is loss of elastic fibers in the papillary and reticular dermis. Mid-dermal elastolysis is clinically characterized by well-circumscribed fine wrinkles or perifollicular papular protrusions usually involving the trunk and upper extremities. Mid-dermal elastolysis is histologically characterized by focal loss of elastic fibers in the mid-dermis.

ACL has been associated with inflammatory dermatoses, including urticaria, systemic lupus erythematosus, dermatitis herpetiformis, and amyloidosis. Cases of ACL due to medication exposure and arthropod bite reactions have been reported [1, 2]. Our patient is most consistent with reports of ACL associated with underlying hematological disorders including multiple myeloma, plasma-cell dyscrasia, and heavy chain deposition disease [3, 4]. The clinical features, treatment, and outcomes of previous cases reported in the literature of ACL associated with plasma-cell dyscrasias and monoclonal gammopathies are summarized in Table 1. There are reports of at least 23 cases, with ~20% reporting acral localization of cutis laxa, ~30% reporting a diagnosis of multiple myeloma associated with amyloidosis, and ~50% describing a preceding cutaneous process. Very few reports describe stabilization of cutis laxa following systemic therapy administered to treat the underlying monoclonal gammopathy. Unlike other connective tissue disorders, ACL has not been associated with vascular fragility, and surgery is not contraindicated since ACL is not thought to affect wound healing. Early management with plastic surgical procedures such as rhytidectomy can be beneficial to mitigate symptoms. However, serial reconstructive procedures are usually required since CL often progresses with time.

Systemic elastolysis has been reported in adult-onset ACL. The most significant internal organs often involved are associated with pulmonary, cardiovascular (i.e., heart failure, ectasia of the aorta, and aortic aneurysms), gastrointestinal (i.e., diverticula and hernias), and urogenital (i.e., hernias, uterine prolapse, and cystocele) systems [25–27]. It is unclear if the aortitis, large vessel vasculitis, and numerous hernias experienced by this patient were related to the paraprotein and elastolysis [4, 8]. Although the exact pathophysiology is unknown, myeloma-associated immunoglobulin deposition is thought to result in a cell-mediated immune response and promotes phagocytic destruction of elastic fiber [4, 28]. In our patient, we suspect that the paraprotein contributed to decreased skin laxity as well as involvement of the vasculature and gastrointestinal system. There is one case report of congenital cutis laxa associated with aortitis in a 17-month-old child [26]. However, to our knowledge, there are no reports of ACL and aortitis secondary to multiple myeloma.

We propose a new term for the dermatological manifestations caused by paraproteinemia: monoclonal gammopathy of dermatological significance or MGODS. This term encapsulates a variety of diagnoses that present with paraproteins and may have significant cutaneous involvement such as nodular and light chain amyloid, cryoglobulinemia, necrobiotic xanthogranuloma, scleromyxedema, papular mucinosis, and POEMS syndrome [29]. Table 2 provides a nonexhaustive list of well-established conditions associated with monoclonal gammopathy and a summary of pertinent cutaneous findings.

MGODS may present in the setting of an otherwise monoclonal gammopathy of undetermined significance (MGUS). Indeed, in our case, the patient was initially diagnosed with MGUS, but the recognition of the likely ACL representing an MGODS prompted further evaluation, including a bone marrow biopsy, resulting in the diagnosis of smoldering myeloma. Given that skin manifestations are not part of diagnostic criteria for progression beyond MGUS, our case report and the term MGODS highlights the utility of recognizing cutaneous manifestations of monoclonal gammopathies as it may guide evaluation and, in some cases, management. End-organ dysfunction is often the impetus to initiate treatment for plasma-cell dyscrasias, with skeletal, renal, and hematological abnormalities being the most common organs triggering induction of therapy. In certain contexts, however, gammopathies of dermatological significance may necessitate initiation of therapy. The types of skin dysfunction that warrant the induction of systemic treatment are far from agreed upon and often require multidisciplinary consultation.

Abbreviations

ACL:	Acquired cutis laxa
CL:	Cutis laxa
CRP:	C-reactive protein
CyBorD:	Cyclophosphamide, bortezomib, and dexamethasone
ESR:	Erythrocyte sedimentation rate
LHCDD:	Light and heavy chain deposition disease
MGODS:	Monoclonal gammopathy of dermatological significance
MGUS:	Monoclonal gammopathy of undetermined significance
POEMS:	Polyneuropathy, organomegaly, endocrinopathy, monoclonal protein, and skin changes
PET-CT:	Positron emission tomography-computed tomography.

Consent

Written informed consent was obtained from the patient for publication of this case report and any accompanying images.

Authors' Contributions

RED, MRN, and DMM managed the patient. SZS wrote the manuscript and provided revisions. All the authors read, critically revised, and approved the final version of the manuscript.

References

[1] F. M. Lewis, S. Lewis-Jones, and M. Gipson, "Acquired cutis laxa with dermatitis herpetiformis and sarcoidosis," *Journal of the American Academy of Dermatology*, vol. 29, no. 5, pp. 846–848, 1993.

[2] D. R. Berk, D. D. Bentley, S. J. Bayliss, A. Lind, and Z. Urban, "Cutis laxa: a review," *Journal of the American Academy of Dermatology*, vol. 66, no. 5, pp. 842 e1–842 e17, 2012.

[3] A. Nikko, M. Dunnigan, A. Black, and C. J. Cockerell, "Acquired cutis laxa associated with a plasma cell dyscrasia," *The American Journal of Dermatopathology*, vol. 18, no. 5, pp. 533–537, 1996.

[4] H. D. New and J. P. Callen, "Generalized acquired cutis laxa associated with multiple myeloma with biphenotypic IgG-λ and IgA-κ gammopathy following treatment of a nodal plasmacytoma," *Archives of Dermatology*, vol. 147, no. 3, pp. 323–328, 2011.

[5] M. A. Scott, Y. C. Kauh, and H. A. Luscombe, "Acquired cutis laxa associated with multiple myeloma," *Archives of Dermatology*, vol. 112, no. 6, pp. 853–855, 1976.

[6] H. C. Ting, M. H. Foo, and D. F. Wang, "Acquired cutis laxa and multiple myeloma," *British Journal of Dermatology*, vol. 110, no. 3, pp. 363–367, 1984.

[7] G. Frémont, D. Kérob, C. Prost-Squarcioni et al., "Cutis laxa acquise généralisée associée à un myélome: découverte de grandes cellules vacuolisées dermiques," *Annales de Dermatologie et de Vénéréologie*, vol. 134, no. 6-7, pp. 548–551, 2007.

[8] A. Gupta and T. N. Helm, "Acquired cutis laxa associated with multiple myeloma," *Cutis*, vol. 69, no. 2, pp. 114–118, 2002.

[9] R. B. Turner, H. A. Haynes, S. R. Granter, and D. M. Miller, "Acquired cutis laxa following urticarial vasculitis associated with IgA myeloma," *Journal of the American Academy of Dermatology*, vol. 60, no. 6, pp. 1052–1057, 2009.

[10] N. Kluger, J. Molès, O. Vanakker, C. Pernet, M. Beylot-Barry, and D. Bessis, "Acral acquired cutis laxa associated with IgA multiple myeloma, joint hyperlaxity and urticarial neutrophilic dermatosis," *Acta Dermato Venereologica*, vol. 94, no. 6, pp. 743-744, 2014.

[11] F. G. Lavorato, M. d. F. G. S. Alves, J. M. P. Maceira, N. Unterstell, L. A. Serpa, and L. Azulay-Abulafia, "Primary systemic amyloidosis, acquired cutis laxa and cutaneous mucinosis in a patient with multiple myeloma," *Anais Brasileiros de Dermatologia*, vol. 88, no. 6 suppl 1, pp. 32–35, 2013.

[12] K. Yoneda, T. Kanoh, S. Nomura, M. Ozaki, and S. Imamura, "Elastolytic cutaneous lesions in myeloma-associated amyloidosis," *Archives of Dermatology*, vol. 126, no. 5, pp. 657–660, 1990.

[13] M. Y. Lee, J. Y. Byun, Y. W. Choi, and H. Y. Choi, "Multiple myeloma presenting with acquired cutis laxa and primary systemic amyloidosis," *European Journal of Dermatology*, vol. 27, no. 6, pp. 654-655, 2017.

[14] T. J. Dicker, J. Morton, R. M. Williamson, and J. Chick, "Myeloma-associated systemic amyloidosis presenting with acquired digital cutis laxa-like changes," *Australasian Journal of Dermatology*, vol. 43, no. 2, pp. 144–146, 2002.

[15] Y. E. Appiah, N. Onumah, H. Wu, R. Elenitsas, and W. James, "Multiple myeloma-associated amyloidosis and acral localized acquired cutis laxa," *Journal of the American Academy of Dermatology*, vol. 58, no. 2, pp. S32–S33, 2008.

[16] C. Ferrandiz-Pulido, M. Serra, S. Bel, B. Ferrer, T. Repiso, and V. Garcia-Patos, "Multiple myeloma-associated amyloidosis presenting with acrolocalized acquired cutis laxa," *Archives of Dermatology*, vol. 146, no. 12, p. 1435, 2010.

[17] L. Silveira, L. Silveria, I. Torres, M. A. Salvino, I. Follador, and A. L Bittencourt, "Acquired cutis laxa with an interstitial granulomatous reaction associated with IgG lambda monoclonal gammopathy," *The American Journal of Dermatopathology*, vol. 35, no. 4, pp. e67–e71, 2013.

[18] J. Gonzalez-Ramos, C. Garrido-Gutiérrez, Y. González-Silva et al., "Relapsing bullous amyloidosis of the oral mucosa and acquired cutis laxa in a patient with multiple myeloma: a rare triple association," *Clinical and Experimental Dermatology*, vol. 42, no. 4, pp. 410–412, 2017.

[19] S. Tan, K. Pon, J. Bargman, and D. Ghazarian, "Generalized cutis laxa associated with heavy chain deposition disease," *Journal of Cutaneous Medicine and Surgery: Incorporating Medical and Surgical Dermatology*, vol. 7, no. 5, pp. 390–394, 2003.

[20] J. T. O'Malley, V. D. D'Agati, W. H. Sherman, and M. E. Grossman, "Acquired cutis laxa associated with heavy chain deposition disease involving dermal elastic fibers," *JAMA Dermatology*, vol. 150, no. 11, pp. 1192–1196, 2014.

[21] C. R. Harrington, T. C. Beswick, J. S. Susa, and A. G. Pandya, "Acquired cutis laxa associated with heavy chain deposition disease," *Journal of the American Academy of Dermatology*, vol. 59, no. 5, pp. S99–S101, 2008.

[22] C. F. de Larrea, M. Rovira, J. M. Mascaró Jr., et al., "Generalized cutis laxa and fibrillar glomerulopathy resulting from IgG Deposition in IgG-lambda Monoclonal Gammopathy: pulmonary hemorrhage during stem cell mobilization and complete hematological response with bortezomib and dexamethasone therapy," *European Journal of Haematology*, vol. 82, no. 2, pp. 154–158, 2009.

[23] R. A. Majithia, L. George, M. Thomas, and N. A. Fouzia, "Acquired cutis laxa associated with light and heavy chain deposition disease," *Indian Dermatology Online Journal*, vol. 9, no. 1, pp. 44–46, 2018.

[24] D. P. Kim and P. A. Klein, "Acquired cutis laxa in a 55-year-old female with multiple myeloma and serologic evidence of systemic lupus erythematosus," *Dermatology Online Journal*, vol. 17, no. 7, p. 8, 2011.

[25] W. B. Reed, R. E. Horowitz, and P. Beighton, "Acquired cutis laxa. Primary generalized elastolysis," *Archives of Dermatology*, vol. 103, no. 6, pp. 661–669, 1971.

[26] C. C. Christensen and F. Gonzalez-Crussi, "Postinflammatory elastolysis and cutis laxa: report of a case with aortitis," *Pediatric Pathology*, vol. 1, no. 2, pp. 199–210, 1983.

[27] A. R. Verhagen and M. J. Woerdeman, "Post-inflammatory elastolysis and cutis laxa," *British Journal of Dermatology*, vol. 92, no. 2, pp. 183–190, 1975.

[28] F. Rongioletti, M. Baldari, M. Burlando, and A. Parodi, "Papular elastolytic giant cell granuloma: report of a case associated with monoclonal gammopathy and responsive to topical tacrolimus," *Clinical and Experimental Dermatology*, vol. 35, no. 2, pp. 145–148, 2010.

[29] M. S. Daoud, J. A. Lust, R. A. Kyle, and M. R. Pittelkow, "Monoclonal gammopathies and associated skin disorders," *Journal of the American Academy of Dermatology*, vol. 40, no. 4, pp. 507–535, 1999.

[30] A. M. Dinneen and C. H. Dicken, "Scleromyxedema," *Journal of the American Academy of Dermatology*, vol. 33, no. 1, pp. 37–43, 1995.

[31] V. Sanchorawala, "Light-chain (AL) amyloidosis: diagnosis and treatment," *Clinical Journal of the American Society of Nephrology*, vol. 1, no. 6, pp. 1331–1341, 2006.

[32] A. O. Moon, K. T. Calamia, and J. S. Walsh, "Nodular amyloidosis: review and long-term follow-up of 16 cases," *Archives of Dermatology*, vol. 139, no. 9, pp. 1157–1159, 2003.

[33] A. Grunenberg and C. Buske, "Monoclonal IgM gammopathy and waldenstrom's macroglobulinemia," *Deutsches Ärzteblatt International*, vol. 114, no. 44, pp. 745–751, 2017.

[34] D. Roccatello, D. Saadoun, M. Ramos-Casals et al., "Cryoglobulinaemia," *Nature Reviews Disease Primers*, vol. 4, no. 1, p. 11, 2018.

[35] D. Lipsker, Y. Veran, F. Grunenberger, B. Cribier, E. Heid, and E. Grosshans, "The schnitzler syndrome," *Medicine*, vol. 80, no. 1, pp. 37–44, 2001.

[36] S. Kossard and R. K. Winkelmann, "Necrobiotic xanthogranuloma with paraproteinemia," *Journal of the American Academy of Dermatology*, vol. 3, no. 3, pp. 257–270, 1980.

[37] G. D. Miralles, J. R. O'Fallon, and N. J. Talley, "Plasma-cell dyscrasia with polyneuropathy," *New England Journal of Medicine*, vol. 327, no. 27, pp. 1919–1923, 1992.

[38] K. Romanska-Gocka, C. Ciescinska, B. Zegarska et al., "Pyoderma gangrenosum with monoclonal IgA gammopathy and pulmonary tuberculosis. Illustrative case and review," *Postepy Dermatologii I Alergologii*, vol. 32, no. 2, pp. 137–141, 2015.

[39] S. Berentsen, E. Ulvestad, R. Langholm et al., "Primary chronic cold agglutinin disease: a population based clinical study of 86 patients," *Haematologica*, vol. 91, no. 1, pp. 460–466, 2006.

[40] E. E. Kasha Jr., and W. W. Epinette, "Subcorneal pustular dermatosis (Sneddon-Wilkinson disease) in association with a monoclonal IgA gammopathy: a report and review of the literature," *Journal of the American Academy of Dermatology*, vol. 19, no. 5, pp. 854–858, 1988.

[41] J. A. Yiannias, R. A. El-Azhary, and L. E. Gibson, "Erythema elevatum diutinum: a clinical and histopathologic study of 13 patients," *Journal of the American Academy of Dermatology*, vol. 26, no. 1, pp. 38–44, 1992.

[42] Z. Adam, P. Szturz, M. Krejci et al., "[Monoclonal immunoglobulin (M-Ig) and skin diseases from the group of mucinoses--scleredema adultorum Buschke and scleromyxedema. Description of four cases and an overview of therapies]," *Vnitřní Lékařství*, vol. 61, no. 12, pp. 1072–1087, 2015.

42

Cutaneous Metastases from Lung Adenocarcinoma

Yu Wang[1,2] **and Ruzeng Xue**[1,2]

[1]*Department of Dermatology, Dermatology Hospital, Southern Medical University, Guangzhou, China*
[2]*Department of Dermatology, Guangdong Provincial Dermatology Hospital, Guangzhou, China*

Correspondence should be addressed to Ruzeng Xue; xueruzeng@163.com

Academic Editor: Jacek Cezary Szepietowski

Cutaneous metastases are unusual presenting symptoms of lung cancer. Therefore, they are prone to be misdiagnosed and missed. The report describes a case of a forty-nine-year-old female with painful zosteriform rashes showing multiple vesicle-like papules localized on the left breast for 10 days. The patient had been diagnosed as lung adenocarcinoma at the department of oncology one year ago. Skin biopsy revealed blue nodular lesions in the dermis, composed of clustered heterogeneous tumor cells with glandular formation. Immunohistochemical stains confirmed the diagnosis of metastatic lung adenocarcinoma.

1. Introduction

Lung cancer can metastasize to almost all organs but more often invades the hilar nodes, liver, adrenal glands, bones, and brain [1]. The incidence of lung cancer with metastases to the skin varies between 1–12% [1]. A lung cancer metastasis is usually classified only as adenocarcinoma, squamous cell carcinoma (SCC), or undifferentiated carcinoma. Until the 1980s, SCC was reported as the most common type of lung cancer. However, adenocarcinoma has replaced SCC as the most common lung cancer subtype, especially in women and in never-smokers. Sun et al. reported that the type of adenocarcinoma was 3.4 times more frequent than that of SCC [2]. Skin metastases can appear on any cutaneous surface, and the most common sites are the chest, abdomen, head, and neck [3, 4]. Cutaneous metastases have various manifestations, such as single papules/nodules or multiple lesions on anywhere of the skin, while other rare forms may show plaque-like lesions, erysipelas-like papules, zosteriform lesions, and scars [3, 5].

2. Case Presentation

A forty-nine-year-old nonsmoker female was admitted to our department with multiple painful papules localized on the left breast. They appeared eruptively for about 10 days and initially diagnosed as herpes zoster in another hospital. The patient had been diagnosed as lung adenocarcinoma at the department of oncology one year ago. She was given oxitinib mesylate, a targeted drug for the treatment of non-small-cell lung cancer. In addition, the patient exhibited symptom of pain, signs of weight loss, anorexia, and fatigue.

Physical examination showed zosteriform vesicle-like papules, measuring 0.5–1.0 cm on the left breast. The lesions were pink or red, firm, and tender (Figure 1). Excisional biopsy was performed revealing blue nodular lesions infiltrating in the dermis, composed of clustered heterogeneous tumor cells with glandular formation. Some tumor cells were detected within vessels or lymphatic vessels. Some cells were transparent. Mitosis was significant (Figures 2(a)–2(c)). In immunohistochemistry, tumor cells were positive for cytokeratin (CK), cytokeratin-7 (CK7), thyroid transcription factor-1 (TTF1), and EMA and negative for cytokeratin-20 (CK20), carcinoembryonic antigen (CEA), and gross cystic disease fluid protein-15 (GCDFP-15) (Figures 3(a)–3(c)). Proliferative index, as measured by Ki-67, was approximately 45–50% of tumor cells. According to the clinical and pathological features, cutaneous metastatic lung adenocarcinoma was made.

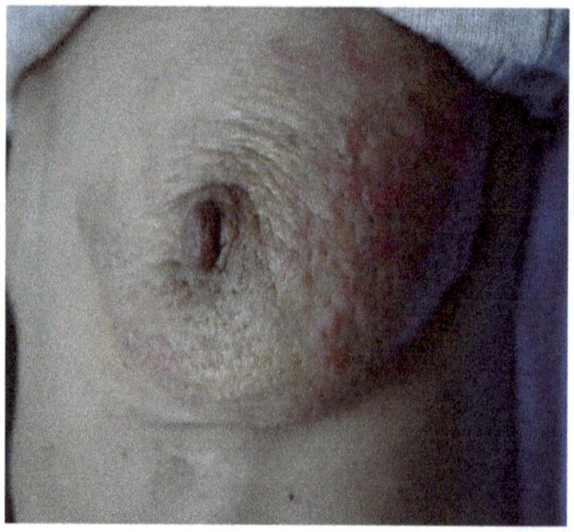

FIGURE 1: Zosteriform vesicle-like papules, measuring 0.5–1.0 cm on the left breast. Pink or red, firm, and tender.

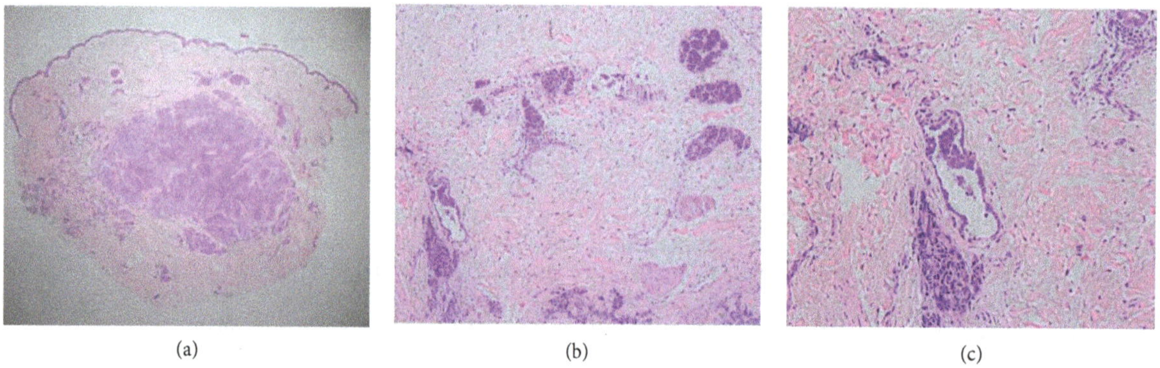

FIGURE 2: Skin biopsy revealed (a) blue nodular lesions infiltrating in the dermis, composed of clustered heterogeneous tumor cells with glandular formation (H&E, magnification: ×20); (b) some tumor cells were detected within vessels or lymphatic vessels (H&E, magnification: ×40); (c) some cells were blue and transparent, and mitosis was significant (H&E, magnification: ×200).

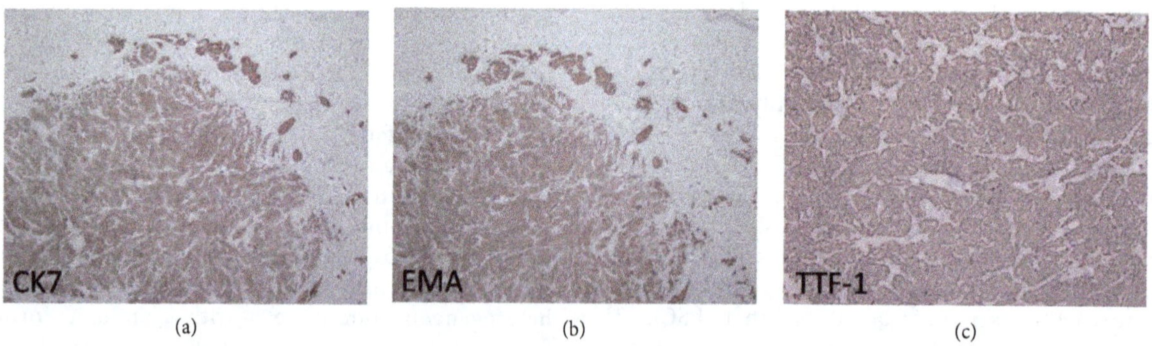

FIGURE 3: Immunohistochemical stain highlighting the tumor cells, showing (a) CK-7, (b) EMA, and (c) TTF-1 positive.

3. Discussion

Skin metastases suggest the progression of primary cancer and portend a poor clinical prognosis. Skin metastases from lung cancer are rare. The percentage of patients with lung cancer that develops cutaneous metastases ranges from 1 to 12 percent [1]. It is seen more often in men than in women [6]. It does not show any specific presentation. It is often painless and less likely to be noticed, making it more difficult to be diagnosed correctly, which may delay treatment. Although described cases show that metastatic nodules are painless, our patient showed severe pain. The presence of zosteriform painful vesicle-like lesions really mimics herpes zoster clinically in our case.

The mechanisms determining the metastasis of lung cancer in skin remain unknown. Pathogenesis is suggested to be by lymphovascular invasion, with poor differentiation and upper lobe tumors increasing the risk [7]. Usually, skin metastasis develops after initial diagnosis of the primary malignancy and late in the course of the disease. Occasionally, skin lesions that arise from lung cancer may develop before the primary tumor is recognized. In our case, skin metastases occurred during the immunotherapy. Histology shows most commonly adenocarcinoma and then squamous/small-cell followed by large-cell carcinoma [1]. Immunohistochemical markers are useful for the identification of the primary cancer or when a shorter differential is desired. Anti-TTF is both sensitive and specific for primary adenocarcinomas, bronchioalveolar carcinomas, and small-cell carcinomas when thyroid primary is excluded [8]. CK7+and CK20− are sensitive but not specific for primary adenocarcinomas and bronchioalveolar carcinomas. The CK7+/CK20−tumors usually include the lung, breast, endometrium, ovary, thyroid, salivary gland, and mesothelioma [8, 9].

Treatment of a single solitary skin lesion usually includes surgery alone or combined with chemotherapy, and/or radiation. If lesions are more disseminated, chemotherapy is the primary option but may elicit an inadequate response [10]. Radiation can also be used alone and/or in combination with chemotherapy, and/or surgery. However, despite the combination of radiotherapy and chemotherapy, patients with lung cancer developing cutaneous metastases have a poor outcome. Mean survival is short, usually 5 to 6 months after diagnosis of cutaneous metastasis [1].

Acknowledgments

This work was supported by a grant from the National Natural Science Foundation of China (81903200).

References

[1] T. W. Mollet, C. A. Garcia, and G. Koester, "Skin metastases from lung cancer," *Dermatology Online Journal*, vol. 15, no. 5, 2009.

[2] S. Sun, J. H. Schiller, and A. F. Gazdar, "Lung cancer in never smokers-a different disease," *Nature Reviews Cancer*, vol. 7, no. 10, pp. 778–790, 2007.

[3] S. Dreizen, H. M. Dhingra, D. F. Chiuten, T. Umsawasdi, and M. Valdivieso, "Cutaneous and subcutaneous metastases of lung cancer," *Postgraduate Medicine*, vol. 80, no. 8, pp. 111–116, 1986.

[4] M. Khaja, D. Mundt, R. A. Dudekula et al., "Lung cancer presenting as skin metastasis of the back and hand: a case series and literature review," *Case Reports in Oncology*, vol. 12, no. 2, pp. 480–487, 2019.

[5] W. T. McSweeney and K. Tan, "Cutaneous metastases as a presenting sign of metastatic NSCLC," *Journal of Surgical Case Reports*, vol. 2019, no. 10, 2019.

[6] M. H. Brownstein and E. B. Helwig, "Metastatic tumors of the skin," *Cancer*, vol. 29, no. 5, pp. 1298–1307, 1972.

[7] R. B. McGrath, S. P. Flood, and R. Casey, "Cutaneous metastases in non-small cell lung cancer," *BMJ Case Reports*, vol. 2014, 2014.

[8] V. Jerome Marson, J. Mazieres, O. Groussard et al., "Expression of TTF-1 and cytokeratins in primary and secondary epithelial lung tumours: correlation with histological type and grade," *Histopathology*, vol. 45, no. 2, pp. 125–134, 2004.

[9] R. Koca, Y. Ustundag, E. Kargi, G. Numanoglu, and H. C. Altinyazar, "A case with widespread cutaneous metastases of unknown primary origin: grave prognostic finding in cancer," *Dermatology Online Journal*, vol. 11, no. 1, p. 16, 2005.

[10] N. A. Babacan, S. Kilickap, S. Sene et al., "A case of multifocal skin metastases from lung cancer presenting with vasculitic-type cutaneous nodule," *Indian Journal of Dermatology*, vol. 60, p. 213, 2015.

43

Primary Cutaneous CD30+ Anaplastic Large T Cell Lymphoma in a Patient Treated with Cyclosporine for Actinic Reticuloid

T. Gambichler[1] **N. Patsinakidis,**[2] **L. Susok,**[1] **M. H. Segert,**[1] **and M. Doerler**[1]

[1]*Skin Cancer Center, Department of Dermatology, Ruhr-University Bochum, Bochum, Germany*
[2]*Division of Experimental Allergy and Immunodermatology, University of Oldenburg, Oldenburg, Germany*

Correspondence should be addressed to T. Gambichler; t.gambichler@klinikum-bochum.de

Academic Editor: Michihiro Hide

Actinic reticuloid (AR)—a subtype of chronic actinic dermatitis—clinically and histopathologically shows lymphoma-like features. We report a male patient initially diagnosed with erythrodermic cutaneous T cell lymphoma (CTCL) who developed severe broadband photosensitivity. Clinical evaluation, histopathology, and phototesting were consistent with AR. The patient was treated with cyclosporine 150–300 mg/d. Under this therapy, he developed several times primary cutaneous anaplastic large cell lymphomas (C-ALCL) which in part tended to regress spontaneously under cyclosporine reduction. The association between cyclosporine treatment and development of C-ALCL and other CD30+ lymphoproliferative disorders has previously been reported in patients with atopic dermatitis, psoriasis, and transplant patients. In conclusion, the present case highlights the difficulties arising in the distinction between AR and CTCL and shows that long-term cyclosporine treatment may cause C-ALCL development in AR as well.

1. Introduction

It has been suggested that photosensitive disorders, including persistent light reaction, photosensitive atopic dermatitis, chronic photosensitivity dermatitis, and actinic reticuloid (AR), should be considered as one entity, so called chronic actinic dermatitis (CAD) [1, 2]. This disorder may develop in healthy skin or on the basis of preceding dermatoses, such as atopic dermatitis, photoallergic dermatitis, allergic contact dermatitis, and drug-induced photosensitivity. CAD is defined on three diagnostic criteria as follows: (1) chronic progressive pruritic dermatitis and lichenification predominantly on ultraviolet- (UV-) exposed skin sites, whereby with disease progression, nonexposed sites may also be affected; (2) on UV testing of previously nonexposed skin reduction of the minimal erythema dose (MED) against UV-A and UV-B including the development of eczematous lesions within a few days; and (3) histology consistent with chronic dermatitis, with or without the presence of lymphoma-like changes [1, 2]. Hence, atopic dermatitis, airborne contact dermatitis, and cutaneous T cell lymphoma (CTCL) are the most important differential diagnoses of CAD. UV protection and immunosuppressive therapy including cyclosporine represent standards in the management of CAD or AR [1, 2]. In patients with inflammatory skin conditions, cyclosporine has been reported to be associated with the occurrence of CD30+ lymphoproliferative diseases [3–7]. We here report a difficult-to-diagnose patient with AR under cyclosporine therapy who developed primary cutaneous CD30+ anaplastic large cell lymphoma (C-ALCL) which spontaneously regressed after reduction of cyclosporine dosage.

2. Case Presentation

We report a male patient with a history of atopic dermatitis and polyvalent type 1-hypersensitivity since childhood. When he was 46 years old, he had erythroderma, palmoplantar hyperkeratosis, alopecia, and lymphadenopathy. The histologic picture of several skin biopsies showed features of CTCL. Lymph node as well as bone marrow biopsy did not demonstrate evidence for lymphoma manifestation. He was initially treated with high-dose corticosteroids and extracorporeal photopheresis (11 cycles) followed by 9 cycles with liposomal-pegylated doxorubicin. Since he did not adequately respond to doxorubicin, his therapy was switched to bexarotene 150 mg/m^2 daily.

At the age of 48 years, he noticed increasing UV sensitivity and worsening of his skin condition, in particular within the sun-exposed skin regions. Notably, he had less skin problems during winter. Clinically, he showed a similar picture as mentioned above. However, the grade of infiltration and induration of skin lesions had significantly increased including impressive tumor-like aggregated papules and nodes mainly affecting the sun-exposed areas (Figure 1). Histology of a papulous lesion on the neck revealed acanthosis and a diffuse lymphocytic infiltrate in the entire dermis. In addition, there was no evident epidermotropism of the T cell dominant infiltrate, resulting in the histologic diagnosis of pseudolymphoma (Figure 1). T cell receptor (TCR) rearrangement was negative. Flow cytometry for lymphocyte subpopulations in the peripheral blood was unremarkable. Again, there was no evidence for lymphoma or other conditions on bone marrow biopsy. Patch-testing including the photopatch test (5 J/cm^2 UV-A; PUVA 180, Waldmann, Villingen-Schwenningen, Germany) did not reveal evidence for airborne contact dermatitis or photocontact allergy [8]. However, the entire test areal on the lower back showed erythema with eczematous changes following the next days.

After a brief warm-up period, the MED for broadband UV-B (280–320 nm) and broadband UV-A (320–400 nm) was determined with a compact previously commercially available phototest device (Multitester SBB LT 400; Saalmann GmbH, Herford, Germany). As generally recommended, phototesting was performed on healthy buttock skin [9]. Twenty-four hours after irradiation (Figure 2), the phototest revealed markedly reduced MEDs both for UV-B (<8 mJ/cm^2) and UV-A (0.9 J/cm^2) based on previously established lower reference limits of 33 mJ/cm^2 and 12.6 J/cm^2, respectively [9]. After 3 days, eczematous lesions were observed in the test sites. Skin biopsies were performed in UV-B as well as UV-A-irradiated sites. Histology revealed dense, in part perivascular or diffuse, infiltrates consisting of monomorph lymphocytes and eosinophils. The infiltrates were predominantly observed in the upper and mid-dermis. On immunohistology, there was a T cell dominant infiltrate (CD8 60%+, CD4 30%+, CD30 negative) and a very low proliferation rate of approximately 5% with Ki-67. TCR rearrangement was negative again. Clinicopathological correlation matched the diagnosis of AR—the lymphoma-like subtype of CAD was made. During the following 9 years, he was predominantly treated with cyclosporine 150–300 mg/d with good control of symptoms, particularly during winter months with almost complete remissions.

At the age of 58 years, he re-attended our department because of new reddish ulcerated nodular lesions (3 × 5 cm in diameter) behind the left ear. Histology and immunohistochemistry was consistent with a CD30+ lymphoproliferative disorder. Given the large and polymorphic lymphocytes and the >90% CD30 positivity, a primary C-ALCL was favored. TCR rearrangement was positive. Tests for EBV were negative. Complete work-up including flow cytometry of peripheral blood, bone marrow biopsy, and thoracic/abdominal/pelvic computed tomography showed no evidence for systemic disease. The lesion could only be excised incompletely. Hence, postsurgery radiotherapy was performed. Five months later, he also developed reddish, partly ulcerated nodules on the scalp as well as upper right arm. Again, histology and immunohistochemistry confirmed the diagnosis of C-ALCL (Figure 3). Interestingly, these lesions completely regressed spontaneously about 4 days after the reduction of cyclosporine from 300 mg/d to 100 mg/d. Following further reduction of cyclosporine, it was finally replaced by azathioprine 100 mg daily. No further C-ALCL lesions reoccurred. Importantly, during his 17-year course of disease, there was no evidence for blood abnormalities (e.g., increase of CD3+ CD4+/CD26− T cells) or the presence of monoclonality.

3. Discussion

As demonstrated by the present case, the action spectrum of CAD and AR is usually very broad, including UV-B, UV-A, and visible wavelength. Even though not tested in our photodermatology unit, our patient had a history for also being highly sensitive to visible light. The clinical and histopathologic features of AR are similar in nature to those of delayed-type hypersensitivity reaction of the allergic contact dermatitis type. For instance, the observation of increased numbers of cutaneous CD8+ T cells in AR indicates a delayed-type immunologic reaction against a cutaneous antigen (e.g., DNA and RNA) likely induced by UV radiation [1, 2]. To distinguish the severe AR subtype of CAD (previously also called pseudolymphomatous chronic actinic dermatitis) from CTCL, the assessment of TCR rearrangements may be used in addition to immunohistochemistry [10–16]. Particularly in erythrodermic CTCL, the CD4/CD8 ratio is frequently increased as a result of an increase of lesional T helper cells. By contrast in AR, there is frequently an increase of lesional CD8+ cells, frequently resulting in inversion of the CD4/CD8 ratio [13, 15]. In contrast to patients with erythrodermic CTCL, a monoclonal TCR rearrangement is usually not found in the skin or blood of patients with AR. As shown in a previous study on patients ($n = 231$) with CAD, the development of genuine lymphomas was not significantly increased compared with the healthy population [1]. Photosensitivity is, however, an infrequent feature of CTCL as well. Agar et al. [17] suggested that, rarely, malignant clonal T cell populations may recognize a unique UV-induced neoantigen, resulting in the clinical features of severe photosensitivity mimicking those seen in CAD or AR [17]. The long benign course of disease with spontaneous improvement during winter and the absence of significant blood alterations or disease progress widely exclude the diagnosis of CTCL in the present case.

Apart from the fact that AR is a serious mimicker of CTCL, the present case also highlights that patients who are

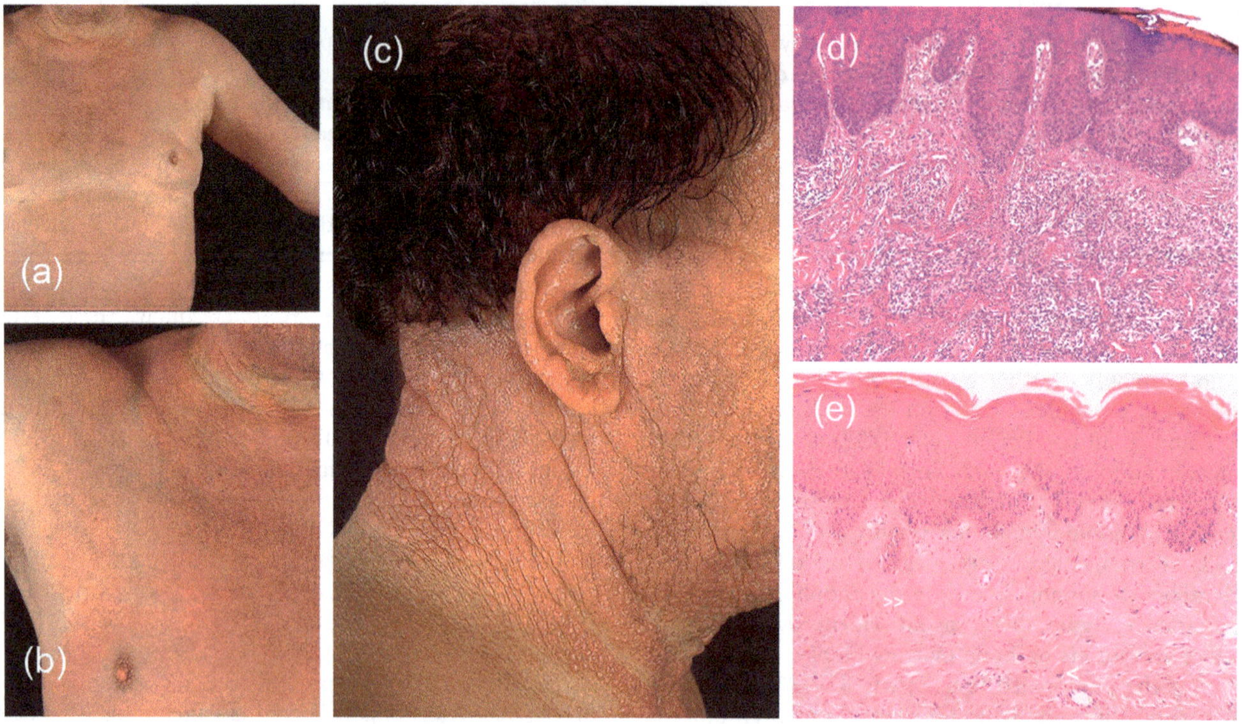

Figure 1: Showing photodistributed erythema (a, b) and massively infiltrated papulous plaques on the face and neck (b) of a patient with actinic reticuloid. Skin biopsy taken from the cheek (c) showing acanthosis and a diffuse lymphocytic infiltrate in the entire dermis. There was no evident epidermotropism of the T cell dominant infiltrate leading to the diagnosis of pseudolymphoma (d). A biopsy taken from eczematous lesions on the trunk (b) showing acanthosis with focal parakeratosis, thickened collagen bundles (>>), and a sparse, mainly lymphocytic infiltrate with hyperchromatic cells (<) in the upper dermis (e). Together, the histologic picture and clinicopathological correlation matched the diagnosis of actinic reticuloid.

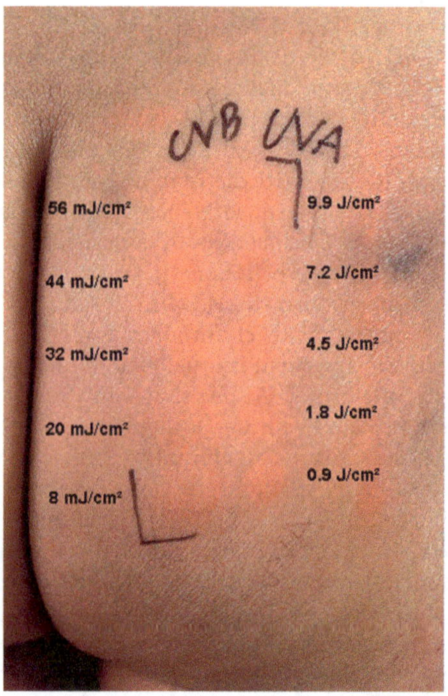

Figure 2: MED testing in a patient with actinic reticuloid showing increased photosensitivity both in the UV-B and UV-A range.

under cyclosporine treatment for inflammatory skin disorders or other conditions are prone to develop C-ALCL. Most patients in such a clinical constellation had atopic dermatitis or psoriasis [18]. Moreover, in organ transplant patients taking immunosuppressants including cyclosporine, the occurrence of CD30+ lymphoproliferative disorders and B cell lymphomas has been observed as well [18–20]. Together, the risk of development of lymphomas in patients with atopic dermatitis or psoriasis on low doses of immunosuppressive therapy (mainly cyclosporine) is considered to be very low [21]. The present case is the first C-ALCL occurrence during cyclosporine therapy for AR. However, our patient previously suffered from long-standing atopic dermatitis that is not infrequently a "precursor" condition of CAD or AR [1, 2]. Indeed, it is barely possible to distinguish C-ALCL from lymphomatoid papulosis (LyP) on histological grounds. Moreover, LyP may manifest clinically with localized or nodular lesions rendering distinction from C-ALCL even more challenging. LyP and C-ALCL, however, differ in their biological behavior and require different treatment approaches. Differentiation between LyP and C-ALCL may succeed by means of immunohistochemistry using markers such as multiple myeloma oncogene 1 and fascin [18–20].

Kirby et al. [7] described a patient with atopic dermatitis who developed C-ALCL during low-dose cyclosporine

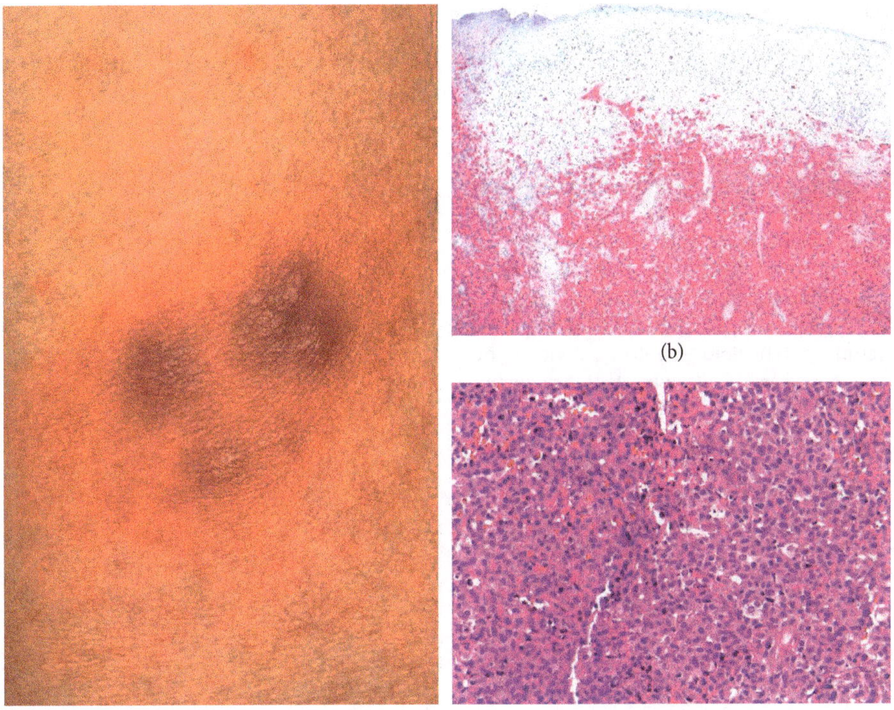

(a) (b) (c)

FIGURE 3: Clinical picture of a histology-proven primary cutaneous anaplastic large T cell lymphoma on the upper right arm (a). CD30 immunohistochemistry showing sheet-like lymphocytic infiltrates of large T cells, which were almost exclusively CD30+ (b, c), consistent with a diagnosis of cutaneous anaplastic large T cell lymphoma.

monotherapy. As similarly observed in the present case, C-ALCL lesions spontaneously resolved after stopping cyclosporine [7]. Fletcher et al. [4] recently reported four cases of CD30+ lymphoproliferative disease in young adult patients with active atopic dermatitis. One of the patients was taking cyclosporine when he developed lymphomatoid papulosis type A that resolved after stopping the drug [4]. Tests for EBV were negative. The authors hypothesize about a link between lymphoproliferative disorder and atopic dermatitis including treatment modalities such as cyclosporine [4]. Possible mechanisms include immunosuppression, chronic antigenic T cell activation, cutaneous bacteria, superantigens, or UV-induced antigens as conceivable in the present case. Cyclosporine inhibits signaling through the TCR to prevent the production of cytokines that would normally stimulate an immune response. This could also theoretically impair T cell activation induced cell death which might prolong lymphocyte survival. Hence, a reduction or cessation of cyclosporine treatment may result in spontaneous regression of CD30+ lymphoproliferative lesions [4, 22].

In conclusion, the present case highlights the difficulties arising in the distinction between AR and CTCL and shows that long-term cyclosporine treatment may cause C-ALCL development in AR as well.

References

[1] T. Gambichler, R. Al-Muhammadi, and S. Boms, "Immunologically mediated photodermatoses," *American Journal of Clinical Dermatology*, vol. 10, no. 3, pp. 169–180, 2009.

[2] H. W. Lim, H. Hönigsmann, and J. L. M. Hawk, *Photodermatology* Informa Healthcare USA, Inc., New York, NY, USA, 2007.

[3] J. Ferguson and J. S. Dover, *Photodermatology*, Manson Publishing, London, UK, 2006.

[4] C. L. Fletcher, G. E. Orchard, V. Hubbard, S. J. Whittaker, R. L. Edelson, and R. Russell-Jones, "CD30 (+) cutaneous lymphoma in association with atopic eczema," *Archives of Dermatology*, vol. 140, pp. 449–454, 2004.

[5] E. Mahe, V. Descamps, M. Grossin, S. Fraitag, and B. Crickx, "CD30+ T-cell lymphoma in a patient with psoriasis treated with ciclosporin and infliximab," *British Journal of Dermatology*, vol. 149, no. 1, pp. 170–173, 2003.

[6] M. Corazza, M. R. Zampino, A. Montanari, E. Altieri, and A. Virgili, "Primary cutaneous CD30+ large T-cell lymphoma in a patient with psoriasis treated with cyclosporine," *Dermatology*, vol. 206, no. 4, pp. 330–333, 2003.

[7] B. Kirby, C. M. Owen, R. W. Blewitt, and V. M. Yates, "Cutaneous T-cell lymphoma developing in a patient on cyclosporin therapy," *Journal of the American Academy of Dermatology*, vol. 47, no. 2, pp. S165–S167, 2002.

[8] J. Geier, A. Bauer, D. Becker et al., "Empfehlungen der arbeitsgruppe "photopatchtest" der deutschen kontaktallergie-gruppe (DKG) zur durchführung des photopatchtests," *JDDG: Journal Der Deutschen Dermatologischen Gesellschaft* vol. 16, no. 11, pp. 1363-1364, 2018.

[9] T. Gambichler, G. Moussa, N. S. Tomi, V. Paech, P. Altmeyer, and A. Kreuter, "Reference limits for erythema-effective UV doses," *Photochemistry and Photobiology*, vol. 82, no. 4, pp. 1097–1102, 2006.

[10] M. Sidiropoulos, J. Deonizio, M. E. Martinez-Escala, P. Gerami, and J. Guitart, "Chronic actinic dermatitis/actinic reticuloid," *The American Journal of Dermatopathology*, vol. 36, no. 11, pp. 875–881, 2014.

[11] D. Pacheco, A. Fraga, A. R Travassos et al., "Actinic reticuloid imitating sézary syndrome," *Acta Dermatovenerologica Alpina, Panonica et Adriatica*, vol. 21, pp. 55–57, 2012.

[12] L. Lugović-Mihić, T. Duvancić, M. Situm, J. Mihić, and I. Krolo, "Actinic reticuloid—photosensitivity or pseudolymphoma?—A review," *Collegium Antropologicum*, vol. 35, no. 2, pp. 325–329, 2011.

[13] P. Heller, R. Wieczorek, E. Waldo et al., "An immunohistochemical study of its T-cell antigenic profile, with comparison to cutaneous T-cell lymphoma," *The American Journal of Dermatopathology*, vol. 16, no. 5, pp. 510–516, 1994.

[14] D. Bilsland, I. K. Crombie, and J. Ferguson, "The photosensitivity dermatitis and actinic reticuloid syndrome: no association with lymphoreticular malignancy," *The British Journal of Dermatology*, vol. 131, no. 131, pp. 209–214, 1994.

[15] P. G. Norris, J. Morris, N. P. Smith, A. C. Chu, and J. L. M. Hawk, "Chronic actinic dermatitis: an immunohistologic and photobiologic study," *Journal of the American Academy of Dermatology*, vol. 21, no. 5, pp. 966–971, 1989.

[16] A. C. Chu, D. Robinson, J. L. M. Hawk, R. Meacham, M. F. Spittle, and N. P. Smith, "Immunologic differentiation of the Sézary syndrome due to cutaneous T-cell lymphoma and chronic actinic dermatitis," *Journal of Investigative Dermatology*, vol. 86, no. 2, pp. 134–137, 1986.

[17] N. Agar, S. Morris, R. Russell-Jones, J. Hawk, and S. Whittaker, "Case report of four patients with erythrodermic cutaneous T-cell lymphoma and severe photosensitivity mimicking chronic actinic dermatitis," *British Journal of Dermatology*, vol. 160, no. 3, pp. 698–703, 2009.

[18] S. Nakamura, K. Takeda, Y. Hashimoto, T. Mizumoto, A. Ishida-Yamamoto, and H. Iizuka, "Primary cutaneous CD30+ lymphoproliferative disorder in an atopic dermatitis patient on cyclosporine therapy," *Indian Journal of Dermatology, Venereology, and Leprology*, vol. 77, no. 2, p. 253, 2011.

[19] F. E. Ravat, M. F. Spittle, and R. Russell-Jones, "Primary cutaneous T-cell lymphoma occurring after organ transplantation," *Journal of the American Academy of Dermatology*, vol. 54, no. 4, pp. 668–675, 2006.

[20] M. Lucioni, G. Ippoliti, C. Campana et al., "EBV positive primary cutaneous CD30+ large T-cell lymphoma in a heart transplanted patient: case report," *American Journal of Transplantation*, vol. 4, no. 11, pp. 1915–1920, 2004.

[21] M. Lebwohl, C. Ellis, A. Gottlieb et al., "Cyclosporine consensus conference: with emphasis on the treatment of psoriasis," *Journal of the American Academy of Dermatology*, vol. 39, no. 3, pp. 464–475, 1998.

[22] M. Hojo, T. Morimoto, M. Maluccio et al., "Cyclosporine induces cancer progression by a cell-autonomous mechanism," *Nature*, vol. 397, no. 6719, pp. 530–534, 1999.

New Onset Granulomatosis with Polyangiitis Associated with COVID-19

Moshe Y. Bressler,[1,2] Naeha Pathak,[2] Kelly Cervellione,[3] Farshad Bagheri,[4] Edward Epstein,[5] Adnan Mir,[6] and Rebecca Tamez[2]

[1]*New York Institute of Technology College of Osteopathic Medicine, Old Westbury, NY, USA*
[2]*Jamaica Hospital, Department of Internal Medicine, Dermatology, New York, NY, USA*
[3]*Jamaica Hospital, Department of Clinical Research, New York, NY, USA*
[4]*Jamaica Hospital, Department of Internal Medicine, Infectious Disease, New York, NY, USA*
[5]*Jamaica Hospital, Department of Internal Medicine, Nephrology, New York, NY, USA*
[6]*Dermpath Diagnostics, New York Medical College Dermatology, Weill Cornell Medicine Dermatology, New York, NY, USA*

Correspondence should be addressed to Rebecca Tamez; rebecca.tamez.md@gmail.com

Academic Editor: Alireza Firooz

The coronavirus disease 2019 (COVID-19) has recently been found to cause cutaneous vasculitis in patients. Granulomatosis with polyangiitis (GPA) is a type of small and medium vessel vasculitis that is often associated with pulmonary issues and has been shown to raise diagnostic complications in COVID-19 infection. In this report, we discuss the first case of new-onset GPA in the setting of active COVID-19 infection. Symptoms often overlap between the two diseases, and while there is no current cure for COVID-19, rapid immunosuppressive initiation can be lifesaving for patients with GPA. Thus, this case is essential in expanding our current knowledge of COVID-19 and its many skin manifestations.

1. Introduction

The coronavirus disease 2019 (COVID-19) pandemic caused by severe acute respiratory syndrome coronavirus 2 (SARS-CoV-2) has rapidly spread across the globe, while clinicians have been compelled to continuously expand their knowledge base of this novel complex disease and its associated symptoms. Several coronavirus patients have been found to have vascular endothelial damage, which is thought to play a role in the development of both skin lesions [1] and strokes [2]. Several dermatologists report seeing a vasculitis-like eruption in COVID patients [3, 4]. Herein, we discuss a case of new onset granulomatosis with polyangiitis (GPA), a small and medium vessel vasculitis, associated with a suspected case of COVID-19.

2. Case Presentation

In April 2020, a 46-year-old man with a past medical history of diabetes presented to the emergency room with symptoms of cough, shortness of breath, and fevers for four weeks. He was treated for suspected pneumonia with azithromycin two weeks prior to presentation and denied any improvement in respiratory symptoms thereafter. In addition, he developed a painful and pruritic rash that was progressively worsening over the last two weeks (see Figure 1 for timeline of patient course).

On physical examination, he was afebrile (36.9 C) with tachycardia (110 bpm), blood pressure 127/77 mm Hg, respiratory rate 20, and O_2 saturation 94% on room air. He had erosions on bilateral nasal mucosa and vermillion lips with overlying crusts. Oropharynx was clear. There were purpuric

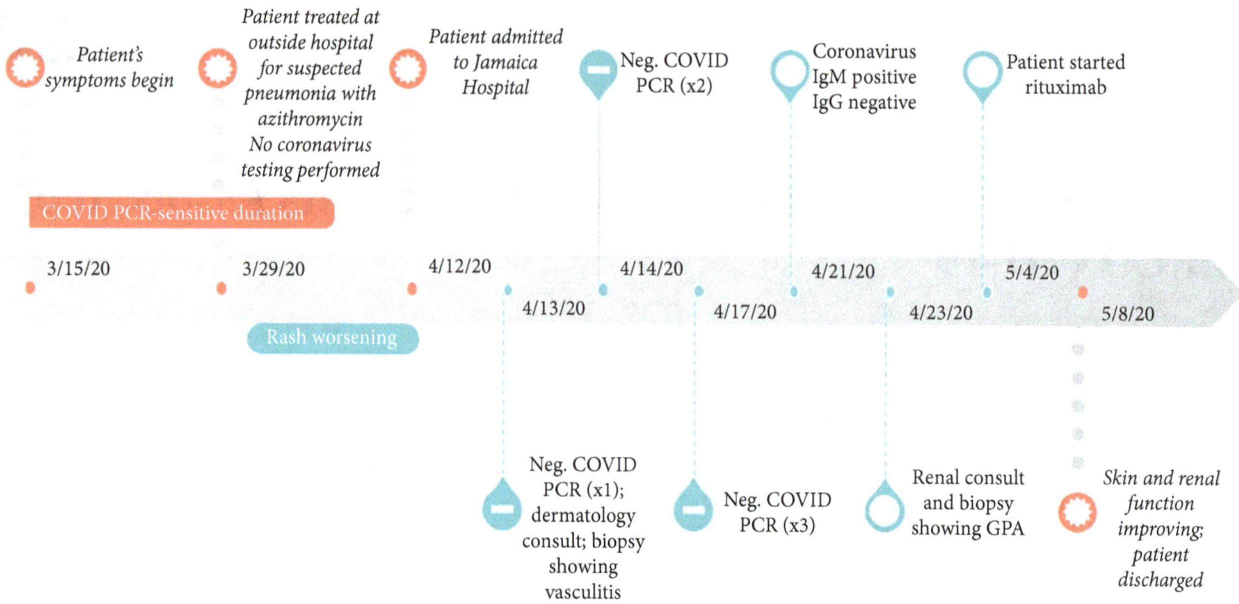

Figure 1: Timeline depicting onset of patient symptoms, test results, and disease course.

macules and papules on bilateral palms, arms, and legs, few with overlying vesicular changes and collarettes of scale (Figures 2(a) and 2(b)). He also had retiform purpuric macules and patches on buttocks and thighs (Figure 2(c)), as well as ulcerations on buttocks at the gluteal cleft.

Laboratory evaluation showed an elevated white blood cell count (15.3K/μL), decreased hemoglobin (10.3 g/dL), elevated blood urea nitrogen (48 mg/dL), creatine (2.9 mg/dL), and D-dimer (8,922 ng/mL). He was cANCA positive, coronavirus PCR negative via nasopharyngeal swab, and coronavirus antibody IgM positive and IgG negative. CT scan of the chest showed patchy ground-glass opacities in the lungs.

Biopsy of skin showed superficial and deep perivascular inflammation with thrombus formation (H&E stain, 10x) (Figure 3(a)). High-power view showed an infiltrate composed of lymphocytes, histiocytes, neutrophils, and eosinophils, with prominent erythrocyte extravasation, leukocytoclasia, and fibrinoid necrosis of vessels (H&E stain, 40x) (Figure 3(b)). Renal biopsy showed interstitial mixed cell infiltrates and intraglomerular thrombi and necrosis, concerning for GPA.

Based upon his clinical presentation, histologic findings, and laboratory studies, the patient was diagnosed with GPA in the setting of suspected coronavirus infection. He was first treated for coronavirus with five-day course of hydroxychloroquine, followed by treatment of GPA with systemic steroids and rituximab infusion. Kidney function improved, and his rash completely resolved. He was discharged on a steroid taper.

3. Discussion

We discuss a case of c-ANCA-positive granulomatosis with polyangiitis possibly triggered by a COVID-19 infection. Our patient presented with four weeks of symptoms and had negative nasopharyngeal PCR test; however, positivity to RT-PCR begins to decline three weeks after initial symptom onset [5]. Furthermore, a review of 8,136 pooled specimens showed RT-PCR positivity using nasopharyngeal swabs to be a mere 45.5% (compared to bronchoalveolar lavage with 91.8%) [6]. Our patient showed positive IgM antibodies to COVID-19, owing to possible recent infection, although there has been a report of cross-reactivity to COVID-19 IgM serological testing in GPA [7]. We are hesitant to conclude this case as a false-positive, rather we hypothesize patient's delayed presentation and low-yield specimen for PCR testing may have missed an active or recent COVID-19 infection (as illustrated in Figure 1).

Infections or viruses can trigger GPA [8], and without treatment, it has a devastatingly high mortality rate [9]. First-line therapies are either rituximab or cyclophosphamide. Glucocorticoids can also be given, especially for maintenance therapy. In the setting of coronavirus, there is a concern that immunosuppressive therapies could increase the likelihood of adverse events including hospitalization and mortality [10, 11]. However, other studies suggest that the increased risk of COVID-19-related adverse events (such as admission to an intensive care unit or requiring mechanical ventilation) is minimal, and outcomes are improved when patients are on immune-modifying medications [10, 12]. Furthermore, patients given

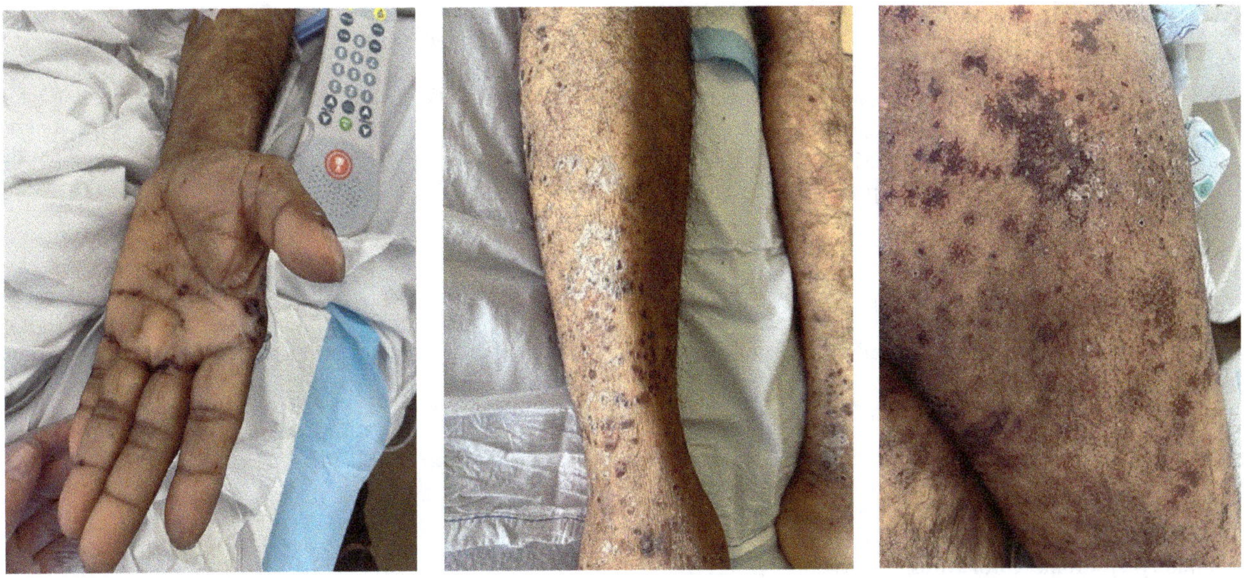

(a) (b) (c)

FIGURE 2: Cutaneous findings in a 46-year-old man with granulomatosis with polyangiitis and an active COVID-19 infection. (a) Purpuric macules and papules on palm and distal arm (b) Purpuric macules and papules with collarettes of scale on lower leg. (c) Retiform purpuric patches on thighs.

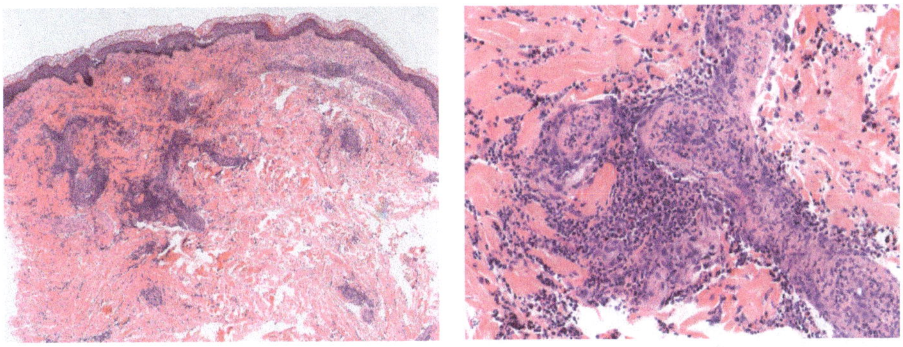

(a) (b)

FIGURE 3: Histopathologic findings of the cutaneous lesions depicting leukocytoclasic vasculitis consistent with granulomatosis with polyangiitis. (a) Superficial and deep dermal perivascular inflammation with thrombus formation (H&E stain, 10x). (b) Extravasated erythrocytes and leukocytoclasia seen in the dermis with fibrinoid necrosis of vessels (H&E stain, 40x) and perivascular infiltrate composed of lymphocytes, histiocytes, neutrophils, and eosinophils.

dexamethasone, a well-known immunomodulatory therapy, had significantly lower mortality and length of hospital stay [11].

4. Conclusion

GPA can mimic the clinical presentation of COVID-19 infection, and cross-reactivity can complicate interpretation of COVID-19 serology results. Prompt treatment for GPA is indicated to prevent irreversible lung and renal damage. While some immunotherapies may increase the risk of a COVID-19 infection, immunosuppressives have overall shown decreased risk of adverse events associated with infection and better patient outcomes. Our patient with biopsy-proven GPA in the setting of coronavirus infection improved clinically with the use of immunosuppressive therapy. We hope that, by presenting his case, we can further expand clinical knowledge about this complicated viral disease and the use of immunotherapy in a setting where the risk of coronavirus infection is high.

Disclosure

The corresponding author had full access to all the data in the study and had final responsibility for the decision to submit for publication.

Authors' Contributions

Moshe Bressler and Naeha Pathak contributed to literature search and writing. Kelly Cervellione, Farshad Bagheri, MD, and Edward Epstein, MD, contributed to case write up. Adnan Mir, MD, and Rebecca Tamez, MD, were responsible for data collection and case write up obtained pathology photos.

Acknowledgments

We thank the patient for granting permission to publish this information.

References

[1] B. Diaz-Guimaraens, M. Dominguez-Santas, A. Suarez-Valle et al., "Petechial skin rash associated with severe acute respiratory syndrome coronavirus 2 infection," *JAMA Dermatology*, vol. 156, no. 7, p. 820, 2020.

[2] T. J. Oxley, J. Mocco, S. Majidi et al., "Large-vessel stroke as a presenting feature of COVID-19 in the young," *New England Journal of Medicine*, vol. 382, no. 20, p. e60, 2020.

[3] L. M. Madigan, R. G. Micheletti, and K. Shinkai, "How dermatologists can learn and contribute at the leading edge of the COVID-19 global pandemic," *JAMA Dermatology*, vol. 156, no. 7, p. 733, 2020.

[4] A. V. Marzano, G. Genovese, G. Fabbrocini et al., "Varicella-like exanthem as a specific COVID-19-associated skin manifestation: multicenter case series of 22 patients," *Journal of the American Academy of Dermatology*, vol. 83, no. 1, pp. 280–285, 2020.

[5] N. Sethuraman, S. S. Jeremiah, and A. Ryo, "Interpreting diagnostic tests for SARS-CoV-2," *JAMA*, vol. 323, no. 22, pp. 2249–2251, 2020.

[6] G. M. Bwire, M. V. Majigo, B. J. Njiro, and A. Mawazo, "Detection profile of SARS-CoV-2 using RT-PCR in different types of clinical specimens: a systematic review and meta-analysis," *Journal of Medical Virology*, vol. 93, no. 2, p. 719, 2020.

[7] A. Tzouvelekis, T. Karampitsakos, A. Krompa, E. Markozannes, and D. Bouros, "False positive COVID-19 antibody test in a case of granulomatosis with polyangiitis," *Frontiers in Medicine*, vol. 7, 2020.

[8] P. M. K. Lutalo and D. P. D'Cruz, "Diagnosis and classification of granulomatosis with polyangiitis (aka Wegener's granulomatosis)," *Journal of Autoimmunity*, vol. 48-49, pp. 94–98, 2014.

[9] N. Nasir, S. A. Ali, and H. M. Mehmood Riaz, "Cutaneous ulcers as initial presentation of localized granulomatosis with polyangiitis: a case report and review of the literature," *Case Reports in Rheumatology*, vol. 2015, Article ID 517025, 7 pages, 2015.

[10] S. Akiyama, S. Hamdeh, D. Micic, and A. Sakuraba, "Prevalence and clinical outcomes of COVID-19 in patients with autoimmune diseases: a systematic review and meta-analysis," *Annals of the Rheumatic Diseases*, vol. 2020, Article ID 218946, 2020.

[11] O. Zahedi Niaki, M. J. Anadkat, S. T. Chen et al., "Navigating immunosuppression in a pandemic: a guide for the dermatologist from the COVID task force of the medical dermatology society and society of dermatology hospitalists," *Journal of the American Academy of Dermatology*, vol. 83, no. 4, p. 1150, 2020.

[12] Z. E. Holcomb, M. R. Santillan, P. C. Morss-Walton et al., "Risk of COVID-19 in dermatologic patients receiving long-term immunomodulatory therapy," *Journal of the American Academy of Dermatology*, vol. 83, no. 4, pp. 1215–1218, 2020.

45

Enigmatic Rapidly Enlarging Nasal Mass that is not Cancer

Trilok Shrivastava,[1] Lin Li,[1] Sonia Tanwar,[1] Rabab Nasim,[1] Vincent Gullas,[1] Jay Pescatore,[1] and Michael Nelson[2]

[1]*Department of Internal Medicine, John H Stroger Hospital of Cook County, Chicago, IL, USA*
[2]*Emergency Department, John H Stroger Hospital of Cook County, Chicago, IL, USA*

Correspondence should be addressed to Trilok Shrivastava; trilok.shrivastava@cookcountyhhs.org

Academic Editor: Sergio A. Cuevas Covarrubias

Cutaneous blastomycosis is not rare, but progressively enlarging nasal mass as the only presentation with nondiagnostic biopsy results, presence of pulmonary fibrosis, nodules and lymphadenopathy, and urinary sediments, as well as ANA and p-ANCA positivity, can make things more cryptic than expected.

1. Introduction

A variety of conditions can lead to deforming skin lesions involving the nose which include granulomatous diseases, vasculitides, fungal infections, atypical bacteria, and neoplasms, but only a few can be rapidly progressing and have systemic involvement. In this report, we present an elderly Hispanic lady who lives in Chicago, Illinois, with no recent travel history presenting with a distorting nasal mass that had been enlarging over a duration of 4 months and accelerated over a period of 2 weeks. She was also found to have left submandibular lymphadenopathy, bilateral pulmonary nodules, hilar and mediastinal lymphadenopathy, and fibrotic pulmonary opacities. The course of investigation was some-what twisted with ANA and p-ANCA positivity, and initial punch biopsy of primary nasal mass was unrevealing but subsequent biopsy being able to demonstrate findings consistent with Blastomyces, reinforced by positive urine Blastomyces antigen.

Blastomycosis is a systemic granulomatous disease caused in majority by *Blastomyces dermatitidis* and *Blastomyces gilchristii* which are dimorphic fungi endemic to North American regions close to Mississippi and Ohio River basins, the Great Lakes, and St. Lawrence River. Transmission is through inhalation of aerosolized conidia leading to a wide range of system involvement [1, 2]. While a majority of cases present with respiratory problems, there have been quite a few presentations with primary extrapulmonary manifestations causing diagnostic dilemma [3–6].

2. Case History and Examination

A 69-year-old lady with a past medical history of diabetes, hypertension, stage-4 chronic kidney disease, and systolic heart failure presented with a rapidly growing nasal mass over a period of 4 months that started out as a pimple which ruptured and started to grow from the nasal bridge up to the tip of nose along columella interiorly into her left nasal cavity. She denied pain, fever, cough, dyspnea, gastrointestinal symptoms, chest pain, visual abnormalities, hematuria, or recent travel. During her admission 3 months back for an episode of decompensated heart failure, the mass was noted to be small, so she was referred to an ENT clinic where a superficial biopsy was done. The histopathology result was nondiagnostic showing squamous mucosa with pseudoepitheliomatous hyperplasia along with acute and chronic inflammatory changes. After this biopsy, the mass enlarged rapidly causing nasal congestion and runny nose, and the patient was admitted to the hospital for further evaluation of the mass. Patient was afebrile throughout admission, and her hemodynamics were stable. Examination showed a large exophytic left nasal mass involving the nasal bridge, columella, ala, philtrum with crusting, areas of hemorrhage, and a few pustules. Left nostril was almost completely occluded during the end of her hospital admission. There was also a 2 cm mobile mildly tender left submandibular lymphadenopathy. Lung exam was unremarkable (Figures 1 and 2).

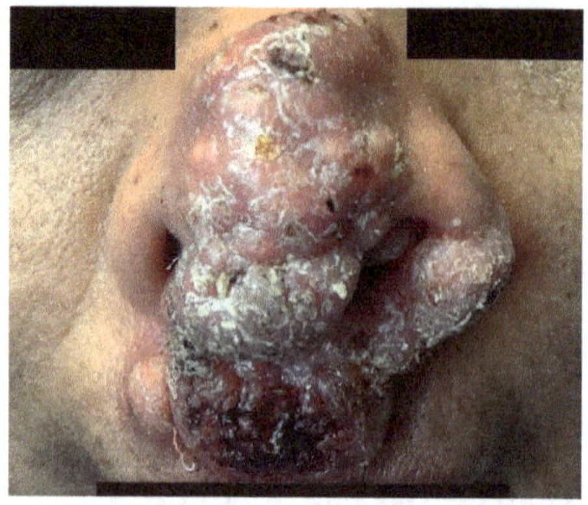

Figure 1: Nasal mass during admission showing involvement of left ala, nasal bridge, columella, philtrum and left nasal cavity with irregular scaly micronodular lesion with pustules, and areas of hemorrhage.

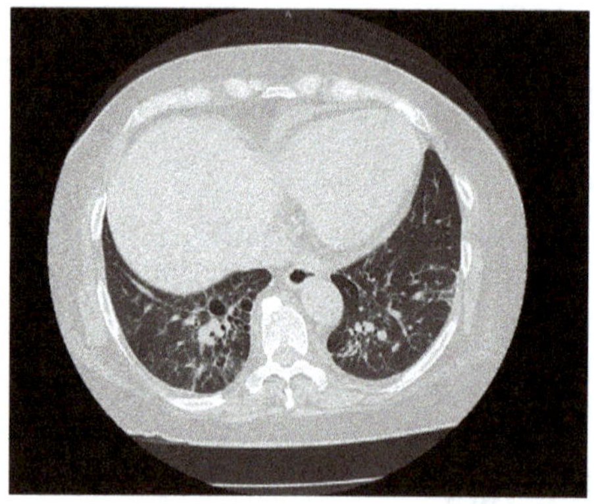

Figure 2: CT chest showing fibrotic parenchyma of both lungs more on the right side with nodules.

2.1. Differential Diagnosis, Investigations, and Treatment. CT neck confirmed the examination findings and also demonstrated inferior nasal turbinate connection of the mass, while CT of the chest showed bilateral pulmonary nodules, bilateral fibrotic opacities, pleural thickening of bilateral pleura, fibrocystic changes of the right lower lobe of the lung, and posterior mediastinal and probable hilar lymphadenopathy. A repeat biopsy of the nasal lesion was again inconclusive demonstrating nonspecific chronic inflammation, fibrosis, and suppurative necrosis. Special stains were negative for fungal infections and acid-fast bacilli. During this time, the differential diagnoses were granulomatous and inflammatory diseases such as sarcoidosis, small vessel vasculitis viz. granulomatosis with polyangiitis, tuberculosis, atypical fungal infections such as rhinosporidiosis, histoplasmosis, blastomycosis, and malignancy; therefore, multidisciplinary discussion was done involving pulmonology, rheumatology, ENT, infectious disease, nephrology, dermatology, and cardiology. On laboratory evaluation, she was noted to have chronic stable anemia with normal white counts, and liver profile was normal except for mild hypoalbuminemia. Her autoimmune panel came back with positive antinuclear antibody (ANA) (<1 : 160) and myeloperoxidase antineutrophil cytoplasmic antibody (MPO-ANCA/p-ANCA) with a titer of 7.6 (ref.: <1). Anti-dsDNA, anti-Smith-Ab, anti-RNP, anti-SSA, and anti-SSB were negative, and C3 and C4 were within normal limits. ESR and CRP were elevated at 103 mm/hr and 8.6 mg/dl, respectively. Her previous urinalysis had few RBC casts, but recent urine was bland; therefore, renal biopsy was deferred. Three sputa smears for acid-fast bacilli, HIV and cryptococcal antigen, and hepatitis A, B, and C serologies were negative. Urine histoplasma and Blastomyces antigen were sent, but results are pending. The left nostril was packed with Merocel impregnated in dexamethasone, and the patient was covered with intravenous ampicillin-sulbactam for possible bacterial superinfection. Bronchoscopy with a biopsy of accessible hilar lymph node was considered, but patient refused the procedure; so, it was withheld. Therefore, a repeat biopsy of the nasal mass and submandibular lymph node was done, and the specimen was sent for special fungal stains, AFB cultures, and histopathology.

The patient was discharged with symptomatic care after the repeat punch biopsy of the nose and cervical lymph node with pending results. Urine antigen came back positive for both Histoplasma and Blastomyces antigens, and the third biopsy demonstrated noncaseating granulomatous inflammation with fungal elements that, on staining with periodic acid-Schiff (PAS) and Grocott-Gomori methenamine silver nitrate (GMS) stains, it showed large round to oval yeasts with double contour and single broad-based buds consistent with blastomycosis. Putting together her clinical picture and laboratory findings, she was diagnosed to have disseminated blastomycosis.

2.2. Outcome and Follow-Up. The patient is being readmitted for systemic antifungal therapy.

3. Discussion

Blastomycosis can present with a wide range of symptoms, and cutaneous manifestations are common representing 40–80% of the cases subdivided into verrucous and ulcerative forms; cases presenting with facial verrucous plaques have been reported [2, 3, 7–9].

What made this case difficult to diagnose was the paucity as well as diversity of pathognomic dermatological findings to any disease; initially, negative biopsy result and positive ANA & MPO-ANCA diverted it towards a vasculitic process, reinforced by presence of RBC casts in one of her previous urinalyses. While granulomatosis with polyangiitis (GPA) is typically associated with c-ANCA/PR3-ANCA, nearly 20% have MPO-ANCA, although the nasal dermatological findings are usually limited to nasal crusting, saddle nose deformity, septal perforation, and sanguineous nasal discharge in these patients and not as extensive as those seen in our patient [10, 11].

Sarcoidosis was another consideration in this patient given her pulmonary nodules, hilar and mediastinal lymphadenopathy, and fibrocystic changes of pulmonary parenchyma. Had the patient allowed bronchoscopy with bronchoalveolar lavage and transbronchial lymph node biopsy, we might have excluded sarcoidosis if the CD4/CD8 ratio was <1 : 1, but if we only found noncaseating granuloma with the ratio in between 1 : 1–4 : 1, it would still be indeterminate, but fungal stains might have still been of essence in that case [12, 13].

Up to 30% of facial basal cell carcinomas (BCC) are found in the nose, and they can invade and obliterate the neighboring anatomy [14]. Squamous cell carcinoma (SCC) is much less common to involve the nose, although possible, and among them, most neoplasms are keratinizing squamous cell carcinomas that usually originate from the sinonasal tract [15]. There has also been a report of lung cancer metastasizing to the nose with "clown nose" as the presenting symptom [16]. However, three sets of biopsies were done in this patient which ruled out any of these malignancies.

Interestingly, the initial skin biopsy results in our patient were similar to the findings in few other reported cases of cutaneous blastomycosis which also displayed pseudoepitheliomatous hyperplasia, an entity that itself represents inflammatory, infectious, and neoplastic conditions [9, 17, 18]. The American Society of Microbiology recommends searching for yeast forms in the biopsy specimens with GMS staining to diagnose blastomycosis, which in fact helped to discover the broad-based buds of Blastomyces in our patient [2]. Her urine antigen positivity for Histoplasma most likely accounts for the cross-reactivity among these two pathogens, which occurs in about 70% of cases [19].

The Infectious Disease Society of America (IDSA) recommends to treat patients with moderate-severe disseminated extrapulmonary blastomycosis as our patient with lipophilic amphotericin B for 1-2 weeks or until clinical improvement that must be followed by oral itraconazole at a tapering-maintenance dose for a total duration of 12 months [20].

References

[1] E. M. Brown, L. R. McTaggart, S. X. Zhang, D. E. Low, D. A. Stevens, and S. E. Richardson, "Phylogenetic analysis reveals a cryptic species *Blastomyces gilchristii*, sp. nov. within the human pathogenic fungus Blastomyces dermatitidis," *PLoS One*, vol. 8, no. 3, Article ID e59237, 2013.

[2] M. Saccente and G. L. Woods, "Clinical and laboratory update on blastomycosis," *Clinical Microbiology Reviews*, vol. 23, no. 2, pp. 367–381, 2010.

[3] A. R. Kuzel, M. U. Lodhi, I. A. Syed et al., "Cutaneous, intranasal blastomycosis infection in two patients from southern West Virginia: diagnostic dilemma," *Cureus*, vol. 10, no. 1, Article ID e2095, 2018.

[4] N. Güler, A. Palanduz, Ü. Önş et al., "Progressive vertebral blastomycosis mimicking tuberculosis," *The Pediatric Infectious Disease Journal*, vol. 14, no. 9, pp. 816–818, 1995.

[5] F. S. Albarillo, G. T. Varma, and S. P. MacLeod, "Mandibular blastomycosis: a case report and review of the literature," *Germs*, vol. 8, no. 4, pp. 207–213, 2018.

[6] S. W. Chapman, A. C. Lin, K. A. Hendricks et al., "Endemic blastomycosis in Mississippi: epidemiological and clinical studies," *Seminars in Respiratory Infections*, vol. 12, no. 3, pp. 219–228, 1997.

[7] S. G. Kapnadak and A. Vinayak, "A case of disseminated blastomycosis presenting as intramuscular abscess," *Respiratory Medicine CME*, vol. 4, no. 1, pp. 9–11, 2011.

[8] J. A. McBride, G. M. Gauthier, and B. S. Klein, "Clinical manifestations and treatment of blastomycosis," *Clinics in Chest Medicine*, vol. 38, no. 3, pp. 435–449, 2017.

[9] A. G. Ortega-Loayza and T. Nguyen, "Cutaneous blastomycosis: a clue to a systemic disease," *Anais Brasileiros de Dermatologia*, vol. 88, no. 2, pp. 287–289, 2013.

[10] R. J. Falk and J. C. Jennette, "ANCA small-vessel vasculitis," *Journal of the American Society of Nephrology*, vol. 8, no. 2, pp. 314–322, 1997.

[11] S. B. Cannady, P. S. Batra, C. Koening et al., "Sinonasal Wegener granulomatosis: a single-institution experience with 120 cases," *The Laryngoscope*, vol. 119, no. 4, pp. 757–761, 2009.

[12] R. H. Winterbauer, J. Lammert, M. Sellami, R. Wu, D. Corley, and S. C. Springmeyer, "Bronchoalveolar lavage cell populations in the diagnosis of sarcoidosis," *Chest*, vol. 104, no. 2, pp. 352–361, 1993.

[13] S. P. Kantrow, K. C. Meyer, P. Kidd, and G. Raghu, "The CD4/CD8 ratio in BAL fluid is highly variable in sarcoidosis," *European Respiratory Journal*, vol. 10, no. 12, pp. 2716–2721, 1997.

[14] U. Wollina, D. Langner, and A. Bennewitz, "Basal cell carcinoma of the outer nose: overview on surgical techniques and analysis of 312 patients," *Journal of Cutaneous and Aesthetic Surgery*, vol. 7, no. 3, pp. 143–150, 2014.

[15] J. S. Lewis Jr., "Sinonasal squamous cell carcinoma: a review with emphasis on emerging histologic subtypes and the role of human papillomavirus," *Head and Neck Pathology*, vol. 10, no. 1, pp. 60–67, 2016.

[16] J. Marcoval, L. Martínez-Molina, M. Bonfill-Ortí, and F. Valentí-Medina, "Clown nose as first manifestation of squamous cell carcinoma of the lung," *Journal of Dermatological Case Reports*, vol. 11, no. 1, pp. 9–11, 2017.

[17] M. Zayour and R. Lazova, "Pseudoepitheliomatous hyperplasia: a review," *The American Journal of Dermatopathology*, vol. 33, no. 2, pp. 112–122, 2011.

[18] N. A. Gray and L. M. Baddour, "Major article: cutaneous inoculation blastomycosis," *Clinical Infectious Diseases*, vol. 34, no. 10, pp. e44–e49, 2002.

[19] P. A. Connolly, M. M. Durkin, A. M. Lemonte, E. J. Hackett, and L. J. Wheat, "Detection of histoplasma antigen by a quantitative enzyme immunoassay," *Clinical and Vaccine Immunology*, vol. 14, no. 12, pp. 1587–1591, 2007.

[20] S. W. Chapman, W. E. Dismukes, L. A. Proia et al., "Clinical practice guidelines for the management of blastomycosis: 2008 update by the infectious diseases society of America," *Clinical Infectious Diseases*, vol. 46, no. 12, pp. 1801–1812, 2008.

Aggressive Acute Marjolin's Ulcer Arising in a Burn Scar

Adela Alvarez Rio, Josep Oriol Roca Mas, Daniel Navarro Sanchez, Ivan Monge Castresana, Gonzalo Joaquin Soroa Moreno, and Jaime Estrada Cuxart

Plastic & Reconstructive Surgery, Hospital Universitario Son Espases, Palma de Mallorca, Spain

Correspondence should be addressed to Adela Alvarez Rio; mariade291@gmail.com

Academic Editor: Sergio A. Cuevas Covarrubias

Marjolin's ulcer is one of the clinical variants of squamous-cell carcinoma. It is a highly aggressive disease that develops from chronic wounds. Almost 65% of these lesions have been diagnosed on underlying burn scars. Although the mean latency time between the primary lesion and the apparition of the ulcer is around 25 years, some cases with an early debut have been described. Squamous-cell carcinomas arising in chronic wounds are typically aggressive and are related with a poor prognosis due to their late diagnosis. Therefore, it is important to recognize symptoms that indicate malignant degeneration of chronic wounds, allowing the clinician to make an early diagnosis in order not to delay the surgical treatment that is required to improve the global survival of the patient. The time elapsed between our patient's burn and the appearance of Marjolin's ulcer was only 7 months, drawing attention to its fast and aggressive progression.

1. Introduction

Squamous-cell carcinoma is a malignant tumour developed from epidermal keratinocytes. A skin biopsy is always required to confirm the diagnosis. Among its clinical variants, we can find Marjolin's ulcer.

Marjolin's ulcer, described for the first time in 1963 by French surgeon Jean-Nicholas Marjolin [1], is considered a highly aggressive disease that develops from chronic wounds and skin scars. Almost 65% of these ulcers have been diagnosed on underlying burn scars, raising the malignancy degeneration rate of a burn to 1.5% [2].

Although other entities have been related with Marjolin's ulcer, the most frequently described histology has always been squamous-cell carcinoma, with rates around 71% [3].

Malignant degeneration is usually slow. Albeit the mean latency time between the primary lesion and the onset of the ulcer is around 25 years, some cases with an exceptionally early debut have been described, with a latency time of around 2 years [2]. Marjolin's ulcers can therefore be described as acute if they appear in the first 12 months since the primary lesion or as chronic if they appear in the posterior 12 months, the latter being the majority [3]. All of these facts indicate that the earlier the primary lesion appears, the more the likelihood of developing this pathology over time.

Squamous-cell carcinomas developed on chronic wounds are typically aggressive and are related with a poor prognosis due to the confusion with a classic wound and the delay in its diagnosis [4].

In our case report, the latency time between our patient's burn and the appearance of Marjolin's ulcer was of only 7 months, drawing attention to its fast and aggressive progression, despite the usually slow development of this disease, as previously described.

2. Case Report

A 48-year-old male patient, on chronic opioid treatment for multiple disc hernias, consulted the emergency room about an extensive 7-month-evolution thermic burn in the dorsum that has presented a torpid evolution.

He presents a large, exophytic, malodorous ulcerated lesion on the back with an approximate length of 15 × 10 cm. In the physical exploration, there are palpable lymph nodes in the left groin, without other alteration. The patient refers to a dermal burn 7 months ago that has worsened gradually despite multiple antibiotic treatments and local dressings with all kinds of antiseptics and bactericides in his primary care centre given by different medical teams (Figure 1). He had never been sent to a specialised centre despite the bad local evolution.

During his stay in the emergency room, two biopsies of the lesion were taken. The histological results are described as moderately differentiated infiltrative squamous-cell carcinoma that invades deep reticular dermis.

Given the results of the biopsy, the case is exposed to the skin cancer committee, and a PET-CT scan is prescribed to complete the case study and get information about the spread of the disease. Results show pathological activity in the left groin and doubtful activity in the right axilla. A fine-needle puncture-aspiration assessment is performed on the right axilla, with negative results for malignancy.

The patient underwent surgery for the first time. We performed a wide resection of the primary tumour with 2 cm lateral margins and including deep lumbar fascia into the resection. A regulated left inguinal lymph node dissection was performed in the same surgery. The lumbar defect was reconstructed with meshed partial-thickness skin grafts.

Histological results evidenced a moderately differentiated infiltrative squamous-cell carcinoma with free surgical margins and a metastatic affectation in 6 out of the 14 lymph nodes extirpated. Postsurgery evolution was favourable, with the results after a 6-month follow-up shown in Figure 2.

7 months after diagnosis, during a routine check-up, 2 axillary lymph nodes become palpable. A new PET-CT scan is performed, and the progression of the disease is acknowledged as the images are positive for malignancy in that axilla (Figure 3).

A second surgery is performed two weeks later. A regulated right axillary lymph node dissection is accomplished. Results inform metastatic affectation in 7 out of 31 lymph nodes extirpated. Due to the aggressiveness of the disease, radiotherapy was elected as an adjuvant treatment for this patient.

6 months after the last surgery and as far as our follow-up has arrived, the patient still continues to be stable without any further progression of the disease either locally or systemically.

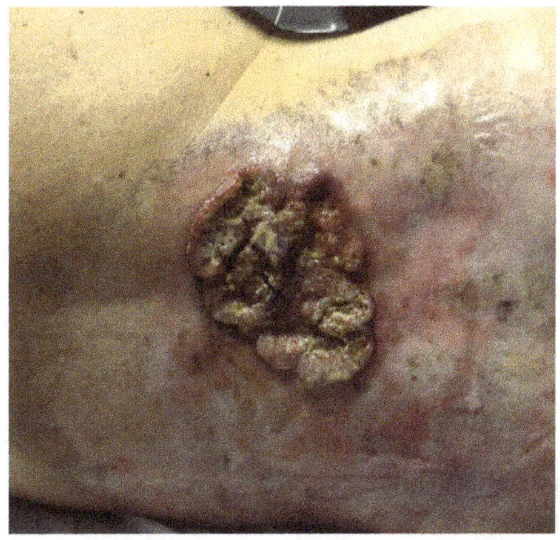

Figure 1: Exophytic ulcer 7-months after a thermic burn in the dorsal region. First patient visit to emergency department.

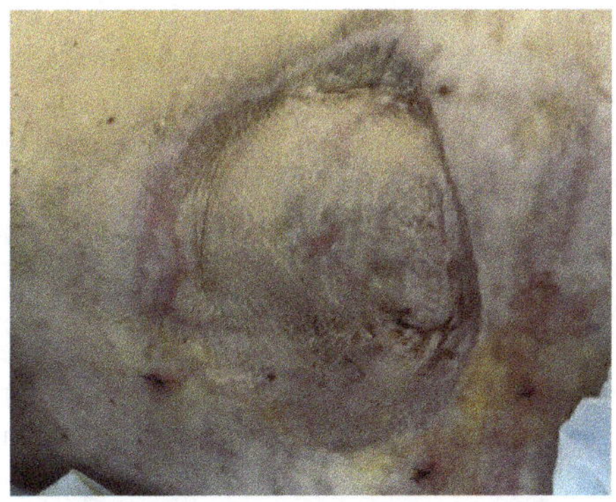

Figure 2: Dorsal region after wide surgical extirpation and reconstruction with meshed split-thickness skin grafts.

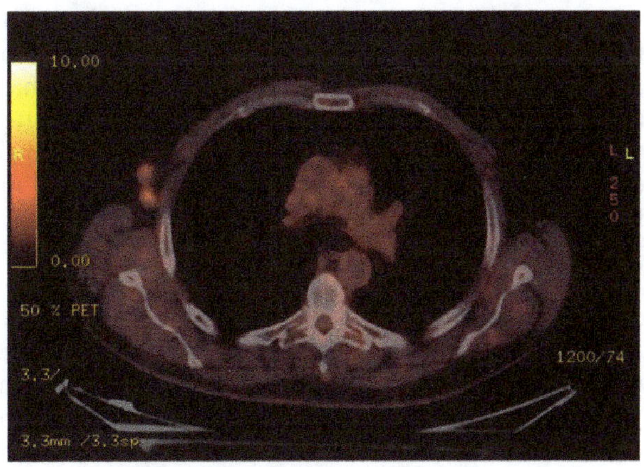

Figure 3: PET-CT scan 6 months after first diagnosis showing two metastasic lymph nodes in the right axilla.

3. Discussion

Malignant degeneration of a burn in the first 12 months since the acute lesion is something unusual. A review of the literature shows that the latency period between initial burn and subsequent malignancy can vary from 20 to 35 years, as shown in most series [5–7]. Xu et al. reported two Marjolin Ulcers arising over chronic foot wounds within 1 and 2 years, and Love RL presented one Marjolin's ulcer arising over a burn scar [8, 9]. There are very few cases with a very low number of patients reported in the literature about acute Marjolin's ulcers with such a fast development, even less about this disease over a recent burn scar, so describing new cases of this entity is important as it tends to be infra-diagnosed and therefore, infratreated [8–10].

In the majority of described cases of acute Marjolin's ulcer, the most frequently isolated histological variant has been basal-cell carcinoma, leading to a more favourable prognosis [11].

Even though Marjolin's ulcer pathogenesis is uncertain, its multifactorial origin is clear, and it is known that genetics and ambience can influence its development. Zones subjected to an acute lesion, such as the bed of a burn, suffer from constant inflammation, which could promote the activation of tumour cells that were already there and trigger DNA mutations [12]. Furthermore, an obliteration of the lymphatic vessels and a decrease in the blood flow accompany the primary lesion, limiting the local tissue's immunological ability to defend from aggressions.

These ulcers tend to be treated on an outpatient basis by different health care professionals who are usually untrained, are inexperienced, and lack diagnostic weapons with this kind of lesions. All of this leads to a delay in this pathology's diagnosis and treatment.

Consequently, all of this translates into a poor prognosis for this disease with a 21% global mortality rate [13]. Undoubtedly, histologic grade of the tumour and lymph node affectation in the moment of diagnosis are the most important prognosis factors. 3 years after diagnosis, the global survival of patients with Marjolin's ulcer is from 65 to 75%, numbers that descend to 35–50% if there is metastasis from the beginning [13].

Hence, it is very important to recognize signs and symptoms that denote a possible malignant degeneration in chronic wounds and burns so an early biopsy can be taken in order to establish the diagnosis as soon as possible.

Despite the fact that developing a Marjolin's ulcer a few months after a primary burn is not very common, if the ulceration is maintained chronically for longer than 3 months and malignancy indicators appear (such as bleeding, excessive pain, or severe exophytic granulation tissue), any clinician must take into account this diagnose and do not delay the biopsy of the lesion.

If a squamous-cell carcinoma is confirmed, due to its high aggressiveness, it is mandatory to start treatment as soon as possible with a radical extirpation with wide margins. An early staging has to be performed, and a regulated lymph node dissection or sentinel lymph node biopsy should be performed if required. Adjuvant chemotherapy and radiotherapy can be added if the case requires it [14].

4. Conclusion

A biopsy of any suspicious lesion should not be delayed even though little time has elapsed since the original burn. Alarm signs and symptoms must be searched for if the evolution of a wound, ulcer, or burn is torpid and more than 3 months have passed. A biopsy should be taken without delay in order to confirm the diagnosis and start medical treatment.

An ample surgical removal must be performed, accompanied by lymph node dissection or sentinel lymph node biopsy when required. After the surgery, every patient should be closely followed up to watch over possible relapses or metastases that can appear.

We want to emphasise in this report the importance of this forgotten entity and remark that, even when the onset is acute, it should be taken into account due to its aggressiveness and fatal consequences if the diagnosis is delayed.

References

[1] A. H. Cruickshank, E. M. McConnell, and D. G. Miller, "Malignancy in scars, chronic ulcers, and sinuses," *Journal of Clinical Pathology*, vol. 16, no. 6, pp. 573–580, 1963.

[2] B. Pekarek, S. Buck, and L. Osher, "A comprehensive review on Marjolin's ulcers: diagnosis and treatment," *The Journal of the American College of Certified Wound Specialists*, vol. 3, no. 3, pp. 60–64, 2011.

[3] C. Tobin and J. R. Sanger, "Marjolin's ulcers: a case series and literature review," *Wounds*, vol. 26, no. 8, pp. 248–254, 2014.

[4] S. M. Al-Zacko, "Malignancy in chronic burn scar: a 20 year experience in Mosul-Iraq," *Burns*, vol. 39, no. 7, pp. 1488–1491, 2013.

[5] F. M. Iqbal, Y. Sinha, and W. Jaffe, "Marjolin's ulcer: a rare entity with a call for early diagnosis," *BMJ Case Reports*, vol. 2015, Article ID bcr2014208176, 2015.

[6] R. Choa, S. Rayatt, and K. Mahtani, "Marjolin's ulcer," *BMJ*, vol. 351, Article ID h3997, 2015.

[7] M. A. Kerr-Valentic, K. Samimi, B. H. Rohlen, J. P. Agarwal, and W. B. Rockwell, "Marjolin's ulcer: modern analysis of an ancient problem," *Plastic and Reconstructive Surgery*, vol. 123, no. 1, pp. 184–191, 2009.

[8] S. Xu, Y. Kang, H. Soeharno, and N. Yeo, "Acute Marjolin's ulcer in chronic foot wounds with previous negative biopsy: report of two cases," *Malaysian Orthopaedic Journal*, vol. 14, no. 3, pp. 194–197, 2020.

[9] J. S. Hammond, S. Thomsen, and C. G. Ward, "Scar carcinoma arising acutely in a skin graft donor site," *The Journal of Trauma, Injury, Infection, and Critical Care*, vol. 27, no. 6, pp. 681–683, 1987.

[10] R. L. Love and A. F. Breidahl, "Acute squamous cell carcinoma arising within a recent burn scar in a 14-year-old boy," *Plastic and Reconstructive Surgery*, vol. 106, no. 5, pp. 1069–1071, 2000.

[11] L. J. Gaughan, J. R. Bergeron, and J. F. Mullins, "Giant basal cell epithelioma developing in acute burn site," *Archives of Dermatology*, vol. 99, no. 5, pp. 594-595, 1969.

[12] M. D. Fleming, J. L. Hunt, G. F. Purdue, and J. Sandstad, "Marjloin's ulcer: a review and reevaluation of a difficult problem," *Journal of Burn Care & Rehabilitation*, vol. 11, no. 5, pp. 460–469, 1990.

[13] M. Saaiq and B. Ashraf, "Marjolin's ulcers in the post-burned lesions and scars," *World Journal of Clinical Cases*, vol. 2, no. 10, pp. 507–514, 2014.

[14] E. Aydogdu, S. Yildirim, and T. Aköz, "Is surgery an effective and adequate treatment in advanced Marjolin's ulcer?" *Burns*, vol. 31, no. 4, pp. 421–431, 2005.

47

Multiple Xanthogranulomas in an Adult Patient with Myelodysplastic Syndrome

Marta Martínez-García,[1] Nicolás Silvestre-Torner,[1] Antonio Aguilar-Martínez,[1] and Fernando Burgos-Lázaro[2]

[1]*Dermatology Service, Severo Ochoa University Hospital, Leganés, Madrid, Spain*
[2]*Pathological Anatomy Service, Severo Ochoa University Hospital, Leganés, Madrid, Spain*

Correspondence should be addressed to Marta Martínez-García; martamgml@yahoo.es

Academic Editor: Sergio A. Cuevas Covarrubias

Adult multiple xanthogranuloma (XG) is a rare late-onset variant of juvenile XG. It is characterized by the appearance of papules or nodules located preferably on the trunk. A case of a 54-year-old man with myelodysplastic syndrome is presented as a history of interest, who consulted due to the appearance of multiple brownish papules distributed mainly in the trunk. So far, there are only 22 cases of this clinical form reported in the literature, 9 of them associated with malignant hematological processes. We highlight the importance of this entity as a possible cutaneous marker of blood dyscrasias.

1. Introduction

Xanthogranuloma (XG) is the most common form of clinical presentation of non-Langerhans cell histiocytosis. Although it can appear at any time of life, XG usually occurs in pediatric age and generally as a single lesion. The appearance of XG in adult patients is very rare and usually occurs in the form of multiple lesions. The association of XG with different blood dyscrasias has been documented both in the juvenile form and in the adult form, although in the latter in a more isolated way.

2. Case Presentation

A 54-year-old male came to the consultation with a 1-year history of clinical history indicating the appearance, spontaneously, of multiple skin lesions distributed on the trunk. The lesions showed a progressive increase in number and size and were not associated with local symptoms. In the personal history, the presence of a myelodysplastic syndrome with low-risk unilinear IPSS-R dysplasia, with an IDH 1 mutation, diagnosed 3 years ago for which he maintained periodic control without treatment, stood out.

A dermatological examination revealed multiple papules between 3 and 5 millimeters in size, yellow-brown in color, distributed mainly in the trunk (Figure 1). The rest of the skin examination showed no data of interest. A histological study was performed that showed dermal occupation by mixed proliferation with elongated cells and multinucleated histiocytic-like cells of large eosinophilic cytoplasms with mild lymphocyte response. No significant atypia, mitosis, or necrosis was observed (Figure 2). The immunohistochemical study showed positivity for histiocytic markers CD 68 (Figure 3), vimentin (Figure 4), and alpha1 antitrypsin (Figure 5) and negativity for S-100, CD1a, factor XIIIa, and cytokeratins.

The hematological study carried out included bone marrow cytology with discrete hypocellularity with dysplasia in 39% of the granulocytic series. Nucleus-cytoplasmic maturation asynchrony was observed in the red series. No increase in the number of blasts was observed. In bone marrow cytometry, hypogranularity was observed in the

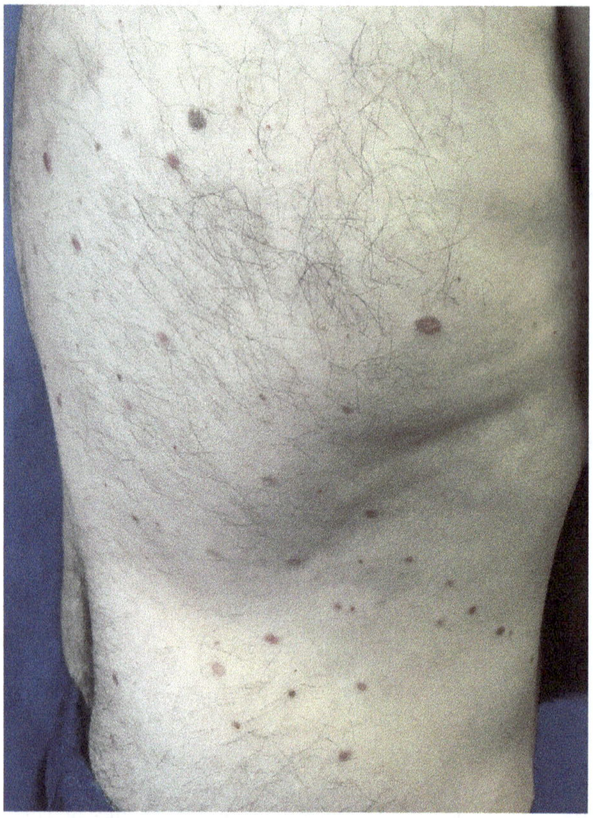

FIGURE 1: Multiple yellow-brown papules in the trunk.

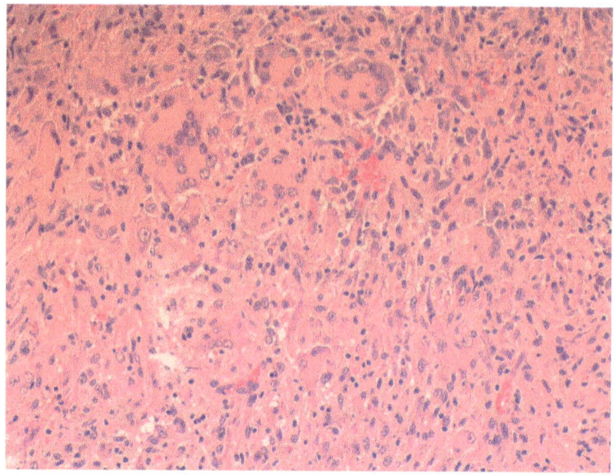

FIGURE 2: Mixed proliferation with elongated cells and multinucleated histiocytic-like cells of large eosinophilic cytoplasms with mild lymphocyte response (H-E ×20).

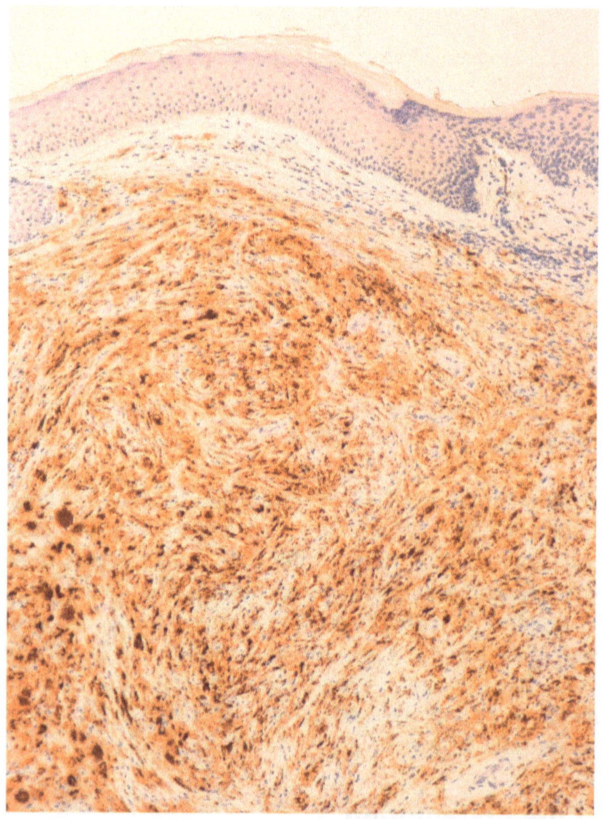

FIGURE 3: Positivity for histiocytic markers CD 68 (×10).

granulocytic series without excess blasts. The following IDH1, TET2, and KMT2A mutations were found in the NGS molecular biology study.

The patient maintains periodic dermatological and hematological control. The skin lesions remained stable, and no type of treatment has been performed.

3. Discussion

XG usually appears in children, mainly in the first year of life, although it can appear at any time of life. The usual form of presentation is a single papule or nodule usually located on the head or neck. The appearance of XG in adults is infrequent, with only 22 cases described in the literature [1–8], being the usual presentation in these cases the multiple forms (10 or more lesions) that are preferably located on the trunk.

Histologically, the findings are similar in both the juvenile and adult forms [9]. A dense foam cell, giant cell, Touton cell, lymphocyte, and eosinophil infiltrate located at the level of the reticular dermis with extension to subcutaneous cell tissue are observed. Immunohistochemistry is positive for macrophage markers such as CD68, HAM56, and factor XIIIa. Negativity for CD 1a and S-100 allows them to be differentiated from Langerhans cell histiocytosis [10–12].

In most patients, XG lesions are located exclusively at the cutaneous level, but the presence of extracutaneous lesions have been described in both juvenile and adult forms [13], with the eyeball being the most frequently affected organ. The association between juvenile XG, neurofibromatosis type 1, and chronic myeloid juvenile leukemia (CMJL) has been documented with approximately 20 patients reported in the literature [14]. A risk of developing CMJL of 0.4%–1.6% has been estimated in children with neurofibromatosis type 1 and juvenile XG [15, 16].

In adult onset forms, association with blood dyscrasias has been described in a total of 9 patients and includes follicular lymphoma, essential thrombocytosis, chronic

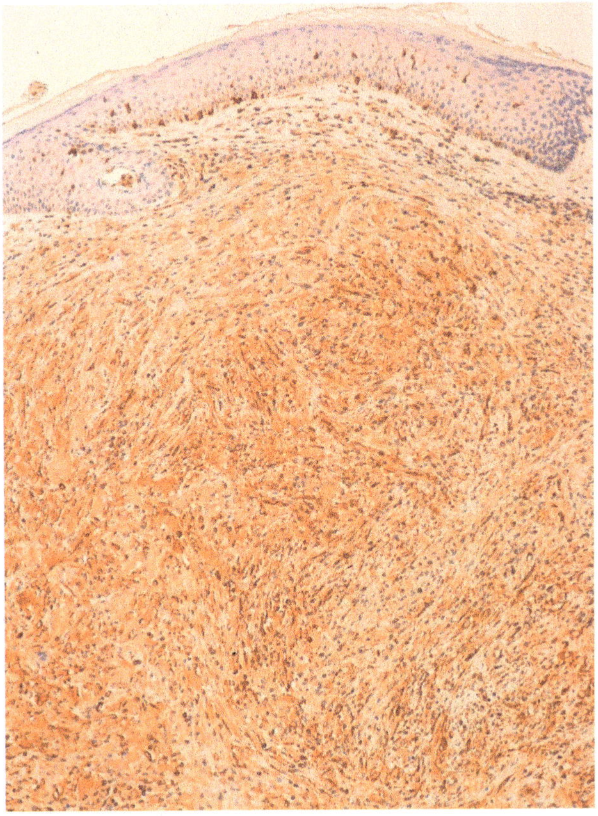

FIGURE 4: Positivity for vimentin (×10).

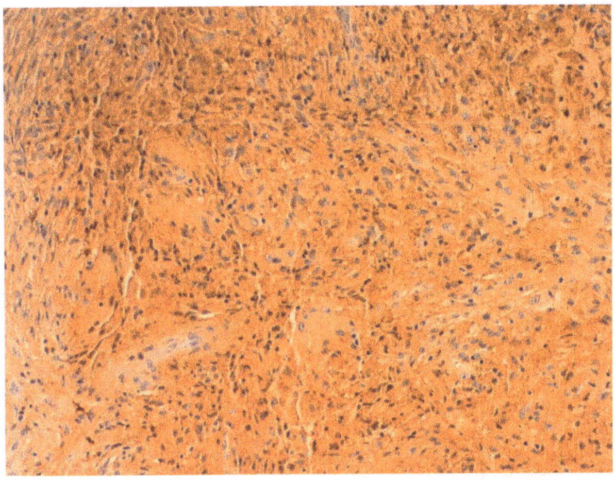

FIGURE 5: Positivity for alpha1 antitrypsin (×20).

lymphatic leukemia B, acute lymphatic leukemia B, large-cell lymphoma b, monoclonal gammopathy, adult T lymphoma/leukemia, and a single patient with myelodysplastic syndrome [3, 4, 6–8, 17, 18]. A case associated with a solid organ tumor has also been documented [19]. We must emphasize that all the patients presented multiple XG and that the development of the cutaneous lesions took place before, during, or after the hematological process. The etiopathogenic mechanism that would justify this association is unknown. Anomalous proliferation of histiocytes from a bone marrow CD 34+ precursor that would be activated against different stimuli such as the induction of cytokines or gammaglobulins produced by the underlying tumor process has been suggested [4, 6, 20–22].

The evolution is usually towards spontaneous regression, less frequently in adults and in multiple forms [12]. In cases associated with blood dyscrasias, a tendency to regression has been observed when treating neoplasia [19]. There is no specific treatment for XG. In most cases, an expectant attitude is recommended, although CO_2 laser, simple excision, and cryotherapy have been used.

Due to the low number of published cases, there is no agreement on the management of XG in adults, although it seems advisable to perform a physical examination together with a periodic hematological study.

In conclusion, we highlight the importance of recognizing these forms of multiple XG in adults as a possible marker of blood dyscrasias, describing a case of multiple XG in an adult patient associated with myelodysplastic syndrome.

References

[1] N. Saad, F. Skowron, S. Dalle, J.-Y. Forestier, B. balme, and L. Thomas, "Multiple adult xanthogranuloma: case report and literature review," *Dermatology*, vol. 212, no. 1, pp. 73–76, 2006.

[2] A. Arun, B. Naskar, P. C. Mondal, and M. Pal, "Multiple generalised xanthogranuloma in adult: case report and treatment," *Indian Journal of Dermatology*, vol. 56, pp. 197–199, 2011.

[3] B. Narváez-Moreno, Á. Pulpillo-Ruiz, T. De Zulueta-Dorado, and J. Conejo-Mir, "Disseminated juvenile xanthogranuloma associated with follicular lymphoma in an adult: successful treatment with chemotherapy and rituximab. A review of the literature," *Actas Dermo-Sifiliográficas (English Edition)*, vol. 104, no. 3, pp. 242–246, 2013.

[4] C.-C. Chiou, P.-N. Wang, L.-C. Yang, T.-T. Kuo, and H.-S. Hong, "Disseminated xanthogranulomas associated with adult T-Cell leukaemia/lymphoma: a case report and review the association of haematologic malignancies," *Journal of the European Academy of Dermatology and Venereology*, vol. 21, pp. 532–535, 2007.

[5] P. Navajas, I. Eguino, O. Trébol, J. Lasa et al., "Multiple adul xanthogranuloma," *Actas Dermosifiliogr*, vol. 96, pp. 171–174, 2005.

[6] A. Biswas, B. Hamid, S. E. Coupland, A. Franks, and N. Leonard, "Multiple periocular adult onset xanthogranulomas in a patient with chronic lymphocytic leukaemia," *European Journal of Dermatology*, vol. 20, pp. 211–213, 2010.

[7] M. J. Larson, C. Bandel, P. J. Eichhorn, and P. D. Cruz Jr., "Concurrent development of eruptive xanthogranulomas and hematologic malignancy: two case reports," *Journal of the American Academy of Dermatology*, vol. 50, no. 6, pp. 976–978, 2004.

[8] G. M. Pino, F. J. Miquel, M. Velasco, J. J. Vilata, and A. Aliaga, "Multiple xanthogranulomas in an adult, associated with essential thrombocytosis," *British Journal of Dermatology*, vol. 132, pp. 1018–1021, 1995.

[9] S.-E. Chang, S. Cho, J.-C. Choi et al., "Clinicohistopathologic comparison of adult type and juvenile type xanthogranulomas

in korea," *The Journal of Dermatology*, vol. 28, no. 8, pp. 413–418, 2001.

[10] A. Hernandez-Martin, E. Baselga, B. A. Drolet, and N. B. Esterly, "Juvenile xanthogranuloma," *Journal of the American Academy of Dermatology*, vol. 36, no. 3, pp. 355–367, 1997.

[11] M. W. Chang, "Update on juvenile xanthogranuloma: unusual cutaneous and systemic variants," *Seminars in Cutaneous Medicine and Surgery*, vol. 18, no. 3, pp. 195–205, 1999.

[12] L. P. Dehner, "Juvenile xanthogranulomas in the first two decades of life: a clinicopathologic study of 174 cases with cutaneous and extracutaneous manifestations," *The American Journal of Surgical Pathology*, vol. 27, no. 5, pp. 579–593, 2003.

[13] E. Cham, D. Siegel, and B. S. Ruben, "Cutaneous xanthogranulomas, hepatosplenomegaly, anemia, and thrombocytopenia as presenting signs of juvenile myelomonocytic leukemia," *American Journal of Clinical Dermatology*, vol. 11, no. 1, pp. 67–71, 2010.

[14] S. Paulus, S. Koronowska, and R. Fölster-Holst, "Association between juvenile myelomonocytic leukemia, juvenile xanthogranulomas and neurofibromatosis type 1: case report and review of the literature," *Pediatric Dermatology*, vol. 34, no. 2, pp. 114–118, 2017.

[15] W. H. C. Burgdorf and B. Zelger, "JXG, NF1, and JMML: alphabet soup or a clinical issue?" *Pediatric Dermatology*, vol. 21, no. 2, pp. 174–176, 2004.

[16] A. Zvulunov, Y. Barak, and A. Metzker, "Juvenile xanthogranuloma, neurofibromatosis, and juvenile chronic myelogenous leukemia: world statistical analysis," *Archives of Dermatology*, vol. 131, no. 8, pp. 904–908, 1995.

[17] T. Namiki, K. Miura, and H. Yokozeki, "Multiple CD163+adult xanthogranuloma associated with myelodysplastic syndrome," *The Journal of Dermatology*, vol. 42, no. 11, pp. 1106-1107, 2015.

[18] B. A. Shoo, K. Shinkai, T. H. McCalmont, and L. P. Fox, "Xanthogranulomas associated with hematologic malignancy in adulthood," *Journal of the American Academy of Dermatology*, vol. 59, no. 3, pp. 488–493, 2008.

[19] S. Vadeboncoeur and N. Provost, "Multiple xanthogranulomas in an adult: known entity, new association," *Journal of Cutaneous Medicine and Surgery*, vol. 20, no. 5, pp. 474–477, 2016.

[20] H. Sueki, T. Saito, M. Iijima, and R. Fujisawa, "Adult-onset xanthogranuloma appearing symmetrically on the ear lobes," *Journal of the American Academy of Dermatology*, vol. 32, no. 2, pp. 372–374, 1995.

[21] H. H. Balfour, C. E. Speicher, D. G. McReynolds, and M. E. Nesbit, "Juvenile xanthogranuloma associated with cytomegalovirus infection," *The American Journal of Medicine*, vol. 50, no. 3, pp. 380–384, 1971.

[22] S. Pérez-Gala, A. Torrelo, I. Colmenero, T. Contra, L. Madero, and A. Zambrano, "Juvenile multiple xanthogranuloma in a patient with Langerhans cell histiocytosis," *Actas Dermo-Sifiliográficas*, vol. 97, no. 9, pp. 594–598, 2006.

48

Perianal Basal Cell Carcinoma Successfully Managed with Excisional Biopsy

Paola C. Aldana[1] **Harris G. Yfantis,**[1,2] **and Preeti R. John**[1,2]

[1] *University of Maryland School of Medicine, Baltimore, MD, USA*
[2] *Baltimore Veterans Affairs Medical Center, Baltimore, MD, USA*

Correspondence should be addressed to Paola C. Aldana; paola.aldana@som.umaryland.edu

Academic Editor: Ioannis D. Bassukas

Basal cell carcinoma (BCC) is the most common cutaneous malignancy in the United States and is often nonaggressive. Its location in the perianal region is very rare and it is estimated that only 0.08% of all BCCs occur in this region. Herein, we present a case of perianal basal cell carcinoma, nodular type. The diagnosis was made using excisional biopsy of a skin lesion. Immunohistochemical staining confirmed the diagnosis: it showed diffuse and strong positivity for smooth muscle actin (SMA) and monoclonal antibody BER-Ep4 and was negative for carcinoembryonic antigen (CEA), pancytokeratin (AE1/AE3), and epithelial membrane antigen (EMA). The treatment of choice has traditionally been local excision to clear margins but the newest guidelines recommend Mohs Micrographic surgery (MMS) or standard 4mm surgical margins for this high-risk BCC. Our patient was successfully treated using excisional biopsy without recurrence. In select patients with lesions smaller than 1cm, excisional biopsy may be sufficient to treat the disease and may be better tolerated than MMS and wider surgical margins. Literature review suggests a predisposition for perianal BCC in individuals susceptible to cutaneous malignancies. Therefore, any history of cutaneous malignancy should further prompt clinicians to examine nonsun exposed areas on full body skin exams.

1. Introduction

Basal cell carcinoma (BCC) is the most common cutaneous malignancy in the United States and mostly frequently occurs on sun exposed areas such as the head and neck [1]. Although it can occur on other areas, involvement of the perianal skin and genitals is extremely rare [2]. It is estimated that perianal BCC accounts for only 0.08% of all BCC and 0.2% of all anorectal neoplasms [1, 3]. In fact, there are less than 200 cases of BCC on the perianal skin and genitals reported in the literature [1]. We present a case of nodular perianal BCC that was diagnosed using immunohistochemical staining, for which excisional biopsy was performed with no subsequent recurrence.

2. Case Presentation

An 89-year-old male with no history of cutaneous malignancies was referred to General Surgery for evaluation of a persistent nodule on the skin of the right perianal region that he had noticed for more than a year. Past medical history was significant for gastric lymphoma (non-Hodgkins follicular type, with spontaneous remission).

He palpated the perianal lesion while cleaning the skin in this region. The lesion was not associated with bleeding, oozing, pain, or itching. He denied any concomitant skin lesion or rashes. He also denied fever, chills, or abdominal symptoms. On physical exam, a single small 0.5 cm cutaneous nodule with central dimpling and no discoloration was visualized in the perianal region. No concerning lesions were palpated on digital rectal exam. An excisional biopsy of the nodule was performed for histopathological examination.

Microscopic exam confirmed the diagnosis of perianal BCC, nodular type (Figure 1(a)). Histopathology revealed a lesion strongly and diffusely positive for immunohistochemical staining of smooth muscle actin (SMA) (Figure 1(b)) and negative for carcinoembryonic antigen (CEA) and pancytokeratin (AE1/AE3), supporting the diagnosis. Staining for epithelial membrane antigen (EMA) was negative in the tumor cells while monoclonal antibody BER-Ep4 displayed

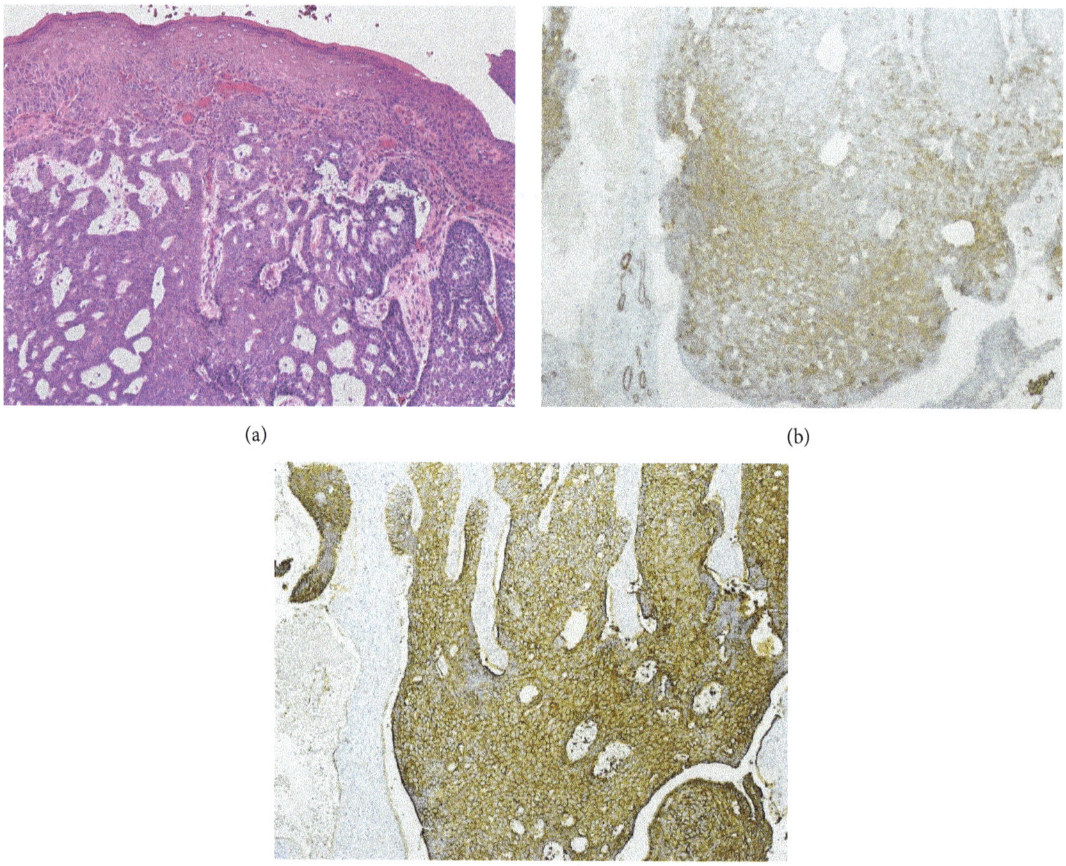

FIGURE 1: *Histopathological analysis of perianal nodule biopsy.* (a) Hematoxylin and Eosin (H&E) stain (original magnification 100x) showing anastomosing cords of basaloid cells with overlying connection to epidermis and stromal retraction. (b) Immunohistochemical staining for smooth muscle actin (original magnification 100x) showing diffuse, strong positivity. (c) Immunohistochemical staining for Ber-EP4 (original magnification 100x) showing diffuse, strong, membranous positivity.

strong and diffuse positivity, further supporting the diagnosis (Figure 1(c)). The patient responded well to excision of the lesion and no further treatment was required.

3. Discussion

Basal cell carcinoma of the perianal skin is a rare entity that is most frequently reported by individual case reports or case series. There is a male predominance and the mean age of onset is 67 years [4]. It may vary in its clinical presentation from erythematous papules and patches to nodules, plaques, and ulcers that may present with bleeding, pain, itching, and mucoid discharge [1, 5]. The majority of these lesions are smaller than 2cm and are located *outside* the anal verge [4]. This location may be useful in distinguishing perianal BCC from basaloid squamous cell carcinoma (BSCL). BSCL is a common anal tumor and most commonly occurs in the anal canal or anorectum (*inside* the anal verge) [6]. Although several subtypes of BCC exist, the nodular type is the most common in the perianal region [6].

The etiology of perianal BCC remains unknown; however chronic irritation, trauma, immunosuppressive medications, and radiation have been suggested as causative factors [1]. Although most patients with perianal BCC do not have a personal history of tanning bed use or nude sunbathing, approximately 1/3 have a history of skin cancer in sun exposed areas [1, 3]. This association suggests a predisposition in individuals susceptible to cutaneous malignancies. Therefore, any history of cutaneous malignancy should further prompt clinicians to examine nonsun exposed areas on full body skin exams. Furthermore, frequent BCC development has been associated with an increased overall cancer risk; therefore occurrence of BCC more than once in the same patient should prompt close surveillance for other malignancies (our patient had a history of gastric lymphoma) [7].

It is important to obtain histologic verification of the disease in order to distinguish it from more aggressive malignancies with higher capacity for metastasis such as BSCL. The classic histology of perianal BCC reveals peripheral palisading and peritumoral slits [4]. Immunohistochemical staining is also useful as perianal BCC usually displays diffuse and strong staining for SMA and Ber-EP4 [6, 8, 9], while BSCL does not [9]. Positive immunohistochemical reactivity with pancytokeratin, EMA, and CEA is not consistent with perianal BCC and may suggest a diagnosis of BSCL [9].

According to The National Comprehensive Cancer Network, a BCC in the perianal region is considered 'high-risk' and Mohs Micrographic surgery (MMS) is recommended, although standard 4mm margin excision can be considered for select tumors [10]. The treatment of choice for perianal BCC has traditionally been local excision to clear margins, especially for lesions that are less than 2cm [4]. Local excision has proven to be the extremely successful since there is usually no recurrence of disease [1, 4]. Larger lesions may require skin grafting for closure and only those involving the anal canal or extending into the surrounding tissues require abdominoperineal resection of the rectum [4, 5]. Our patient exhibited a lesion that was 0.5cm in size and excisional biopsy was sufficient treatment for his disease.

Since perianal BCC is so uncommon and is located in an inconspicuous skin area, it may be easily overlooked by clinicians. Therefore, we recommend that gluteal and genital areas be included in full body skin exams, particularly in higher risk individuals. Suspicious lesions should be biopsied and immunohistochemical staining performed to establish the diagnosis.

In summary, perianal BCC is a nonaggressive malignancy with excellent prognosis following local excision to clear margins. Specifically, for perianal lesions smaller than 1cm, excisional biopsy may be sufficient and better tolerated than MMS or standard local excision with 4mm margins. This case report supports the notion that proper clinical vigilance and early detection of perianal BCC can result in excellent prognosis.

Acknowledgments

We thank the patient for granting permission to publish this information.

References

[1] G. E. Gibson and I. Ahmed, "Perianal and genital basal cell carcinoma: a clinicopathologic review of 51 cases," *Journal of the American Academy of Dermatology*, vol. 45, no. 1, pp. 68–71, 2001.

[2] R. Betti, C. Bruscagin, E. Inselvini, and C. Crosti, "Basal cell carcinomas of covered and unusual sites of the body," *International Journal of Dermatology*, vol. 36, no. 7, pp. 503–505, 1997.

[3] M. L. Welton and M. G. Varma, "Anal cancer," in *The ASCRS Textbook of Colon and Rectal Surgery*, B. G. Wolff, J. W. Fleshman, D. E. Beck, J. H. Pemberton, and S. D. Wexner, Eds., pp. 482–500, Springer, New York, NY, USA, 1st edition, 2007.

[4] C. A. Paterson, T. M. Young-Fadok, and R. R. Dozois, "Basal cell carcinoma of the perianal region: 20-year experience," *Diseases of the Colon & Rectum*, vol. 42, no. 9, pp. 1200–1202, 1999.

[5] O. V. Nielsen and S. L. Jensen, "Basal cell carcinoma of the anus—a clinical study of 34 cases," *British Journal of Surgery*, vol. 68, no. 12, pp. 856-857, 1981.

[6] D. T. Patil, J. R. Goldblum, and S. D. Billings, "Clinicopathological analysis of basal cell carcinoma of the anal region and its distinction from basaloid squamous cell carcinoma," *Modern Pathology*, vol. 26, no. 10, pp. 1382–1389, 2013.

[7] H. Cho, K. Kuo, S. Li et al., "164 Frequent basal cell cancer development is a clinical marker for inherited cancer susceptibility," *Journal of Investigative Dermatology*, vol. 138, no. 5, p. S28, 2018.

[8] M. M. Christian, R. L. Moy, R. F. Wagner, and A. Yen-Moore, "A correlation of alpha-smooth muscle actin and invasion in micronodular basal cell carcinoma," *Dermatologic Surgery*, vol. 27, no. 5, pp. 441–445, 2001.

[9] M. C. Alvarez-Cañas, F. A. Fernández, I. G. Rodilla, and J. F. Val-Bernal, "Perianal basal cell carcinoma: a comparative histologic, immunohistochemical, and flow cytometric study with basaloid carcinoma of the anus," *American Journal of Dermatopathology*, vol. 18, no. 4, pp. 371–379, 1996.

[10] J. Y. Kim, J. H. Kozlow, B. Mittal et al., "Guidelines of care for the management of basal cell carcinoma," *Journal of the American Academy of Dermatology*, vol. 78, no. 3, pp. 540–559, 2018.

49

Cutaneous Metastasis vs. Isolated Skin Recurrence of Invasive Breast Carcinoma after Modified Radical Mastectomy

Reza Hosseinpour[1,2] **and Mohammad Javad Yavari Barhaghtalab**[2]

[1]*Cancer institute, Imam Khomeini Hospital, Tehran University of Medical Sciences, Tehran, Iran*
[2]*Department of General Surgery, Shahid Beheshti Hospital, Yasuj University of Medical Sciences, Yasuj, Iran*

Correspondence should be addressed to Reza Hosseinpour; reza.hosseinpour@yums.ac.ir and Mohammad Javad Yavari Barhaghtalab; mj.yavari.barhaghtalab@gmail.com

Academic Editor: Jacek Cezary Szepietowski

Background. Five to ten percent of the patients with operable breast cancer develop a chest wall recurrence within 10 years following the mastectomy. One of the most distressing presentations of locally recurrent breast cancer is the appearance of cutaneous metastases. To the best of authors' knowledge, there is no study distinguishing skin metastasis from local recurrence, so the main aim of this report was to elucidate if these two features are important in the prognosis and management of the disease. *Case Presentation.* A 51-year-old woman referred to the breast clinic due to a painful mass in the left breast. The patient underwent the modified radical mastectomy (MRM) and left axillary lymph node dissection followed by 30 sessions of radiotherapy and 8 sessions of chemotherapy (T3N1M0, ER−, and HER2+). About 15 months after the surgery, she presented with redness and eruptive lesions over the mastectomy scar that increased in size within a three-month follow-up. *Conclusion.* Mastectomy is not an absolute cure in the treatment of an invasive breast cancer because almost always, there is a recurrence risk and possibility of metastasis. It is vital to differentiate between local recurrence and skin metastasis because it would alter the overall treatment decision, prognosis, and patient outcomes.

1. Background

Five to ten percent of patients with operable breast cancer develop a chest wall recurrence within 10 years following the mastectomy [1]. One of the most distressing presentations of locally recurrent breast cancer is the appearance of cutaneous metastases [2]. It usually presents as a firm nodule at the site of the primary cancer that can be associated with ulceration, bleeding, and pain [3]. Cutaneous breast metastases most commonly present on the chest wall [4]. The abdomen, back, head and neck, scalp, and upper extremities are also common sites [5, 6]. Cutaneous metastases show that the underlying tumor has infiltrated into the skin, blood capillaries, and lymph vessels [1]. The presence of skin metastases signifies widespread systemic disease and a poor prognosis [6]. To the best of authors' knowledge, there is no study distinguishing skin metastasis from local recurrence, so in this study, our main concerns are if we could distinguish the skin lesions which are presented after the mastectomy as cutaneous metastasis or isolated skin recurrence, and if we could consider these lesions as metastasis or recurrence, it would change the prognosis or management of the disease.

2. Case Presentation

A 51-year-old woman referred to the breast clinic due to a painful bulging in the left breast. The patient had no past medical history and family history of any cancer within her family. On the initial presentation, she had two palpable, 6×4 cm and 4×2 cm, well-circumscribed hard masses at the upper outer quadrant of the left breast with no skin changes or attachment to the underlying muscle. The left axilla had several palpable lymph nodes with the maximum diameter of 2 cm. Core needle biopsy of the breast mass revealed an invasive ductal carcinoma, estrogen and progesterone receptors (ER/PR) negative, human epidermal growth factor receptor 2 (HER2) positive 3+, and Ki-67 25% nuclear labeling. The patient underwent the modified radical mastectomy (MRM) and left axillary lymph node dissection followed with 30 sessions of radiotherapy and 8 sessions of chemotherapy. Pathological examination of the mastectomy specimen revealed a 6 cm tumor nodule with the invasive ductal carcinoma, solid and comedo type, grade 2, ER/PR negative, and HER2 positive. All surgical margins were uninvolved by the tumor, and 16 out of 19 lymph nodes were involved by invasive carcinoma (T3N1M0, ER−, and HER2+).

About 15 months after the surgery, she presented with redness and eruptive lesions over the mastectomy scar that increased in size within a three-month follow-up in the clinic. On the physical examination, the skin lesion was a localized, well-defined, 7 × 5 cm, indurated erythematous ulcerative papulonodular plaque on the left anterior chest and also abdominal wall over the previous MRM scar (Figure 1).

An incisional biopsy of the skin from the MRM site was taken and was sent for pathology evaluation. The patient was revealed to have an invasive ductal carcinoma with apocrine features with invasion to the papillary dermis (grade three or high grade), ER/PR negative, HER2 positive 3+, Ki-67 15%, and E-cadherin positive. The patient underwent whole-body bone scintigraphy or technetium 99m-methyl diphosphonate (Tc99m-MDP) and spiral chest, abdomen, and pelvic CT-scan with intravenous (IV) contrast, and both studies had normal findings. The patient received 24 sessions of chemotherapy afterward.

3. Discussion

Recovery or recurrence is the natural history of a patient with breast cancer who undergoes the mastectomy procedure. Recurrence occurs as local or local and distant metastases. Local isolated skin recurrence without concomitant metastatic disease after the mastectomy has been rarely reported [7]. More than 20% of all cutaneous metastases are arising from the breast cancer, and this is more than any other malignancies in women. If a patient has skin metastases, a systemic disease might be inevitable, and it shows a poor prognosis [6, 8]. The most common sites which could be involved are the chest wall, the abdomen, the back, the head and neck, and the upper extremities [5, 6, 8].

It has been shown that a small percentage of local recurrences after treatment for ductal carcinoma in situ (DCIS) has a component of invasive disease, which may increase the risk of distant metastases and have a reduced rate of survival [9]. Young patient age, incomplete breast tissue resection (residual breast tissue and inadequate margin resection during surgery), presence of occult invasive focus, size of the tumor, multiquadrant tumors, comedo type and high nuclear grade, and diffuse necrosis are reported as risk factors for local recurrence [10].

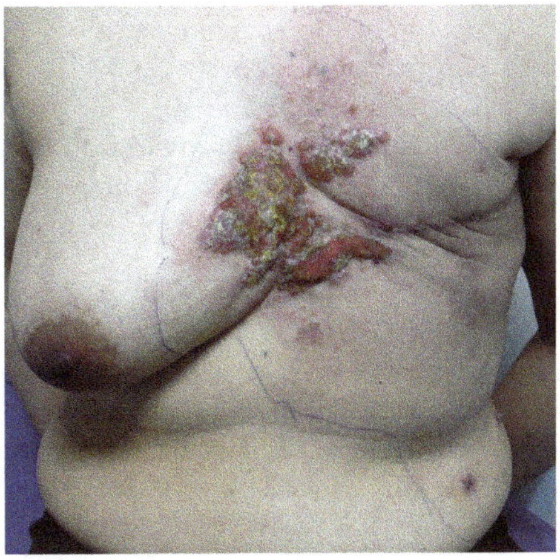

Figure 1: Indurated erythematous ulcerative papulonodular plaque appearance lesion on the previous MRM scar.

It is difficult to cure an advanced metastatic breast cancer as there may be an ultimate resistance to cytotoxic treatment. Progression of cutaneous metastases to a fungating ulcerative mass could destruct psychological well-being, grow social isolation, and reduce the quality of life [8]. In the advanced stages of the breast cancer with cutaneous metastasis, it is not possible to do the surgery; so, limited surgeries are done, and this is the reason for why the recognition of breast cancer at an early stage is very important for the therapeutic approach [8].

If locoregional recurrence occurs within the same quadrant as the initial tumor, it does not affect the outcome [11]. On the contrary, diffuse locoregional recurrence involving the breast skin or presenting as axillary recurrence has a poorer prognosis than isolated breast involvement [12]. Patients with locoregional recurrence involving the skin have a 50% rate of local failure compared with only a 14% failure rate in patients without skin involvement [13]. Skin involvement at locoregional recurrence increases the incidence of distant metastases from 14% to 44% [14]. It has also been shown that patients with locoregional recurrence involving the skin have a 44% to 83% risk for distant metastases simultaneously or within 2 months of locoregional recurrence, compared with 5% for those patients without skin involvement at recurrence [15, 16]. Locoregional recurrence involving the skin portends a poor overall survival of 13% to 18% between 5 and 10 years after recurrence [13, 17].

Mastectomy is not an absolute cure in the treatment of an invasive breast cancer because almost always, there is a recurrence risk and possibility of metastasis. As it is impossible to perform the surgery, if the breast cancer progresses to the advanced stages with cutaneous metastasis, the recognition and management of the disease at earlier stages are very important, so it is vital to differentiate between local recurrence and skin metastasis because it would alter the overall treatment decision, prognosis, and patient outcomes.

Abbreviations

MRM: Modified radical mastectomy
ER/PR: Estrogen and progesterone receptors

CT-scan: Computed tomography scan
IV: Intravenous contrast
DCIS: Ductal carcinoma in situ
HER2: Human epidermal growth factor receptor 2
Tc99m-MDP: Technetium 99m-methyl diphosphonate.

Consent

Written informed consent was obtained from the patient for publication of this case report and any accompanying images. A copy of written consent is available for review by the Editor-in-Chief of this journal.

Authors' Contributions

RH evaluated the patient clinically, operated the patient, and revised the paper. MJYB prepared the first draft and revised the paper. Both authors read and approved the final manuscript.

Acknowledgments

The authors express their gratitude to the patient who kindly gave consent for this case to be presented in this paper.

References

[1] B. Kalmykow and S. Walker, "Cutaneous metastases in breast cancer," *Clinical Journal of Oncology Nursing*, vol. 15, no. 1, pp. 99–101, 2011.

[2] S. Moore, "Cutaneous metastatic breast cancer," *Clinical Journal of Oncology Nursing*, vol. 6, no. 5, pp. 255–260, 2002.

[3] A. M. Nasralla, M. A. Al-Duhileb, A. J. Arini, and S. S. Amr, "Cutaneous erythema at scar site of modified radical mastectomy: an unexpected manifestation of recurrent carcinoma," *Case Reports in Surgery*, vol. 2017, Article ID 6879626, 2017.

[4] S. Vano-Galvan, P. Moreno-Martin, I. Salguero, and P. Jaen, "Cutaneous metastases of breast carcinoma: a case report," *Cases Journal*, vol. 2, no. 1, p. 71, 2009.

[5] S.-S. Hu, G.-S. Chen, Y.-W. Lu, C.-S. Wu, and C.-C. Lan, "Cutaneous metastases from different internal malignancies: a clinical and prognostic appraisal," *Journal of the European Academy of Dermatology and Venereology*, vol. 22, no. 6, pp. 735–740, 2008.

[6] M. R. A. Hussein, "Skin metastasis: a pathologist's perspective," *Journal of Cutaneous Pathology*, vol. 37, no. 9, pp. e1–e20, 2010.

[7] F. Jaffre, V. Lavoue, H. Mesbah et al., "Prognosis for isolated skin recurrence after breast cancer treated by mastectomy," *Anticancer Research*, vol. 29, no. 5, pp. 1697–1701, 2009.

[8] G. Kamińska-Winciorek and J. Wydmański, "Dermoscopy of skin metastases from breast cancer and of the orange peel type ("peau d'orange"): a report of two cases," *International Journal of Dermatology*, vol. 54, no. 3, pp. 343–346, 2015.

[9] C. Vargas, L. Kestin, N. Go et al., "Factors associated with local recurrence and cause-specific survival in patients with ductal carcinoma in situ of the breast treated with breast-conserving therapy or mastectomy," *International Journal of Radiation Oncology∗Biology∗Physics*, vol. 63, no. 5, pp. 1514–1521, 2005.

[10] B. Kaya, B. H. Bakkal, and M. Sayın, "Chest wall relapse of ductal carcinoma in situ after mastectomy: a case report," *The Journal of Breast Health*, vol. 9, no. 1, pp. 35–37, 2013.

[11] A. L. Abner, A. Recht, T. Eberlein et al., "Prognosis following salvage mastectomy for recurrence in the breast after conservative surgery and radiation therapy for early-stage breast cancer," *Journal of Clinical Oncology*, vol. 11, no. 1, pp. 44–48, 1993.

[12] T. L. Huston and R. M. Simmons, "Locally recurrent breast cancer after conservation therapy," *The American Journal of Surgery*, vol. 189, no. 2, pp. 229–235, 2005.

[13] A. Fortin, M. Larochelle, J. Laverdière, S. Lavertu, and D. Tremblay, "Local failure is responsible for the decrease in survival for patients with breast cancer treated with conservative surgery and postoperative radiotherapy," *Journal of Clinical Oncology*, vol. 17, no. 1, p. 101, 1999.

[14] B. G. Haffty, N. B. Goldberg, D. Fischer et al., "Conservative surgery and radiation therapy in breast carcinoma: local recurrence and prognostic implications," *International Journal of Radiation Oncology∗Biology∗Physics*, vol. 17, no. 4, pp. 727–732, 1989.

[15] A. Recht, S. J. Schnitt, J. L. Connolly et al., "Prognosis following local or regional recurrence after conservative surgery and radiotherapy for early stage breast carcinoma," *International Journal of Radiation Oncology∗Biology∗Physics*, vol. 16, no. 1, pp. 3–9, 1989.

[16] I. Gage, S. J. Schnitt, A. Recht et al., "Skin recurrences after breast-conserving therapy for early-stage breast cancer," *Journal of Clinical Oncology*, vol. 16, no. 2, pp. 480–486, 1998.

[17] S. J. Schnitt, J. L. Connolly, A. Recht, B. Silvers, and J. R. Harris, "Breast relapse following primary radiation therapy for early breast cancer. II. detection, pathologic features and prognostic significance," *International Journal of Radiation Oncology∗Biology∗Physics*, vol. 11, no. 7, pp. 1277–1284, 1985.

50

Blue Nevus of the Hard Palate: The Importance of a Careful Examination in an Emergency Setting

Ana Teresa Tavares,[1] André Pereira,[1] João Pimentel,[2] Marcelo Prates,[1] Luís Fonseca,[1] Maria Rosário Marques,[1] and Francisco Proença[1]

[1]*Stomatology Department, Centro Hospitalar Universitário de Lisboa Central, Lisbon, Portugal*
[2]*Pathology Department, Centro Hospitalar Universitário de Lisboa Central, Lisbon, Portugal*

Correspondence should be addressed to Ana Teresa Tavares; anatetavares@gmail.com

Academic Editor: Ioannis D. Bassukas

Oral common blue nevus is an asymptomatic, benign, rare, pigmented lesion and sometimes clinically indistinguishable from other pigmented lesions such as the cellular blue nevus or early-stage malignant melanoma. Since it shows clinical similarities with a malignant lesion and with cellular blue nevus that can itself suffer malignant transformation, the decisive diagnosis is crucial for adequate treatment, follow-up, and prognosis. Diagnosis confirmation is given by histological analysis, the reason why most oral pigmented lesions are excised. The following case presents an asymptomatic oral pigmented lesion of the hard palate discovered during observation in an emergency setting due to an abscess of dental origin. The lesion was fully excised, and histological examination reported a "common blue nevus." In this case, we intend to present a rare lesion of the oral cavity and the importance of performing a routine oral examination when given a chance as a preventive approach.

1. Introduction

Oral melanocytic nevi (OMN) are rare, benign tumors of melanocytes [1–7]. The pathogenesis and etiology of OMN are still poorly understood [1, 2, 4, 5, 8, 9]; the most consensual theory is that they arise from latent dendritic melanocytes, which remain trapped in the dermis, from the embryologic migration of melanoblasts, their precursors, and from the neural crest to the epidermis [1, 3, 4, 10–12]. OMN can be congenital or acquired with higher prevalence of the latter [4, 5, 9, 13] and are histologically classified as junctional, compound, intradermic (intramucosal), combined, and blue [1–3, 7]. This classification depends on distribution, localization, and morphology of the nevus cells [1–3]. The most common OMN is the intramucosal nevus followed by the blue nevus (19–36%) [1–7, 14]. Blue nevus itself has several histological classifications from which can be clinically indistinct: common blue nevus, cellular blue nevus (CBN), and atypical nevus [1, 3, 5, 7, 9, 10, 13, 15].

Oral blue nevus has a prevalence of 0.1% in the general population, appears mainly from the third to the fifth decades, and women tend to be more affected than men [2, 4, 7, 14]. It develops more frequently in the hard palate (69%), followed by the labial mucosa and vermillion border [1–3, 5–7, 14]. Most lesions are asymptomatic, and therefore, its oral presentation is mostly discovered during routine dental examinations [2, 15]. Clinically, the common blue nevus usually presents as a solitary, smooth-surfaced, well-defined, flat, or elevated papule with a diameter of less than 10 mm, though wider lesions have been described [1, 2, 5, 7, 9, 11, 13]. Its color varies from brown to blue, depending on the pigment quantity and depth or location [2–5, 13]. Histologically, the diagnostic cell of the blue nevus is a pigmented, spindle-shaped dendritic melanocyte with a slender, branching network of dendritic processes without atypia or mitotic figures [1–3, 7, 10–13]. The nuclei are small, elongated, and hyperchromatic [2, 11, 13]. Blue nevus' cells are frequently positive to S100, MelanA (MART-1), and HMB-45 [2, 4, 11, 13]. Literature states that the risk of malignant transformation of CBN into oral malignant melanoma (OMM) is estimated to be between 5.2% and 6.3% [9]. Because of multiple reports of tumors with features combined between CBN and OMM, the controversial designation of "atypical blue nevus" or "atypical cellular blue nevus" was created for these borderline lesions [8, 10, 14, 15]. However, despite the efforts, there is still no uniform histological criteria to differentiate atypical CBN from OMM [14, 16].

The following case presents a 40-year-old male with an asymptomatic pigmented lesion located in the left hard palate, discovered during an emergency visit due to a dental abscess. The lesion was fully excised with the histological diagnosis of "common blue nevus of the oral mucosa." This case report presents a rare lesion of the oral cavity that has a risk of malignant transformation, thus highlighting the importance of the routine oral examination as a preventive approach.

2. Case Presentation

A 40-year-old male presented in the Stomatology Emergency Room with chief complaint of toothache in the fourth quadrant. He had a history of treated pulmonary tuberculosis, high blood pressure, abdominal surgery after trauma, and obstructive sleep apnea-hypopnea syndrome, treated with continuous positive airway pressure (CPAP). He was medicated with nebivolol, valproic acid, bromazepam, and risperidone and slept with continuous positive airway pressure. He denied any history of alcohol intake or smoking habits. Regarding family history, he alleged to have had an aunt with oral cancer.

While being diagnosed with an acute apical periodontitis of the inferior right first molar, during oral examination, it was found a black melanocytic-type lesion on the posterior half of the left hard palate (Figure 1). The lesion measured 5 mm × 2.5 mm, was flat, homogeneous, well-defined, nonulcerated, and painless. The patient had no recollection of its existence. No masses or nodes were palpable in the cervical or preauricular areas.

The acute dental infection was primarily addressed. Regarding palatal lesion, given the fact that he was unaware of the palatal lesion, and therefore there was no way of knowing if it had a recent growth and due to his alleged family history, an excisional biopsy was scheduled and blood analysis was requested.

The blood tests revealed normal, besides slightly elevated hemoglobin (17.9 × 10 g/L).

The biopsy was performed under local anesthesia with lidocaine + adrenaline (1 : 80000) and a number 15 scalpel blade. The lesion was excised with a 2 mm margin, and local hemostasis was obtained with a periodontal dressing.

Histological examination of the lesion revealed a "common blue nevus of oral mucosa" (Figures 2 and 3).

Upon follow-up, the patient remains asymptomatic, and the surgical wound is fully closed (Figure 4), with no signs of clinical recurrence.

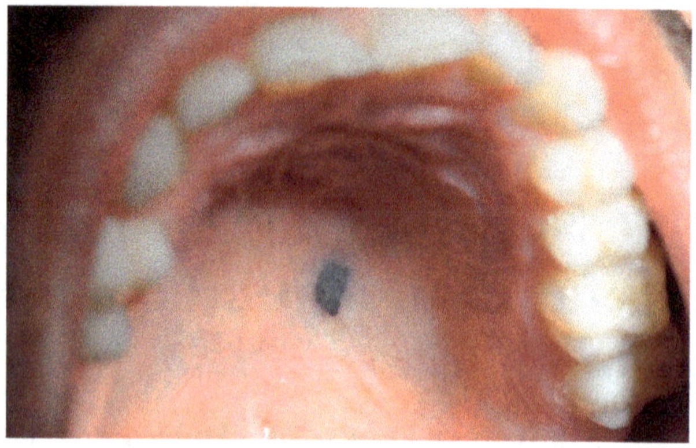

FIGURE 1: Palatal lesion during oral examination.

3. Discussion

Blue nevus is very rarely seen in the oral cavity [2, 3, 7, 14]. Since they are usually asymptomatic, their finding in a routine oral examination is frequent [2, 5].

Although the ABCDE system may be a helpful tool in considering malignancy in the oral cavity, clinical impression is insufficient for definite diagnosis and most pigmented lesions end up excised [2, 17]. This procedure should also be considered in these local findings: pain, swelling, recent growth, color changes, bleeding, and ulceration [2].

Due to the fact that most oral pigmented lesions are benign, excision usually is required only when the patient reports discomfort [2]; however, performing an incisional biopsy of oral pigmented lesions with malignant potential is an area of controversy among researchers [2, 3]. Some authors defend that cutting into malignant lesions when performing an incisional biopsy can result in increased risk of local recurrence or regional or distant metastasis, but several studies have also refuted this hypothesis [2, 3, 17, 18]. The extent of the surgical margins when excising oral pigmented lesions is still in debate [2]. Australia and New Zealand guidelines for cutaneous melanoma recommend an initial excisional biopsy with 2 mm margins whenever possible [2, 19], but no OMM parallel has yet been established.

Around 30% of all OMM develop from previous existing pigmented lesion, while most are *de novo* [20]. Still, primary OMM is an infrequent but very aggressive lesion, accounting for 0.5% of all oral malignancies [2, 4, 6, 13, 14, 17] and less than 1% of all melanomas [13, 19, 20]. Its 5-year survival rate ranges from 10–45% [7]. Malignant transformation or recurrence of a blue nevus, though extremely rare, can in fact develop [2, 7, 16, 21]; most often, if not always, its stated that it occurs in cellular types, although this is still subject to debate [2, 3, 6, 7, 11, 15].

Some oncogenic protein mutations have been described in common nevi and in both cutaneous and oral melanoma; the most consensual finding is a mutation in Bioinformatics Resources and Applications Facility (BRAF). The suggested mechanism for this association is that BRAF mutations trigger the proliferation of melanocytic cells, thus forming a nevus. When a growth-arrest response occurs, the

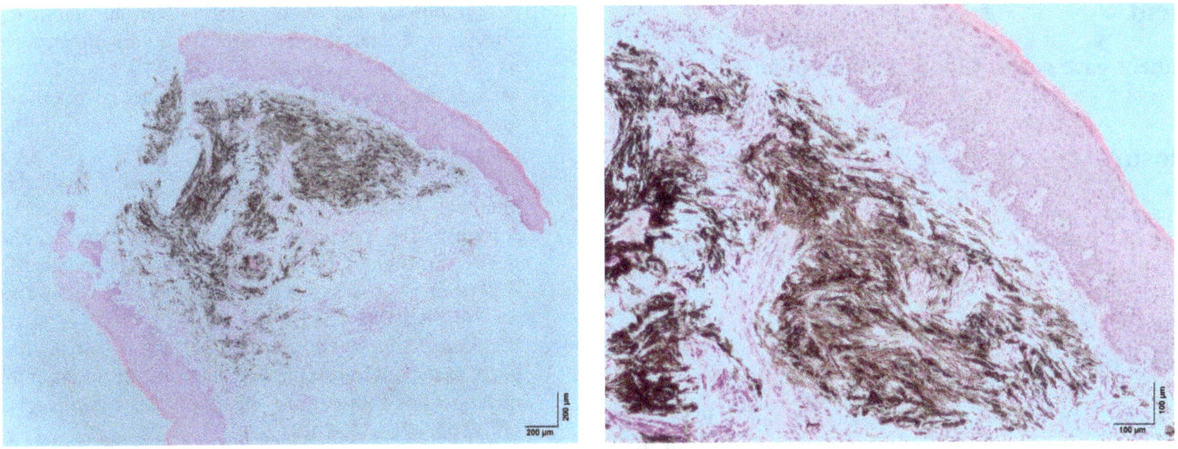

(a) (b)

FIGURE 2: Microscopic examination at magnifications 40x (a) and 100x (b) with hematoxylin and eosin. There is a noncircumscribed submucosal proliferation of elongated spindle-shaped melanocytes that are grouped in short fascicles some of them arranged parallel to the overlying epithelium. The melanocytes contain a variable amount of melanin pigments in the cytoplasm. Some fibrosis is observed in between the fascicles of pigmented cells. There is no atypia or areas of necrosis. No mitoses were observed.

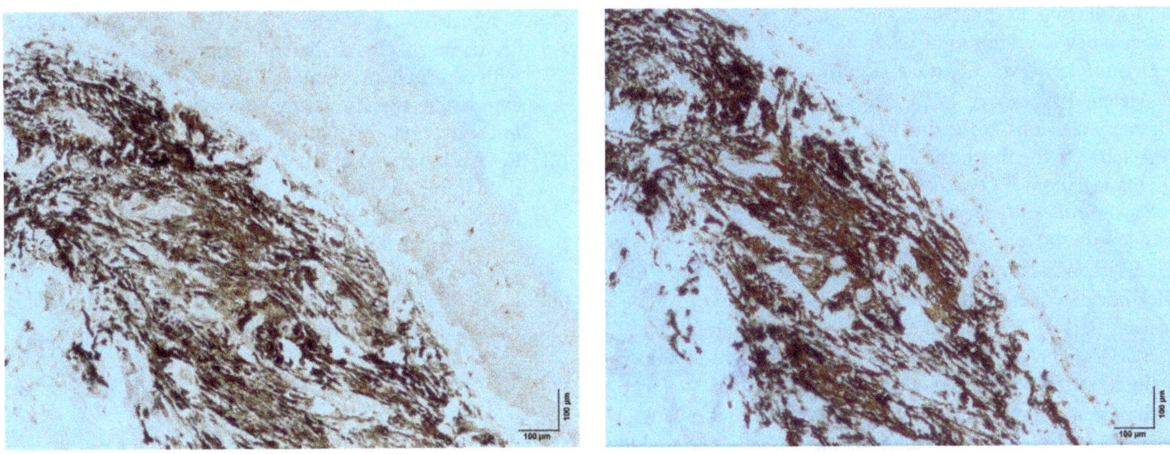

(a) (b)

FIGURE 3: Microscopic examination at magnification 100x. Nevus cells stain for MelanA (a) and S100 (b).

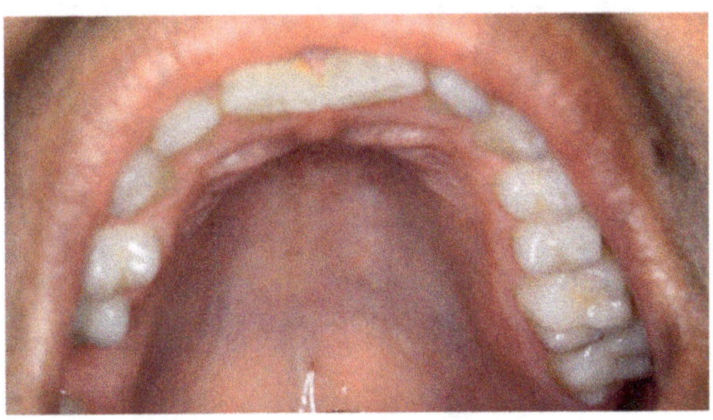

FIGURE 4: Surgical wound 4 months after biopsy.

proliferation ceases. This mutation, however, is only found in less than 10% of OMM compared to 80% found in cutaneous melanoma; furthermore, some studies suggest that blue nevus rarely has such mutation, which may imply that they represent a distinct type of melanocytic neoplasms [1, 5, 11, 22].

The final diagnosis is therefore of utmost relevance since treatment and prognosis of benign pigmented lesions are far different from OMM [3, 8].

This case presents the uncertainty of malignancy of an oral pigmented lesion which is, by itself, very rare, and data are scarce regarding its proper approach. An oral examination in an emergency setting regarding dental problems revealed the lesion. An excision was performed, with the positive reassurance that only an excisional biopsy can provide, that no malignancy was found associated with the palatal lesion.

Consent

The patient gave consent for this article publication.

Disclosure

The research was part of the author's employment at Hospital de São José–Centro Hospitalar Universitário de Lisboa Central.

References

[1] L. Ferreira, B. Jham, R. Assi, A. Readinger, and H. P. Kessler, "Oral melanocytic nevi: a clinicopathologic study of 100 cases," *Oral Surgery, Oral Medicine, Oral Pathology and Oral Radiology*, vol. 120, no. 3, pp. 358–367, 2015.

[2] Y. Toeda, K. Uzawa, Y. Yamano et al., "Blue nevus of the hard palate: a case report," *Journal of Oral and Maxillofacial Surgery, Medicine, and Pathology*, vol. 28, no. 5, pp. 406–409, 2016.

[3] T. d. S. Santos, R. Frota, P. R. S. Martins-Filho, J. R. Cavalcante, R. d. C. Raimundo, and E. S. d. S. Andrade, "Extenso nevo azul intraoral: relato de caso," *Anais Brasileiros de Dermatologia*, vol. 86, no. 4 suppl 1, pp. 61–65, 2011.

[4] M. Meleti, P. Vescovi, W. J. Mooi, and I. van der Waal, "Pigmented lesions of the oral mucosa and perioral tissues: a flow-chart for the diagnosis and some recommendations for the management," *Oral Surgery, Oral Medicine, Oral Pathology, Oral Radiology & Endodontics*, vol. 105, no. 5, pp. 606–616, 2008.

[5] M. Meleti, W. J. Mooi, M. K. Casparie, and I. van der Waal, "Melanocytic nevi of the oral mucosa–No evidence of increased risk for oral malignant melanoma: an analysis of 119 cases," *Oral Oncology*, vol. 43, no. 10, pp. 976–981, 2007.

[6] A. Buchner, P. W. Merrell, and W. M. Carpenter, "Relative frequency of solitary melanocytic lesions of the oral mucosa," *Journal of Oral Pathology and Medicine*, vol. 33, no. 9, pp. 550–557, 2004.

[7] A. Pinto, S. Raghavendra, R. Lee, S. DeRossi, and F. Alawi, "Epithelioid blue nevus of the oral mucosa: a rare histologic variant," *Oral Surgery, Oral Medicine, Oral Pathology, Oral Radiology & Endodontics*, vol. 96, no. 4, pp. 429–436, 2003.

[8] C. Hasney, R. B. Butcher, and R. G. Amedee, "Malignant melanoma of the head and neck: a brief review of pathophysiology, current staging, and management," *The Ochsner Journal*, vol. 8, pp. 181–185, 2008.

[9] K. Kesty and O. Zargari, "Eruptive blue nevi," *Indian Journal of Dermatology, Venereology and Leprology*, vol. 81, pp. 198–201, 2015.

[10] K. Scheller, C. Scheller, S. Becker, H.-J. Holzhausen, and J. Schubert, "Cellular blue nevus (CBN) lymph node metastases of the neck with no primary skin lesion: a case report and review of literature," *Journal of Cranio-Maxillofacial Surgery*, vol. 38, no. 8, pp. 601–604, 2010.

[11] A. Zembowicz and P. A. Phadke, "Blue nevi and variants: an update," *Archives of Pathology & Laboratory Medicine*, vol. 135, no. 3, pp. 327–336, 2011.

[12] A. Moshaver, L. Puttagunta, and H. Seikaly, "Malignant blue nevus of the parotid gland: a case report," *Head & Neck*, vol. 28, no. 10, pp. 960–962, 2006.

[13] A. Zembowicz and M. C. Mihm, "Dermal dendritic melanocytic proliferations: an update," *Histopathology*, vol. 45, no. 5, pp. 433–451, 2004.

[14] M. J. Hicks and C. M. Flaitz, "Oral mucosal melanoma: epidemiology and pathobiology," *Oral Oncology*, vol. 36, no. 2, pp. 152–169, 2000.

[15] R. L. Barnhill, Z. Argenyi, M. Berwick et al., "Atypical cellular blue nevi (cellular blue nevi with atypical features): lack of consensus for diagnosis and distinction from cellular blue nevi and malignant melanoma ("malignant blue nevus")," *The American Journal of Surgical Pathology*, vol. 32, no. 1, pp. 36–44, 2008.

[16] B. S. Shumway, Y. B. Rawal, C. M. Allen, J. R. Kalmar, and C. M. Magro, "Oral atypical cellular blue nevus: an infiltrative melanocytic proliferation," *Head and Neck Pathology*, vol. 7, no. 2, pp. 171–177, 2013.

[17] M. Meleti, C. R. Leemans, W. J. Mooi, P. Vescovi, and I. van der Waal, "Oral malignant melanoma: a review of the literature," *Oral Oncology*, vol. 43, no. 2, pp. 116–121, 2007.

[18] J. L. Bong, R. M. Herd, and J. A. A. Hunter, "Incisional biopsy and melanoma prognosis," *Journal of the American Academy of Dermatology*, vol. 46, no. 5, pp. 690–694, 2002.

[19] C. P. Guidelines and N. Zealand, *Management Melanoma*, 2008.

[20] S. A. Castillo, A. K. Pham, J. A. Lefferts, S. Yan, and J. Bridge, "A diagnostically-challenging case of melanoma ex blue nevus with comprehensive molecular analysis, including the 23-gene expression signature (myPath melanoma)," *Journal of Cutaneous Pathology*, vol. 46, no. 3, pp. 226–230, 2018.

[21] R. Andrei, S. Zurac, C. Socoliuc, P. Mandisodza, and F. Staniceanu, "Problems of differential diagnosis in melanoma arising from blue naevus," *Romanian Journal of Internal Medicine = Revue Roumaine de Medecine Interne*, vol. 53, pp. 95–101, 2015.

[22] P. M. Zito, "Cancer," *Oral Melanoma Pathophysiology Histopathology Treatment/Management*, pp. 1–6, 2019.

Permissions

All chapters in this book were first published by Hindawi Publishing Corporation; hereby published with permission under the Creative Commons Attribution License or equivalent. Every chapter published in this book has been scrutinized by our experts. Their significance has been extensively debated. The topics covered herein carry significant findings which will fuel the growth of the discipline. They may even be implemented as practical applications or may be referred to as a beginning point for another development.

The contributors of this book come from diverse backgrounds, making this book a truly international effort. This book will bring forth new frontiers with its revolutionizing research information and detailed analysis of the nascent developments around the world.

We would like to thank all the contributing authors for lending their expertise to make the book truly unique. They have played a crucial role in the development of this book. Without their invaluable contributions this book wouldn't have been possible. They have made vital efforts to compile up to date information on the varied aspects of this subject to make this book a valuable addition to the collection of many professionals and students.

This book was conceptualized with the vision of imparting up-to-date information and advanced data in this field. To ensure the same, a matchless editorial board was set up. Every individual on the board went through rigorous rounds of assessment to prove their worth. After which they invested a large part of their time researching and compiling the most relevant data for our readers.

The editorial board has been involved in producing this book since its inception. They have spent rigorous hours researching and exploring the diverse topics which have resulted in the successful publishing of this book. They have passed on their knowledge of decades through this book. To expedite this challenging task, the publisher supported the team at every step. A small team of assistant editors was also appointed to further simplify the editing procedure and attain best results for the readers.

Apart from the editorial board, the designing team has also invested a significant amount of their time in understanding the subject and creating the most relevant covers. They scrutinized every image to scout for the most suitable representation of the subject and create an appropriate cover for the book.

The publishing team has been an ardent support to the editorial, designing and production team. Their endless efforts to recruit the best for this project, has resulted in the accomplishment of this book. They are a veteran in the field of academics and their pool of knowledge is as vast as their experience in printing. Their expertise and guidance has proved useful at every step. Their uncompromising quality standards have made this book an exceptional effort. Their encouragement from time to time has been an inspiration for everyone.

The publisher and the editorial board hope that this book will prove to be a valuable piece of knowledge for researchers, students, practitioners and scholars across the globe.

List of Contributors

Kamran Balighi and Arghavan Azizpour
Autoimmune Bullous Diseases Research Center, Tehran University of Medical Sciences, Tehran, Iran

Kambiz Kamyab Hesari
Autoimmune Bullous Diseases Research Center, Tehran University of Medical Sciences, Tehran, Iran
Department of Dermatopathology, Razi Hospital, Tehran University of Medical Sciences, Tehran, Iran

Xiao Yan Wang, Juliandri, Zi Jing Liu, Jia Wen Zhang, Yun Yi Liu, Da-Guang Wang and Yang Xu
Department of Dermatology, The First Affiliated Hospital of Nanjing Medical University, Nanjing 210029, China

Fadi A. Alghamdi
Department of Dermatology, King Fahad Armed Forces Hospital, Jeddah, Saudi Arabia

Shahad T. Khayyat
College of Medicine and Surgery, King Abdulaziz University, Jeddah, Saudi Arabia

Mohammed M. Alshareef
Department of Dermatology, King Abdulaziz Hospital, Makkah, Saudi Arabia

Wala'a Felemban
Department of Pathology, King Fahad Armed Forces Hospital, Jeddah, Saudi Arabia

Carina G. Colossi
Institute of Cardiology/University Cardiology Foundation and Post-Graduation Program, Ivo Corréa Meyer Institute of Ophthalmology, Porto Alegre-RS, Brazil

Juliano Mondadori, Pedro K. M. Barreto, Felipe M. Valença and Rodrigo Duquia
Federal University of Health Sciences of Porto Alegre, Brazil

Manuel A. P. Vilela
Institute of Cardiology/University Cardiology Foundation and Post-Graduation Program, Ivo Corréa Meyer Institute of Ophthalmology, Porto Alegre-RS, Brazil
Federal University of Health Sciences of Porto Alegre, Brazil

Maria Tzardi
Department of Pathology, University Hospital of Heraklion, 71500 Heraklion, Greece

Eirini Kavvalou, Maria Stefanidou, Sabine Elke Krueger-Krasagakis, George Evangelou, Dimitra Koumaki and Konstantinos Krasagakis
Department of Dermatology, University General Hospital of Heraklion, 71500 Heraklion, Greece

Chanidapa Wongtada
M.D., Graduated from Chulalongkorn University, Bangkok, Thailand

Pravit Asawanonda and Marisa Pongprutthipan
Division of Dermatology, Department of Medicine, King Chulalongkorn Memorial Hospital, Bangkok, Thailand

T. Iqbal and V. Mudaliar
Department of Dermatology, Leighton Hospital, Mid Cheshire Hospitals NHS Foundation Trust, Crewe, UK
Department of Pathology, University Hospital of North Midlands NHS Trust, Stoke-on-Trent, UK

Jarett J. Casale, Mikél E. Muse, Tara J. Snow, Karen P. Gould and Natalie D. Depcik-Smith
Campbell University at Sampson Regional Medical Center, Clinton 28328, NC, USA

Zahra Nikyar
Autoimmune Bullous Diseases Research Center, Tehran University of Medical Sciences, Tehran, Iran
Department of Dermatology, School of Medicine, Razi Hospital, Tehran University of Medical Sciences, Tehran, Iran
Department of Dermatology, Skin Diseases and Leishmaniasis Research Center, School of Medicine, Isfahan University of Medical Sciences, Isfahan, Iran

Parvaneh Hatami
Autoimmune Bullous Diseases Research Center, Tehran University of Medical Sciences, Tehran, Iran

Azadeh Goodarzi
Department of Dermatology, School of Medicine, Rasoul Akram Hospital, Iran University of Medical Sciences, Tehran, Iran
Department of Dermatology, Rasool Akram Medical Complex Clinical Research Development Center, School of Medicine, Iran University of Medical Sciences, Tehran, Iran
Skin and Stem Cell Research Center, Tehran University of Medical Sciences, Tehran, Iran

Anahita Borzouei
Department of Dermatology, Mashhad University of Medical Sciences, Mashhad, Iran

Georgios Gaitanis and Ioannis D. Bassukas
Department of Skin and Venereal Diseases, Faculty of Medicine, School of Health Sciences, University of Ioannina, Ioannina, Greece
Department of Dermatology, University Hospital of Ioannina, Ioannina, Greece

Alexandra Papoudou-Bai
Department of Pathology, Faculty of Medicine, School of Health Sciences, University of Ioannina, Ioannina, Greece

Leonidas Marinos
Department of Haematopathology, Evaggelismos General Hospital of Athens, Ipsilantou 45-47, 10676, Athens, Greece

Amalia Vassou and Eleni Kapsali
Department of Hematology, Faculty of Medicine, School of Health Sciences, University of Ioannina, Ioannina, Greece

Panagiotis Kanavaros
Department of Anatomy-Histology-Embryology, Faculty of Medicine, School of Health Sciences, University of Ioannina, Ioannina, Greece

Sebo Gene Wang and Nicholas C. Hsu
Top IVF USA, Hacienda Heights, CA, USA

Sebo Michelle Wang
Loma Linda University School of Medicine, Loma Linda, CA, USA

Fu Nan Wang
Stem Cell Life Science Corp., New Taipei City, Taiwan

Jerey L. Dobrzynski
University of Iowa Roy J. and Lucille A. Carver College of Medicine, 375 Newton Rd, Iowa City, IA 52242, USA

Blake E. Vest and Brian L. Swick
University of Iowa Hospitals and Clinics, Dermatology, 200 Hawkins Drive, Iowa City, IA 52242, USA

Masafumi Ishibashi and Rie Shiiyama
Department of Dermatology, Nippon Kokan Hospital, Kawasaki, Japan

Neha Singh
Virginia Tech Carilion School of Medicine, Roanoke, VA, USA

Kiley K. Fagan
Section of Dermatology, Department of Internal Medicine, Virginia Tech Carilion School of Medicine, Roanoke, VA, USA

Douglas J. Grider
Department of Basic Science Education, Virginia Tech Carilion School of Medicine, Roanoke, VA, USA
Carilion Clinic and Virginia Tech Carilion School of Medicine, Department of Internal Medicine, Section of Dermatology, Roanoke, VA, USA
Virginia Tech Carilion School of Medicine, Department of Basic Science Education, Roanoke, VA, USA

Yuri Sugita, Teruhiko Makino, Kotaro Matsui and Tadamichi Shimizu
Department of Dermatology, Graduate School of Medicine and Pharmaceutical Sciences, University of Toyama, Toyama 930-0194, Japan

Amresh Kumar Singh, Ankur Kumar, Jayesh Pandey, Vivek Gaur and Pratima Tripathi
Department of Microbiology, Baba Raghav Das Medical College, Gorakhpur, Uttar Pradesh 273013, India

Indra Prasad Adhikari
Department of Biochemistry, Baba Raghav Das Medical College, Gorakhpur, Uttar Pradesh 273013, India

Yaritza Serrano Gomez
Department of Family Medicine, Northwell Health Glen Cove Hospital, Glen Cove, New York, USA

Brittney Grella
Department of Medicine, Northwell Health Huntington Hospital, Huntington, New York, USA

Hongbei Wang
Department of Pathology, Northwell Health, New Hyde Park, New York, USA

Segametsi Mary-Jane Mthanti
Prime Cure Medical Centre, 1843 Tsubaki Street, Dube, Soweto 1801, Johannesburg, South Africa

Gloria Pelle
Safarmex, 85 Newton Road, Meadowdale, Germiston 1614, Johannesburg, South Africa

Niels A. J. Cremers
Maastricht University Medical Centre, Department of Gynecology and Obstetrics, 6202AZ Maastricht, Netherlands
Triticum Exploitatie BV, Sleperweg 44, 6222NK Maastricht, Netherlands

Hideyuki Kinoshita, Takeshi Ishii, Hiroto Kamoda, Toshinori Tsukanishi and Tsukasa Yonemoto
Department of Orthopedic Surgery, Chiba Cancer Center, 666-2 Nitonacho, Chuo-ku, Chiba 260-8717, Japan

Sumihisa Orita, Kazuhide Inage and Seiji Ohtori
Department of Orthopaedic Surgery, Graduate School ofMedicine, Chiba University, 1-8-1 Inohana, Chuo-ku, Chiba 260-8670, Japan

Sharleen St. Surin-Lord
Howard University College of Medicine, 520 W St NW, Washington, DC 20059, USA
Visage Clinical Research LLC, 1400 Mercantile Lane, Suite 110, Largo, MD 20774, USA

Judi Miller
Strategic Pharmaceutical Advisors, 1750 Tysons Boulevard, Suite 1500 McLean, VA, USA

Shohei Iida, Kyoko Sugioka, Makoto Kondo, Yoshiaki Matsushima, Kento Mizutani, Koji Habe and Keiichi Yamanaka
Department of Dermatology, Mie University, Graduate School of Medicine, 2-174 Edobashi, Tsu, Mie 514-8507, Japan

Vikash Paudel
Department of Dermatology, National Medical College, Birgunj, Parsa, Nepal

Eric Bessell
Department of Clinical Oncology, Nottingham City Hospital, Nottingham, UK

Martin Dalton and John David Parry
The Surgery, Ravenshead, Nottinghamshire, UK

V. Thadchanamoorthy and Markandu Thirukumar
Faculty of Health Care Sciences, Eastern University, Sri Lanka

Kavinda Dayasiri
Base Hospital, Mahaoya, Sri Lanka

N. Thamilvannan and Judy Jeyakumar
Teaching Hospital, Batticaloa, Sri Lanka
Department of Psychiatry, Base Hospital, Valaichenai, Sri Lanka

Cameron Moattari
State University of New York Downstate Medical Center, Brooklyn, NY 11203, USA

Richard A. Giovane
Regional Medical Center of Central Alabama, Family Medicine, 29L V Stabler Drive, Greenville, AL 36037, USA

Stephanie DiGiovanni Kinsely
University of Alabama, Department of Family Medicine, 801 Campus Drive, Tuscaloosa, AL 35487, USA

Drew C. Mitchell
University of Rochester School of Medicine & Dentistry, 601 Elmwood Avenue Box 400, Rochester, NY 14642, USA

Gina J. Kuehn and Francisco Tausk
Department of Dermatology, University of Rochester Medical Center, 40 Celebration Drive, Rochester, NY 14642, USA

Glynis A. Scott
Department of Dermatology, University of Rochester Medical Center, 40 Celebration Drive, Rochester, NY 14642, USA
Department of Pathology, University of Rochester Medical Center, 601 Elmwood Avenue Box 626, Rochester, NY 14642, USA

Timothy D. Doerr
Department of Otolaryngology, University of Rochester Medical Center, 601 Elmwood Avenue Box 629, Rochester, NY 14642, USA

Amanda Walker
University of Utah, School of Medicine, Salt Lake City, UT 84132, USA

Vikram Nath Sahni
Drexel University, College of Medicine, Philadelphia, PA 19129, USA

Dev Ram Sahni and Julia Curtis
University of Utah School of Medicine, Department of Dermatology, Salt Lake City, UT 84132, USA

Andjela Egger, Andrea Maderal, Hadar Lev-Tov and Olivera Stojadinovic
Dr Phillip Frost Department of Dermatology and Cutaneous Surgery, University of Miami Miller School of Medicine, 1600 NW 10th Ave #1140, Miami, FL 33136, USA

Hafsa Abbas
Department of Medicine, Division of Gastroenterology, Bronxcare Hospital Center, Bronx, NY 10457, USA

Ahsan Aslam
Department of Medicine, IU Health University Hospital, Indianapolis, IN 46202, USA

Muhammad Saad and Sridhar Chilimuri
Department of Medicine, Bronxcare Hospital Center, Bronx, NY 10457, USA

Masooma Niazi
Department of Pathology, Bronxcare Hospital Center, Bronx, NY 10457, USA

J. B. Ntihebuwayo, F. Hali, A. Kerouach, H. Rachadi and S. Chiheb
Dermatology and Venereology Department, Ibn Rochd University Hospital-Casablanca, Casablanca, Morocco

F. Marnissi
Laboratory of Pathological Anatomy, Ibn Rochd University Hospital-Casablanca, Casablanca, Morocco

Niraj Parajuli, Shraddha Shrestha, Laila Lama, Rushma Shrestha and Anupama Karki
Department of Dermatology & Venereology, National Academy of Medical Sciences, Bir Hospital, Kathmandu, Nepal

Sumida Tiwari
Department of Pathology, National Academy of Medical Sciences, Bir Hospital, Kathmandu, Nepal

Ambika Pradhan
Jigmi Dorji Wangchuck National Referral Hospital, imphu, Bhutan

Tashi Tobgay and Sithar Dorjee
Khesar Gyalpo University of Medical Sciences of Bhutan, Thimphu, Bhutan

Tenzin Wangdi
Vector-borne Disease Control Programme, Ministry of Health, Thimphu, Bhutan

Guofa Zhou
Program in Public Health, University of California, Irvine, CA, USA

Nadira D. Karunaweera
Department of Parasitology, Faculty of Medicine, University of Colombo, Colombo, Sri Lanka

Sanusi Umar
Department of Medicine, Dermatology Division, University of California at Los Angeles, Los Angeles, CA, USA
Division of Dermatology, Harbor-UCLA Medical Center, Torrance, CA, USA
Dr. U Hair and Skin Clinic, Manhattan Beach, CA, USA

Marissa J. Carter
Strategic Solutions, Inc., Bozeman, MT, USA

Zeinab Aryanian
Autoimmune Bullous Diseases Research Center, Tehran University of Medical Sciences, Tehran, Iran
Department of Dermatology, Babol University of Medical Sciences, Babol, Iran

Soheila Sotoudeh
Department of Dermatology, Children's Medical Center, Center of Excellence, Tehran University of Medical Sciences, Tehran, Iran

Vahid Ziaee
Pediatric Rheumatology Research Goroup, Rheumatology Research Center, Tehran University of Medical Sciences, Tehran, Iran
Department of Pediatrics, Tehran University of Medical Sciences, Tehran, Iran

Narciss Mobini
University of Nevada, School of Medicine, Reno and Las Vegas, NV, USA
Director of Dermatopathology, Associated Pathologists, Chartered, Las Vegas, NV, USA
4230 Burnham Ave., Las Vegas, NV, 89119, USA
Associated Pathologists Chartered, Las Vegas, Nevada, USA

Kaviyon Sadrolashrafi
University of California, Los Angeles (UCLA), Department of Life Sciences, Los Angeles, CA, USA

Susun Michaels
Touro College of Osteopathic Medicine, Las Vegas, NV, USA
Las Vegas Skin and Cancer Clinics, Las Vegas, NV, USA

Younes Benyamna, Farah Marraha, Ibtissam Al Faker, Hanane Chahoub, Najlae Rahmani, Yasmine Rkiek, Soukayna Kabbou and Salim Gallouj
Department of Dermatology, University Hospital Center of Tangier, Tetouan, Al Hoceima, Morocco
Faculty of Medicine and Pharmacy Tangier, Abdelmalek Essaadi University, Tangier, Morocco

Driss Soussi Tanani
Faculty of Medicine and Pharmacy Tangier, Abdelmalek Essaadi University, Tangier, Morocco
Department of Pharmacology and Pharmacovigilance, University Hospital Center of Tangier, Tetouan, Al Hoceima, Morocco

Rummit Dhillon and Jason Dickey
College of Osteopathic Medicine, Touro University, Henderson, Nevada, USA

Jordan Spoon
Thomas Dermatology, Las Vegas, Nevada, USA

Alex C. Holliday, Mohammed I. Khan and Sean E. Mazloom
Carilion Clinic and Virginia Tech Carilion School of Medicine, Department of Internal Medicine, Section of Dermatology, Roanoke, VA, USA

Rahul N. Chavan
Alabama College of Osteopathic Medicine, Dothan, AL, USA

Panagiota Spyridonos
Department of Medical Physics/Informatics, Faculty of Medicine, School of Health Sciences, University of Ioannina, Ioannina, Greece

Vasiliki Zampeli
Department of Skin and Venereal Diseases, Faculty of Medicine, School of Health Sciences, University of Ioannina, Ioannina, Greece

Sophia-Nefeli Rapti
Department of Dermatology, University Hospital of Ioannina, Ioannina, Greece

Sophia Z. Shalhout and David M. Miller
Division of Hematology/Oncology and Department of Dermatology, Massachusetts General Hospital, Harvard Medical School, Boston, MA 02114, USA

Myrna R. Nahas and Reed E. Drews
Division of Hematology/Oncology, Beth Israel Deaconess Medical Center, Harvard Medical School, Boston, MA 02215, USA

Yu Wang and Ruzeng Xue
Department of Dermatology, Dermatology Hospital, Southern Medical University, Guangzhou, China
Department of Dermatology, Guangdong Provincial Dermatology Hospital, Guangzhou, China

T. Gambichler, L. Susok, M. H. Segert and M. Doerler
Skin Cancer Center, Department of Dermatology, Ruhr-University Bochum, Bochum, Germany

N. Patsinakidis
Division of Experimental Allergy and Immunodermatology, University of Oldenburg, Oldenburg, Germany

Moshe Y. Bressler
New York Institute of Technology College of Osteopathic Medicine, Old Westbury, NY, USA
Jamaica Hospital, Department of Internal Medicine, Dermatology, New York, NY, USA

Naeha Pathak and Rebecca Tamez
Jamaica Hospital, Department of Internal Medicine, Dermatology, New York, NY, USA

Kelly Cervellione
Jamaica Hospital, Department of Clinical Research, New York, NY, USA

Farshad Bagheri
Jamaica Hospital, Department of Internal Medicine, Infectious Disease, New York, NY, USA

Edward Epstein
Jamaica Hospital, Department of Internal Medicine, Nephrology, New York, NY, USA

Adnan Mir
Dermpath Diagnostics, New York Medical College Dermatology, Weill Cornell Medicine Dermatology, New York, NY, USA

Trilok Shrivastava, Lin Li, Sonia Tanwar, Rabab Nasim, Vincent Gullas and Jay Pescatore
Department of Internal Medicine, John H Stroger Hospital of Cook County, Chicago, IL, USA

Michael Nelson
Emergency Department, John H Stroger Hospital of Cook County, Chicago, IL, USA

Adela Alvarez Rio, Josep Oriol Roca Mas, Daniel Navarro Sanchez, Ivan Monge Castresana, Gonzalo Joaquin Soroa Moreno and Jaime Estrada Cuxart
Plastic & Reconstructive Surgery, Hospital Universitario Son Espases, Palma de Mallorca, Spain

Marta Martínez-García, Nicolás Silvestre-Torner and Antonio Aguilar-Martínez
Dermatology Service, Severo Ochoa University Hospital, Leganés, Madrid, Spain

Fernando Burgos-Lázaro
Pathological Anatomy Service, Severo Ochoa University Hospital, Leganés, Madrid, Spain

Paola C. Aldana
University of Maryland School of Medicine, Baltimore, MD, USA

Harris G. Yfantis and Preeti R. John
University of Maryland School of Medicine, Baltimore, MD, USA
Baltimore Veterans Affairs Medical Center, Baltimore, MD, USA

Reza Hosseinpour
Cancer institute, Imam Khomeini Hospital, Tehran University of Medical Sciences, Tehran, Iran
Department of General Surgery, Shahid Beheshti Hospital, Yasuj University of Medical Sciences, Yasuj, Iran

Mohammad Javad Yavari Barhaghtalab
Department of General Surgery, Shahid Beheshti Hospital, Yasuj University of Medical Sciences, Yasuj, Iran

Ana Teresa Tavares, André Pereira, Marcelo Prates, Luís Fonseca, Maria Rosário Marques and Francisco Proença
Stomatology Department, Centro Hospitalar Universitário de Lisboa Central, Lisbon, Portugal

João Pimentel
Pathology Department, Centro Hospitalar Universitário de Lisboa Central, Lisbon, Portugal

Index

www.ingramcontent.com/pod-product-compliance
Lightning Source LLC
LaVergne TN
LVHW082223200926
848484LV00008B/2293